Social Indicators Research Series

Volume 56

This new series aims to provide a public forum for single treatises and collections of papers on social indicators research that are too long to be published in our journal *Social Indicators Research*. Like the journal, the book series deals with statistical assessments of the quality of life from a broad perspective, It welcomes the research on a wide variety of substantive areas, including health, crime, housing, education, family life, leisure activities, transportation, mobility, economics, work, religion and environmental issues. These areas of research will focus on the impact of key issues such as health on the overall quality of life and vice versa. An international review board, consisting of Ruut Veenhoven, Joachim Vogel, Ed Diener, Torbjorn Moum, Mirjam A.G. Sprangers and Wolfgang Glatzer, will ensure the high quality of the series as a whole.

More information about this series at http://www.springer.com/series/6548

Ronald E. Anderson

Editor

World Suffering
and Quality of Life

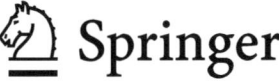 Springer

Editor
Ronald E. Anderson
Department of Sociology
Emeritus Faculty of Sociology
University of Minnesota
Minneapolis, MN, USA

ISSN 1387-6570   ISSN 2215-0099   (electronic)
Social Indicators Research Series
ISBN 978-94-017-9669-9   ISBN 978-94-017-9670-5   (eBook)
DOI 10.1007/978-94-017-9670-5

Library of Congress Control Number: 2015930254

Springer Dordrecht Heidelberg New York London

Springer Science+Business Media B.V. Dordrecht is part of Springer Science+Business Media (www.springer.com)

Foreword

On Suffering: What We Do Not See

David B. Morris, Author of *The Culture of Pain*, and Emeritus Professor of English, University of Virginia, Charlottesville, VA, USA

> We all believe in life.
> We feel a certain devotion.
> We feel called upon to live as good a life as we can.
> We feel that we are in the dark and that even in darkness we must
> struggle to know what is best to do.
>
> —Agnes Martin (1979)

"The philosophers have only *interpreted* the world in various ways," as Marx wrote in his well-known "Theses on Feuerbach" (1888); "the point is to *change* it."[1] Some suffering is certainly political and social in the sense that politics and societies create it—or create the conditions that permit it to arise and continue; with significant effort and luck, good politics and wise societies can help to un-create it.[2] *Praxis* here trumps *gnosis*. It is not necessary to define suffering perfectly or to understand suffering perfectly in order, no matter how imperfectly, to relieve suffering. Or, realistically, to relieve some suffering. We can relieve the suffering of a child who does not have enough food, for example, or who cannot afford life-saving medications or who has no access to disease-free drinking water. The ethical and pragmatic question is whether we, as individuals, will act. The political and social question is whether—and how—organizations and nations will act. It is the great virtue demonstrated by specific foundations, churches, doctors, social workers, teachers, students and ordinary citizens that they see a particular instance of suffering and—without waiting for politicians, philosophers, or perfect knowledge— they act effectively to relieve what they can.

---

[1] Marx, K. (1983).

[2] See, for just two examples, Kleinman et al. (1997) and Sayad (2004).

   Politics, while important, is never more than the art of the possible and never
sufficient to address the full spectrum of human suffering, and in addition it encounters one near-fatal, but possibly preventable, blindness to which individual ethics
also is subject: that is, politics, ethics, and good intentions can *address* suffering
only where they *recognize* suffering. This is an implication in painter Agnes Martin's
provocative prose meditation—a fragment of which appears as the epigraph to this
foreword—entitled *What We Do Not See if We Do Not See*. The medical name *sco-*
toma applies to a visual-field defect that we all possess: a blindness of which the
individual is unaware. *Anosognosia* is a rare deficit of self-awareness, usually the
result of brain damage following a stroke, in which patients who suffer an impairment seem unaware that they are impaired. What don't we see, it seems fair to ask,
in the suffering that we do not and cannot see?

   I thought, for example, that I knew something about AIDS, but I was wrong. I
knew something about AIDS in the developed world. I knew nothing about AIDS in
Africa. I simply did not see it. My abrupt wake up came as a visiting faculty member
on the Spring 2013 Semester at Sea voyage, where more than 600 undergraduates
spend 4 months taking classes aboard ship and visiting countries from Asia and
India through Africa. As I prepared my classes, I encountered the amazing book by
Stephanie Nolen entitled *28: Stories of AIDS in Africa* (2007). Nolen—award-
winning Africa bureau chief for Toronto's *Globe and Mail* newspaper—lived and
traveled extensively in Africa, reporting from more than 40 countries. Her book
offers 28 brief individual stories representing the 28 million Africans (at the time
she wrote) infected by HIV/AIDS. Her book was my introduction to some of the
confusing cultural, geopolitical, and global complexities attached to suffering. I
began to see what I had not seen.

   We see to some extent only what we are willing to acknowledge. HIV, as Nolan
says, targets the topics that people generally "least like to discuss—the drugs we
inject, the sex we have, especially the sex with people we aren't supposed to have
sex with—and the interactions least open to honest discussion or to change."[3]
Traditional African societies often treat the discussion of sex as taboo, so that the
link between eros and HIV/AIDS lends extra difficulties to prevention and treatment. Most important, however, Nolen emphasizes that HIV thrives on imbalances
of power. It got its foothold among sex workers, drug users, gay men, and migrants—
the poorest and most marginalized members of African society—but once established it found power imbalances and routes of transmission (like the highways
traveled by long-distance truckers) almost everywhere. Rawanda in 1986 was the
first country to do a national survey of HIV prevalence. The nightmare results:
17.8 % of people in cities were infected. In 1990, nearly one in five adults in Uganda
had the virus. By 2005, at least 20 million Africans had died from AIDS. This was
devastation on a scale like nothing I had seen or could envision. Similar losses
would depopulate the entire state of New York.

---

[3] Nolen, S. (2007). Facts and figures cited in my discussion are directly indebted to Nolen's account.

What I learned aboard ship added another layer of complication. Among my new shipmates was Desmond Tutu, the Nobel-prize winning Emeritus Archbishop of Cape Town. Tutu played a major role in the peaceful transition from apartheid rule in South Africa as head of the Truth and Reconciliation Commission. He is far less well known, however, for his contributions in establishing The Desmond Tutu HIV Foundation, which he developed in the early 1990s and which is justly acclaimed as among the first public clinics in Africa to offer the (then) controversial and inaccessible anti-retroviral therapy.[4] As our unofficial informant about African life and culture, Tutu advised his largely Western colleagues and students about the key African concept known as *Ubuntu*. *Ubuntu*—a Bantu word—refers to a traditional African alternative to the deeply entrenched Western tendency to identify humanness in our capacity for thought. *Ubuntu*, unlike the Cartesian *cogito ergo sum,* situates our basic human-ness in social connections.[5] As Tutu once wrote, "*Ubuntu* says that we cannot exist as a human being in isolation. We are interconnected. We are family. If you are not well, I am not well."[6] On board ship, for the benefit of students and faculty, he translated it in the brief, simple, strikingly resonant statement "*I am because you are*."

Suffering, among its multiple impacts, certainly helps to strain the affective social bonds that hold individuals together, and HIV/AIDS as a source of both illness and suffering struck the world of *Ubuntu* as much more than a sexually transmitted infectious disease. As it attacked the individual immune system, it simultaneously attacked and undermined the social cohesion at the heart of African identity. *Ubuntu*, unfortunately, can come undone or work in reverse. Nolen offers grim accounts of gaunt villagers demonized and left alone to die because fellow villagers suspect them of wasting away with Slim—the local name for AIDS. The widely shared stigma isolated patients, fractured families, and disrupted the ancient fabric of village life: as the number of AIDS victims increased among young parents, the number of AIDS orphans mounted. Villages could no longer look after the hungry children increasingly left to fend for themselves. In short, HIV/AIDS in Africa held a distinctively African profile, unlike anything I knew in the West.

My own work with pain required me to think too about suffering, and at a purely conceptual level we can tease them apart.[7] I feel pain when I stub my toe, but I do not suffer. I might suffer from the loss of a spouse but not feel pain. Neurosurgeon John D. Loeser, internationally respected specialist in pain medicine, described the distinctive conceptual relations among pain, nociception, and suffering in a now-famous diagram reproduced in numerous medical texts.

---

[4] See Desmond Tutu HIV Foundation (2015).

[5] For additional discussion, see Battle, M. (2009) and Gade, C. B. N. (2012).

[6] Tutu, D. (2014).

[7] See Morris, D. B. (1991, 2010).

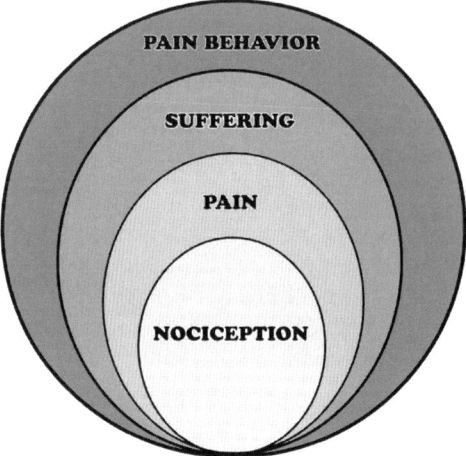

Fig. 1 John D. Loeser's biopsychosocial model for the components of pain (Reproduced courtesy of John D. Loeser)

From a different perspective, my thinking about pain produced an hourglass diagram that places individual consciousness in the center, where a clean, conceptual demarcation between pain and suffering is harder to maintain. "Our concepts of pain, impairment, and disability," Loeser's colleague Wilbert E. Fordyce writes, "must consider environmental factors as well as the person."[8] The extensive sociocultural environment, as solid as a medieval cathedral and as diffuse as Augustinian theology, affects pain in complex ways, mediated by multiple biological systems, but, no matter how complex its organic processes, no matter how fully we sympathize with the pain of others, we experience pain only in and through an individual consciousness. When we temporarily turn off consciousness, via anesthesia, sleep, or drugs, we turn off pain. Consciousness, therefore, is at the center of the hourglass:

So too suffering. In an integrative, biocultural model, the focus moves both inward and outward: inward toward the micro-level processes of cell biology (good nutrition can work wonders) and outward toward the macro-level sociocultural environments: families, villages, states, religions, media, and international agencies or multinational corporations. Intervention at any level in such an interconnected model is likely to have an impact at other levels.

---

[8] Fordyce, W. E. (1995).

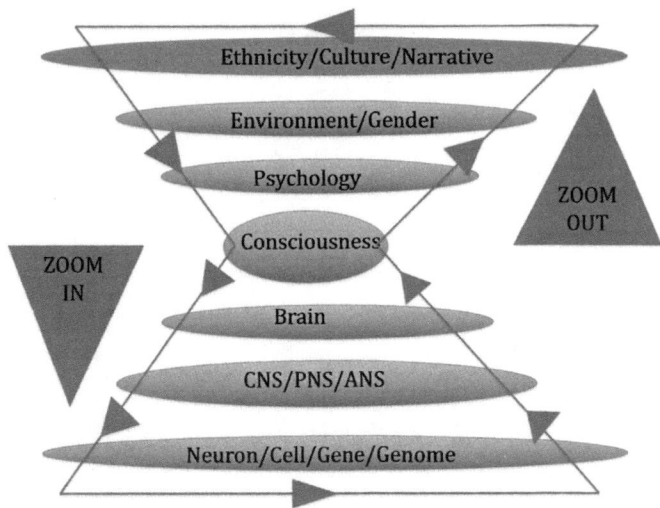

Fig. 2 An integrative model of pain (Reproduced Courtesy of David B. Morris)

A truly integrative and biocultural model should be three-dimensional and spin, but at least a flat, static version marks a significant distance from the popular belief that pain is an electrochemical signal that registers a direct one-to-one relation with tissue damage. Human suffering, like pain, involves complex interrelations among social and biological dimensions as they play out, inescapably, in a single consciousness. Even collective trauma, as in the Holocaust or in the forced marches of Native Americans, register their added cultural burden in the consciousness of each individual member of the group.

"The brain," as John Loeser puts it, "is the organ responsible for all pain."[9] Suffering too requires the human brain in all its complex biological networks. *What we do not see if we do not see*, on the other hand, is how suffering plays out in an individual consciousness situated within a particular culture. A global perspective cannot afford to overlook the ways in which cultures and consciousness, at the level of single individuals, rework the experience of suffering. Agnes Martin, in her writing, certainly recognizes the difficulties and darkness in which most of us struggle to know what is best to do. Her paintings, however, confront us with almost the opposite of anguish and confusion: a serene and geometrical perfection that hovers somewhere above or beyond the materiality of everyday life with its almost inescapable pain and suffering.

---

[9] Loeser, J.D. (1991).

Fig. 3 Agnes Martin. *Untitled #7*. 1992. Acrylic on canvas. 72″ × 72″ (Photo credit: Davis Museum at Wellesley College / Art Resource, NY)

"My paintings," she wrote in 1966, "have neither objects nor space nor time not anything—no forms. They are light, lightness, about merging, about formlessness, breaking down form."[10] Such a vision may seem to ignore the awful facts of human suffering, but perhaps it also recognizes suffering or a dimension of suffering in ways that we do not see if we do not see. That is, did Nelson Mandela during his 27 year imprisonment—18 years on brutal Robben Island—imagine patterns of racial and social harmony that others perhaps did not see? Did such a vision help sustain him in times, such as the death of his son, when daily suffering reached a crescendo pitch?

The value of a global perspective on suffering may lie less in its power to reveal a sameness in suffering, exposing core similarities or universal responses, than in awakening us to its subtle differences within a particular culture and an individual consciousness, its potential for radical strangeness, even its almost inexplicable and limitless possibilities, as in ancient Greek tragedy or in the abstract paintings of Agnes Martin, for recognizing (where others see only evident turmoil, hunger, privation, and sorrow) larger and perhaps mostly invisible patterns: God's will, Fate's unseen hand, Zen emptiness, Ubuntu connectedness, the geometry of a harmonious life. The ultimate goal of course is to relieve suffering. From a global perspective, however, such a goal requires not only that we address the suffering we see but also that we strive to recognize suffering in the lives of individuals who may not closely resemble us, who may not suffer in ways that we are familiar with, and thus—accounting for our own scotomic blindnesses or built-in cognitive and visual-field defects—to address the suffering that we do not see.

Charlottesville, VA, USA   David B. Morris

---

[10] Martin, A. quoted in Wilson, A. (1966).

References

Battle, M. (2009). *Reconciliation: The Ubuntu theology of Desmond Tutu* (Rev. ed.). Cleveland: The Pilgrim Press.

Desmond Tutu HIV Foundation. (2015). *Who we are.* http://www.desmondtutuhivfoundation.org. za/page/about/. Accessed 14 Jan 2015.

Fordyce, W. E. (Ed.). (1995). *Back pain in the workplace: Management of disability in nonspecific conditions.* Seattle: IASP Press.

Gade, C. B. N. (2012). What is Ubuntu? Different interpretations among South Africans of African Descent. *South African Journal of Philosophy, 31*, 484–503.

Kleinman, A., Das, V., & Lock, M. (Eds.). (1997). *Social suffering.* Berkeley: University of California Press.

Loeser, J. D. (1991). What is chronic pain? *Theoretical Medicine, 12*(3), 213–225.

Martin, A. (1979). Excerpts from 'What we do not see if we do not see.' In A. Glimcher (Ed.). (2012). *Agnes Martin: Paintings, writings, remembrances* (p. 34). New York: Phaidon Press.

Marx, K. (1983). Theses on Feuerbach. In E. Kamenka (Ed.), *The portable Karl Marx* (p. 158). New York: Penguin.

Morris, D. B. (1991). *The culture of pain.* Berkeley: University of California Press.

Morris, D. B. (2010). Sociocultural dimensions of pain management. In J. C. Ballantyne, J. P. Rathmell & S. M. Fishman (Eds.), *Bonica's management of pain* (4th ed., pp. 133–145). New York: Lippincott Williams & Wilkins.

Nolen, S. (2007). *28: Stories of AIDS in Africa.* New York: Walker & Company.

Sayad, A. (2004). *The suffering of the immigrant* (D. Macey, Trans.). New York: Polity Press.

Tutu, D. (2014). *The Politics of Ubuntu. HuffingtonPost.com, Inc.* http://www.huffingtonpost.com/desmond-tutu/the-politics-of-ubuntu_b_5125854.html. Accessed 12 Apr 2014.

Wilson, A. (1966). Linear webs. *Art and Artists, 1*(7), 49.

Preface

Goals This book grew out of a desire to compile in one place the ideas, perspectives, and findings of researchers who are pioneers in understanding human suffering around the world. Though suffering is a universal experience, these reports reveal surprising diversity in approach, emphasis and findings. Some conceptualizations highlight close associations between suffering and various worldviews including humanitarianism, human rights, caring, and healing.

"Global" and "suffering" may be household words, but not until this collection has a book explicitly tackled the topic of *world suffering*. In this pioneering book project, I sought to build momentum for a research tradition that might ultimately help reduce world suffering. Toward this end, I assembled leaders who have explored the fields of suffering and quality of life (QOL) to write exemplary essays and reports showing examples of what is known, how to improve methods to study suffering, how to collect new and better data, and otherwise how to expand knowledge about suffering around the world. Those reporting research results used quite different methodologies: case studies, surveys, in-depth interviews, participant observations, and secondary data analysis. Not only do these pages explicate the concept of world suffering, they show how it can be investigated on a global scale, and, perhaps most importantly, reveal how suffering relief remains central to the purpose of human societies.

As we link the notion of freedom from suffering with indicators of QOL, we achieve a new depth of knowledge. In taking this approach, progress in research on suffering or QOL spills over from one to the other, offering new perspectives for both. This collaborative writing project explores ways to improve research on suffering by using paradigms and methodologies from QOL research. It also offers improvements to QOL research by taking into account pain and suffering. The reader will gain a wealth of insights about the interaction between suffering and quality of life, the most up-to-date characterization of worldwide suffering, and a grasp of the implications of these data for local and global policy on health and social well-being.

Processes Over the past several years, in preparation for writing a short book, *Human Suffering and Quality of Life* (Anderson 2014), I digested hundreds of articles and books on suffering. In reviewing the bodies of literature on suffering, pain and quality of life, I found the diversity of approaches and opinions startling. Such divergence made the mission for this book even more compelling.

To obtain the chapters for this volume, I emailed invitations to about 100 authors of academic books or articles related to suffering. Each was charged with writing something important pertaining to *world suffering* in 5,000–7,000 words. I received about 70 good abstracts and asked for the authors to write chapter drafts.

Over a 9-month period, I worked with these authors and obtained reviews in order to create high quality, in-depth but succinct essays or reports for this volume. Together, the 32 chapters assembled here represent the best of contemporary thought and cutting edge research on world suffering and quality of life. The authors live in 16 countries and represent each major continent except Antarctica. The authors don't necessarily agree on precisely how to define suffering, but their work contributes to a cumulative body of knowledge on suffering that ultimately will be enormous.

The authors chose to focus on one or more of these types of suffering:

- Physical suffering, especially what we typically call pain
- Mental suffering, including depression, anxiety, existential suffering, other severe mental illness
- Interpersonal suffering, that suffering caused by social rejection, social isolation, and deficits in social interaction
- Social suffering (resulting from local or global social institutions that harm specific categories of people, such as the poor, the disabled, etc.)
- Co-occurrences of all these four types of suffering, which I call "total suffering"

By bringing a more precise and complete vocabulary of suffering into every day and humanitarian discourse, we have the basic tools to collaborate to alleviate suffering and reduce its future occurrence.

Audiences As I assembled the chapters, I divided them in many different ways, including by study methods used and key themes. From this process, the principal audience communities became more apparent. Anticipated audiences include:

- Those concerned with understanding pain and suffering and their effects
- Researchers wanting to assess the ongoing quality of life of different groups or sectors of the world
- Those studying community, including online community, and the role social suffering and interpersonal deficits, such as isolation, have on members of these communities
- Those supporting or participating in humanitarian activities, including human rights, development and otherwise improving the human condition
- Healthcare providers and informal caregivers, especially those who struggle with suffering

- Anyone who wants to alleviate suffering, including reduction of global inequality from which many people live with life-consuming, intense suffering

Challenges In today's world, it is nearly impossible to escape images showing violence, famine, disease, and other calamities. As noted in Chap. 6, media scholars tend to agree that social media and other new technology, combined with narcissist marketing of humanitarian aid, produces half-hearted concern for global suffering. Thus, the public sees second-hand a barrage of disasters, epidemics, wars, and terrorism. Existing institutions such as human rights organizations and humanitarian relief agencies rally support for relief from these calamities. But often their appeals fall flat because the giving public has not been socialized in the humane values that demand social responsibility for all tragically suffering human beings.

Avoiding preventable suffering is an ultimate human concern. This means that human beings must come to terms with it and understand it as a central social responsibility in exchange for life. Research on suffering will help us identify and evaluate how best to act responsibly.

In contrast, unpreventable suffering, such as natural death, can be a tragedy that we learn to approach with serenity and accept as part of life. Toward that end, some of the chapters here offer enlightenment on how suffering can become a source of meaning and an aid to making peace in a cruel world.

Minneapolis, MN, USA   Ronald E. Anderson

Acknowledgments

A book this size—with 46 authors, 32 chapters, and a foreword—requires a village to conceive, produce, and deliver a new, literary life. My mixed metaphor, if nothing else, hints that the book's production had its moments of excitement and pain as well as hard, tedious but challenging work.

The book project began in Buenos Aires at an ISQOLS (International Society for Quality of Life Studies) in July 2012, when I met Esther Otten, editor of health, well-being and sociology publications at Springer Science + Business Media (commonly known as Springer) in Dordrecht, The Netherlands. She expressed interest in my work on the topic of suffering, and by the end of the year, I had presented two successful book proposals to Springer. After finishing the first book in June 2013, I immediately initiated the 12 months required to assemble the contributions to this book.

During that time, I sent dozens of email requests for help to Esther Otten, as well as Tuerlings Hendrikje and Miranda Dijksman, both editorial assistants in social sciences at Springer in Dordrecht. Without their guidance and help, it would have taken twice as long. I am very grateful for their support throughout.

Here in Minnesota, I began the project doing everything myself, but as the number of authors and potential authors of chapters expanded toward 100, I found local support for the editorial and administrative work. Letta Page and Sherri Hildebrandt provided excellent copy editing of every document, and they also gave invaluable advice on content and presentation of ideas. Kathryn Albrecht served as the project's expert on citations and references, checking every chapter and helping to fill in the missing details. Carol Miller managed the time-consuming process of communicating with every author to get their approvals of the edited papers as well as the authors' signed consent forms. It is amazing what can be done with highly skilled assistants working together using only email communication.

While the writing, reviewing, and editing process took only a year, it seemed much longer, because the authors and I learned so much in the process. I will forever feel grateful to my new friends and what they contributed to this work. I predict that the authors of this volume's chapters will evolve into a community of scholars and researchers who will continue to generate theoretical and practical knowledge—both qualitative and quantitative—about global, human suffering.

Many authors helped by reviewing papers and finding additional prospective authors. Special thanks to authors Iain Wilkinson, Nancy Johnston, and Daina Harvey in this regard. The preface that immediately follows this page gives additional details about collaborating with the authors and implications for the future.

Several well-known scholars, whose tight schedules made it impossible to contribute to the book itself, nonetheless gave their enthusiastic moral support, boosting my morale with the encouragement they gave for the book. They include: Craig Calhoun, president, London School of Economics; Paul Farmer, professor and global health leader, Harvard University; Richard Estes, professor emeritus, University of Pennsylvania; and Alex C. Michalos, professor emeritus, Brandon University and editor, *Social Indicators Research*.

This research and writing project benefited greatly by two small grants to Ronald Anderson from the University of Minnesota Office of the Vice President for Research and the University of Minnesota Retirees Association (UMRA).

Finally, I wish to thank my wife, Nancy Kehmeier, for her ongoing support for the project. Not once did she claim to suffer from social rejection due to my preoccupation with this intense and time-consuming project.

Contents

Part I   World Suffering: A Challenge to Humanity, Humanitarianism and Human Rights

1   Implications of World Suffering for Human Progress   3
Ronald E. Anderson

2   Suffering in Silence? The Silencing of Sexual Violence Against Men in War Torn Countries   31
Élise Féron

3   Social Suffering and Critical Humanitarianism   45
Iain Wilkinson

4   Compassion, Cruelty, and Human Rights   55
Natan Sznaider

5   Making Sense of Suffering: Insights from Buddhism and Critical Social Science   65
Ruben Flores

6   Distant Suffering and the Mediation of Humanitarian Disaster   75
Johannes von Engelhardt and Jeroen Jansz

Part II   Professional and Informal Caregiving

7   Suffering and Identity: "Difficult Patients" in Hospice Care   91
Cindy L. Cain

8   Healing Suffering: The Evolution of Caring Practices 101
Nancy E. Johnston

9   Meaning in Bereavement 115
Robert A. Neimeyer

10 **Coping with the Suffering of Ambiguous Loss** 125
    Pauline Boss

11 **Social Suffering and an Approach to Professionals' Burnout** 135
    Graciela Tonon, Lia Rodriguez-de-la-Vega, and Inés Aristegui

12 **The Invisible Suffering of HIV and AIDS Caregivers
    in Botswana** 147
    Gloria Jacques

13 **Loneliness as Social Suffering: Social Participation,
    Quality of Life, and Chronic Stroke** 159
    Narelle Warren and Darshini Ayton

Part III Quality of Life: Global, Community, and Personal

14 **Child Well-Being and Child Suffering** 173
    Kenneth C. Land, Vicki L. Lamb, and Qiang Fu

15 **Felt-Suffering and Its Social Variations in China** 187
    Yanjie Bian and Jing Shen

16 **Suffering Ailments and Addiction Problems in the Family** 203
    Mariano Rojas

17 **Suffering and Good Society Analysis Across African Countries** 217
    Ferdi Botha

18 **Lifetime Suffering and Capabilities in Chile** 233
    Francisca Dussaillant and Pablo A. González

19 **Shame, Humiliation and Social Isolation: Missing Dimensions
    of Poverty and Suffering Analysis** 251
    China Mills and Diego Zavaleta

Part IV Suffering and Community: Online and Offline Contexts

20 **The Cultural Geography of Community Suffering** 269
    Daina Cheyenne Harvey

21 **Social Organization of Suffering and Justice-Seeking
    in a Tragic Day Care Fire Disaster** 281
    Eric C. Jones and Arthur D. Murphy

22 **Community Quality-of-Life Indicators to Avoid Tragedies** 293
    Rhonda Phillips

23 **Community Action to Alleviate Suffering from Racism:
    The Role of Religion and Caring Capital in Small City USA** 305
    Meg Wilkes Karraker

24 **Suffering in Online Interactions** 317
   Katrin Döveling and Katrin Wasgien

25 **Cosmopolitan Perspectives on Suffering** 331
   Laura Robinson

26 **Iconography of Suffering in Social Media: Images
   of Sitting Girls** 341
   Anna Johansson and Hans T. Sternudd

Part V   Research and Policy Challenges for the Future

27 **The Neurosociology of Social Rejection and Suffering** 359
   David D. Franks

28 **Collaborative Humanitarianism: Information
   Networks that Reduce Suffering** 367
   Louis-Marie Ngamassi Tchouakeu and Andrea H. Tapia

29 **A New Method for Measuring and Analyzing Suffering:
   Comparing Suffering Patterns in Italian Society** 385
   Marco Fattore and Filomena Maggino

30 **Hurricane Katrina, Family Trouble, and the Micro-politics
   of Suffering** 401
   Ara Francis and Daina Cheyenne Harvey

31 **Emotions, Empathy, and the Choice to Alleviate Suffering** 413
   Caitlin O. Mahoney and Laura M. Harder

32 **How Suffering Challenges Our Future** 427
   Ronald E. Anderson

Contributors

Ronald E. Anderson Department of Sociology, Emeritus Faculty of Sociology, University of Minnesota, Minneapolis, MN, USA

Inés Aristegui Psychology Program, Faculty of Social Sciences, Universidad de Palermo, Ciudad Autonoma de Buenos Aires, Argentina

Darshini Ayton School of Public Health and Preventive Medicine, Monash University, Clayton, VIC, Australia

Yanjie Bian Department of Sociology, Faculty of Sociology, University of Minnesota, Minneapolis, MN, USA

Faculty of Sociology, Xi'an Jiaotong University, Xi'an, China

Pauline Boss Family Social Science Department, University of Minnesota, Minneapolis, MN, USA

Ferdi Botha Department of Economics and Economic History, Rhodes University, Grahamstown, South Africa

Cindy L. Cain Division of Health Policy and Management, University of Minnesota, Minneapolis, MN, USA

Katrin Döveling Institute of Communication and Media Studies, Department of Empiric Research in Communication and Media, University of Leipzig, Dresden, Germany

Francisca Dussaillant School of Government, Universidad del Desarrollo, Santiago, Chile

Marco Fattore Department of Statistics and Quantitative Methods, Università degli Studi di Milano – Bicocca, Milan, Italy

Élise Féron Conflict Analysis Research Centre, University of Kent, Canterbury, UK

Ruben Flores Faculty of Social Sciences, National Research University – Higher School of Economics, Moscow, Russian Federation

Ara Francis Department of Sociology and Anthropology, College of the Holy Cross, Worcester, MA, USA

David D. Franks Department of Sociology, Emeritus Professor of Sociology, Virginia Commonwealth University, Richmond, VA, USA

Qiang Fu Department of Sociology, Duke University, Durham, NC, USA

Pablo A. González Department of Industrial Engineering, Faculty of Physical and Mathematical Sciences, Universidad de Chile, Santiago, Chile

Laura M. Harder Department of Psychology, Metropolitan State University, St Paul, MN, USA

Daina Cheyenne Harvey Department of Sociology and Anthropology, College of the Holy Cross, Worcester, MA, USA

Gloria Jacques Department of Social Work, University of Botswana, Gaborone, Botswana

Jeroen Jansz Erasmus Research Centre for Media, Communication and Culture, Erasmus University Rotterdam, Rotterdam, The Netherlands

Anna Johansson HUMlab, Umeå University, Umeå, Sweden

Nancy E. Johnston Faculty of Health, School of Nursing, York University, Toronto, ON, Canada

Eric C. Jones Faculty of School of Public Health, University of Texas-Houston, El Paso, TX, USA

Meg Wilkes Karraker Department of Sociology, Faculty of Sociology, Family Studies and Women's Studies, University of St. Thomas, St. Paul, MN, USA

Vicki L. Lamb Department of Human Sciences, Faculty of Human Sciences, North Carolina Central University, Durham, NC, USA

Kenneth C. Land Department of Sociology, Faculty of Sociology, Duke University, Durham, NC, USA

Filomena Maggino Department of Statistics, Informatics, Applications "G. Parenti" (DiSIA), Università degli Studi di Firenze, Florence, Italy

Caitlin O. Mahoney Faculty of Psychology, Metropolitan State University, St Paul, MN, USA

China Mills Faculty of Education, University of Sheffield, Sheffield, UK

David B. Morris Writer and Emeritus Professor of English, University of Virginia, Charlottesville, VA, USA

Arthur D. Murphy Department of Anthropology, UNC Greensboro, Greensboro, NC, USA

Robert A. Neimeyer Department of Psychology, Faculty of Psychology, University of Memphis, Memphis, TN, USA

Rhonda Phillips Professor, Department of Agricultural Economics and Dean, Honors College, Purdue University, West Lafayette, IN, USA

Laura Robinson Santa Clara University, Santa Clara, USA

Lia Rodriguez-de-la-Vega CICS-Faculty of Social Sciences, Universidad de Palermo, Ciudad Autonoma de Buenos Aires, Argentina

Mariano Rojas FLACSO-México and UPAEP, Mexico, D.F., Mexico

Jing Shen The Prentice Institute for Global Population and Economy, University of Lethbridge, Lethbridge, AB, Canada

Hans T. Sternudd Department of Music and Art, Faculty of Art History and Visual Culture, Linnaeus University, Växjö, Sweden

Natan Sznaider Faculty, School of Behavioral Sciences, The Academic College of Tel Aviv-Yaffo, Tel Aviv, Israel

Andrea H. Tapia Faculty of College of Information Sciences and Technology, Pennsylvania State University, State College, PA, USA

Louis-Marie Ngamassi Tchouakeu Faculty of College of Business, Prairie View A&M University, Prairie View, TX, USA

Graciela Tonon CICS-Faculty of Social Sciences, Universidad de Palermo, Ciudad Autonoma de Buenos Aires, Argentina

Johannes von Engelhardt Erasmus Research Centre for Media, Communication and Culture, Erasmus University Rotterdam, Rotterdam, The Netherlands

Narelle Warren School of Social Sciences, Monash University, Clayton, VIC, Australia

Katrin Wasgien Institute of Communication and Media Studies, Department of Empiric Research in Communication and Media, University of Leipzig, Dresden, Germany

Iain Wilkinson Faculty of Sociology, University of Kent, Canterbury, Kent, UK

Diego Zavaleta Oxford Poverty and Human Development Initiative, Queen Elizabeth House, University of Oxford, Oxford, UK

About the Editor

Ronald (Ron) Anderson is Professor Emeritus at the University of Minnesota. He received his Ph.D. in sociology from Stanford University in 1970. From 1968 until retiring in 2005, he served on the faculty of sociology at the University of Minnesota. From 1990 to 2005, he coordinated several international studies of the social and learning effects of information technology within primary and secondary education in 20 or more countries in each study. From that and earlier work, he wrote or edited seven books and over 100 articles. Since retirement, his research interests have focused on suffering and caring.

Part I
World Suffering: A Challenge to Humanity, Humanitarianism and Human Rights

Chapter 1
Implications of World Suffering for Human Progress

Ronald E. Anderson

1.1 Introduction

Suffering ranks high on the list of what it means to be human, yet the desire and action to alleviate our suffering, and that of others, ranks even higher. However, for many historic reasons, suffering tends to be repressed and largely ignored. This escape from suffering may account in part for the ease by which large numbers of people can be indifferent to the tragic suffering around the world.

Despite each individual's unique suffering, it is possible to study suffering among not only individuals, but families, groups, communities, nations, and the world. Study after study, conducted in different communities and countries, reveals that despite small cultural differences, the structure, patterns, and oftentimes meanings of suffering, ring true across all social contexts around the globe (Anderson 2014). I had expected that many of the most interesting findings would be comparative (across communities or countries), but this was not the case. Instead, the most intriguing results were from the uniqueness of a study's methodology. Progress on social policies regarding suffering requires multiple methods: subjective and objective measurements; qualitative and quantitative data collection; formal and informal analytical approaches, in both research and policy.

A comprehensive discussion of suffering naturally leads to considerations of alternative strategies for the relief of suffering. Separating chapters into the categories of humanitarianism, caregiving, quality of life (QOL), community systems, and human rights, led to the realization that to some extent, these are parallel types of strategies for the relief of suffering. And while funding is a prerequisite for solving

R.E. Anderson (✉)
Department of Sociology, Emeritus Faculty of Sociology, University of Minnesota, Minneapolis, MN 55455, USA
e-mail: rea@umn.edu

© Springer Science+Business Media Dordrecht 2015
R.E. Anderson (ed.), *World Suffering and Quality of Life*,
Social Indicators Research Series 56, DOI 10.1007/978-94-017-9670-5_1

many problems of human suffering, changes in basic social and political institutions are the real requirements for long-term solutions to the enormous amount of human suffering worldwide.

1.2   Defining and Delineating World Suffering

In his classic book on suffering for the caregiving professions, Cassell (1991) defined suffering as severe distress that interfered with one's personhood. I followed Cassell in defining suffering as distress resulting from threat, major loss, or damage to one's body and/or self-identity (Anderson 2014). Cassell distinguished not only the body and mind but also the conceptions that a person holds of time, causation, and most of all, meanings of life. We all agree that suffering can vary in intensity, duration, awareness, source, and preventability, but Cassell as a physician was curious to understand why his patients responded so differently to not only trauma but treatment. While his analysis produced in-depth insights into the suffering of specific individuals, making generalizations about global suffering requires more precision and succinctness in conceptualizing and defining suffering.

There are times, particularly in ethnographic studies, when one should focus on the meanings (principally for the sense of self) that suffering has, or does not have, for different individuals. But for large-scale comparisons, it is important to focus upon the principal source of the suffering: physical, mental, interpersonal or social. *Physical suffering* is the subset of distress resulting from threat or damage to one's physical being, whereas *mental suffering* is distress perceived as originating in one's cognitive or affective self-identity (Anderson 2014). Physical suffering is equated with pain, even though it often co-occurs with mental suffering (Black 2005; Carr et al. 2005; Livingston 1998; Morris 2002; Wilson et al. 2009). Mental suffering includes cognitive suffering (thoughts that produce suffering) and affective or emotional suffering (Francis 2006). Mental suffering does not necessarily have an origin in painful sensory events, and is more elusive. Depression and anxiety, perhaps the most persistent varieties of mental suffering, when combined with other mental maladies such as grief, serious mental illness, and existential suffering, together form a major type of suffering labeled here as mental suffering.

Physical suffering, typified by chronic pain, usually depends upon neurological paths between a sensory organ and the brain as a communication system. However, recent neuroscience research discovered a number of ways that pain arises without following the simple neurological pathways (Borsook 2012).

The more extreme the suffering, the more likely the sufferer is to experience multiple types of suffering. In fact, it is not uncommon for sufferers to simultaneously feel all types of suffering: physical, mental, social, and interpersonal. Cicely Saunders (2006), the founder of the modern hospice movement, called this type of suffering, "total pain." To be specific, she defined total pain as the intersection of physical, mental, spiritual (existential), and social. Some people prefer to equate the word suffering to situations of "total pain"; I prefer to reserve the label *total suffering* for deep distress that intersects all the major types of suffering.

1.2.1 Social Suffering and Social Pain

The third major class of suffering, *interpersonal suffering*, constitutes another name for what many call "social pain." Common examples of interpersonal suffering would be social rejection, forced social isolation, and withdrawal of affection or interaction privileges. It can also be defined as distress inflicted by a primary group: family, friends, or people with whom one might have had regular contact. In Chap. 27, David Franks summarizes the research in neuroscience on social pain (interpersonal suffering). Principal findings include (1) the potential for highly traumatic responses to social isolation and rejection, and (2) the discovery that interpersonal suffering and physical suffering affect the identical areas of the brain.

In contrast to interpersonal suffering, *social suffering* results from social institutions, especially from community or societal norms that encourage discrimination or harm against members of social groups toward which stigma has been directed, e.g., minority belief groups, disability or racial groups. These negative effects are legitimized and maintained by powerful organizational institutions like governments and religions.

In the past two decades, the label 'social suffering' has come to mean suffering produced primarily by social conditions that damage a collective's sense of self-worth and heightens powerlessness produced from socially shared traumas (Kleinman et al. 1997; Wilkinson 2005). One frequent consequence of social suffering is the loss of caring for self and others as valued human beings. Good examples of social suffering are victims of social discrimination, disability, poverty, and others treated as second-class citizens. Social institutions typically maintain the status quo that perpetuates the stigma and the socially shared suffering (Bourdieu et al. 2000).

Social suffering as a concept concerns more than trauma produced by social forces. Those who continue to write about social suffering seek to convey that those who experience social suffering, and in some instances, those who perpetuate it, come to understand the interconnectedness of all involved. Such illumination of the full reality of the imposition on those persecuted presumably leads to awareness of the moral-immoral aspects of the social relations in play.

Another way of thinking about social suffering is that it exposes the role of the larger community and society in maintaining unequal social trauma ranging from a structure of violence to subtle disparaging of others (Wilkinson 2012, 2013). Social suffering is generally studied using ethnographic, case study methods (Wilkinson 2005). Classic case studies applying this approach include community violence in Fiji (Trnka 2008), street drug addicts (Singer 2006) and religious persecution in India and Pakistan (Nagappan 2005). In this book, Chaps. 2, 11, 12, 13, 23, and 30 apply the notion of social suffering.

Some social suffering occurs in the form of genocide and massive atrocities against socially defined groups. Sociologist Alexander (2012) developed a theory to explain how individual suffering gets transformed into cultural traumas. His theory essentially outlines "cultural work," such as speeches and campaigns, as the critical force behind the social definition of horrific cultural traumas. Sometimes the cultural work lacks adequate power to define a trauma; for example, in the United States, there remains considerable disagreement over whether mainstream culture discriminates against African-Americans. Thus, the social suffering of African-Americans goes unrecognized by a large sector of the society.

1.2.2 The Language of Suffering

Thernstrom (2010) found a word for "headache" in almost every language, but the definitions for the word "torture" not only differ across cultures, but the amount of pain felt from specific forms of torture depends on the culture as well as specific social situations. Cultural differences account not only for variation in emotional expressiveness but the assignment of meanings to a wide variety of situations involving pain and suffering. Thus the actual intensity of pain and suffering varies extensively by cultural context (Davidhizar and Giger 2004; Narayan 2010).

Not surprisingly, those who think about the concepts of pain or suffering, or work with those trying to manage their pain or suffering, lack a common vocabulary (Thernstrom 2010). This greatly constrains discourse on the subject and blocks the emergence of theory and research, and curtails the building of a global knowledge base.

A typology of suffering from the perspective of both the social sciences and public health and development could facilitate communication as well as empirical research on suffering. My general-purpose taxonomy of suffering, detailed in the previous section, addresses research as well as practice needs. To illustrate, statistics from a large, national health survey reported in the second column of Table 1.1 provide a portrait of suffering in America in 2010.

One of the most important findings from the suffering prevalence analysis of the American health study was that the most common type of suffering found was the co-occurrence of two or three types rather than one type (physical, mental, or social) alone. Finally, of all the different types of suffering, the only type of suffering that dramatically increased with age was physical. Those 60 or older were three times more likely than adults in their 20s to report significant pain (Anderson 2014).

1.2.3 Qualitative Depth and Quantitative Breadth in Suffering Research

Statistical estimates of suffering prevalences are useful for comparing suffering across events, places, and conditions. But comparing in-depth, subjective perceptions is critical for understanding suffering, its idiosyncratic nature, and its perceived meaning to the individual. Without such qualitative information, it would be nearly impossible to assess how any given type of suffering affects a person's

Table 1.1 A preliminary typology of global suffering, prevalences and associated emotions[a]

Types of suffering	Prevalence in USA 2010[b]	Associated emotions
1.0 Physical (aka pain)	19 %	Hurt, aching, torture, agony
2.0 Mental/Affective (any)	14	See four subtypes below
2.1. Depression	9	Misery, desolation, melancholy
2.2 Anxiety	8	Agitation, affliction, obsession, craving
2.3 Existential suffering	5	Purposeless, hopeless, angst, helpless
2.4 Grief	3	Loss, sorrow, heartbreak, immobilizing
2.5 Major mental illnesses	–	Rage, desolation, dread
3.0 Interpersonal suffering	–	Isolation, interpersonal rejection or neglect
4.0 Social suffering	–	Humiliation, shame, stigma-based discrimination

– The dash refers to a category that was not included in this analysis
[a]This typology and the data were first published in Anderson (2014) using data from 2010 Integration Health Interview Study in the United States in 2010
[b]Prevalences overlap categories, thus they cannot be summed to 100 %. Prevalence of any type of suffering in the study was estimated as 36 %

identity, which in turn changes his or her social relationships. The accumulation of such shifts in identity affects entire communities and societies.

For example, Rummel (1994) estimated that more than 100,000 reputed female witches were burned alive "at the stake" between the fifteenth and eighteenth centuries. This exemplifies how throughout much of recorded history, due to their lower status, women tended to suffer greater persecution and torture than men.

1.2.4 The Prevention of Suffering

The focus of most research on suffering continues to be on suffering that can be prevented, such as torture and other inhumane punishment. Unpreventable suffering, such as the plague and other infectious diseases, will be considered, but only in terms of reducing suffering. For preventable suffering, our goal as caring persons should be to try to eliminate the cause as well as the suffering itself. With global climate change caused primarily by human choices, the distinction between preventable and unpreventable suffering increasingly becomes more complex and cloudy. Floods, hurricanes, and other catastrophic, climate-related events could formerly be considered acts of nature, but undoubtedly they increasingly arise from both natural and anthropogenic (man-made) sources.

Suffering comes from three places: individuals, social institutions, and forces of nature. Suffering that arises strictly from "acts of God," such as earthquakes and tornadoes, does not fall within our primary concern because it is largely unpreventable. Suffering is preventable when it follows from human choices, such as driving

Table 1.2 Examples of preventable and unpreventable suffering

Types of suffering	Preventable suffering	Unpreventable suffering
Physical pain	Self-injury	Lightning strikes
Mental suffering	Self-pity	Congenital brain damage
Grief	Unrecoverable mourning	Short-term mourning
Social suffering	Incarceration for possession of illegal drugs	Earthquakes

too fast and playing with a loaded gun. With disasters such as hurricanes, we do not know to what extent the ensuing suffering is preventable because hurricanes now gain their force from both natural and man-made forces. Table 1.2 gives examples to illustrate both preventable and unpreventable instances of each major type of suffering.

Many of the atrocities described in past eras consisted of preventable suffering. However, much of suffering was unpreventable—specifically, that caused by natural disasters and infectious diseases such as the plague. Before the invention of anesthesia, surgery produced unpreventable suffering as well. Here is the narrative of a woman in France in 1810 who underwent removal of a breast tumor:

> When the dreadful steel was plunged into my breast, I released an unremitting scream.... I felt the knife rackling against the breast bone, scraping it while I remained in torture. (Hemlow 1975)

While one might be tempted to dismiss this as a problem we no longer face because of modern medicine, anesthetics, and pain relievers, in the twenty-first century, many people in remote, impoverished areas of the world cannot afford the anesthetics and pain relievers that the Western world has come to expect as an everyday part of life. Illness and suffering remain two very relevant issues in almost every corner of the globe.

1.2.5 Global Traumatic Suffering: Estimating Quantity and Quality

Global violence may have declined over the past 3,000 years on a per capita basis, but it is doubtful that the absolute number of people killed each year has declined because the population has been rising so rapidly, particularly in agrarian societies. The global population tripled in the twentieth century alone. At some point between the distant past and the twentieth century, typical but cruel punishments came to be called atrocities. Furthermore, as record-keeping systems improved, the volume of deaths, injuries, diseases, and displacements could be estimated with increasing precision. Based upon UN and World Health Organization (WHO) statistics, Table 1.3 provides estimates of unnatural deaths and other events producing traumatic world suffering in 2010.

Table 1.3 Global traumatic suffering estimates, 2010

Deaths, starvations, assaults, self-injuries, displacements & HIV/AIDS counts[a]	Estimates
Unintended starvation (energy-deprived diets)	766,229,726
Non-lethal assaults (officially reported)	380,746,682
Natural disasters (deaths & displacements)[a]	257,272,601
HIV/AIDS prevalence	33,446,568
Suicides and attempted suicides[b]	20,000,000
Needless deaths from non-infectious diseases[c]	14,281,370
Pollution-related deaths	5,030,203
Homicides	302,093
Civil war deaths	103,437
Grand Total (22 % of world population)	1,477,412,680

Source: United Nations Development Program (2010) and Human Development Report
[a]WHO suicide database
[b]Displacements were those relocated due to lost housing
[c]This death count was calculated from HDR (2010) data by comparing the top 40 (HDI) nations with the remaining 130 less developed nations

Keep in mind that these statistical estimates contain error and only approximate the number of people actually suffering for a considerable amount of time during the year. The table says that at least 22 % of the global population (one in five persons) had a major suffering event such as those listed in Table 1.3 during the year 2010. However, only about one third of these "suffering events" include actual deaths during the year. If you were to add in serious war injuries to these counts, which currently add up to about three persons per war death, this amounts to well over a half-billion persons left suffering from wars since 1900 (White 2011). And this does not include those suffering grief over one or more war dead. This numeric picture of suffering significantly underestimates the total suffering in another ways: some physical suffering, e.g., deaths from infectious diseases other than HIV did not get included because many countries do not count them separately from other deaths.

In the past 25 years the population of the developed world sector rose 0.6 % per year, while the 40 least-developed countries increased in size by 2.5 % per year.[1] Meanwhile, the life expectancy in the top 40 countries increased to 22 years longer than those living in the 40 least-developed countries (80 versus 58 years life expectancy at birth). Therefore, rising global inequality leads to greater worldwide suffering except in so far as greater longevity may increase total suffering.

Normally, longevity is seen as a sign of good health, but in fact those who live to a very old age tend to report a much higher prevalence of reoccurring illnesses, such as stroke. Thus, some affluent individuals may suffer more in general than the poor who do not live so long. Furthermore, those who live in societies with high life

---

[1] These demographic statistics were derived from the World Health Organization's online data files, accessed 25 June 2014.

expectancies also tend to suffer from "affluenzas" (Graaf et al. 2014) – ailments such as obesity, diabetes, and depression with associated suicide risk. The estimates of suffering in Table 1.3 do not include any direct estimates of social suffering. Instances of severe racial discrimination, constant bullying, slavery, severe poverty, and disabilities have not been included. Including such prevalences might double the number of sufferers.

1.3   The Humanitarian System and Human Rights Activities

1.3.1   Humanitarian Versus Human Rights Activities

Humanitarian and human rights activities often overlap, and sometimes they can be confused. Human rights are standards of behavior to which any person is entitled, simply because of being a human (Wronka 2008). Both humanitarian and human rights concepts have been formalized into law. However, as already noted, International Humanitarian Law (IHL) applies to armed conflict, while International Human Rights Law (IHRL) protects people in peacetime as well.

Both humanitarianism and human rights primarily play a role of social action in the world rather than as instigators of legal statutes. Humanitarian aid focuses on delivery of assistance and tries to be as neutral as possible in conflict situations. Human rights workers engage in activism, specifically getting political bodies to adopt human rights principles and offer solutions to human rights issues such as freedom, education, and health. Therefore, humanitarian thought considers immediate causes of suffering, while human rights thought looks for root causes of suffering and ways that social justice can be achieved, as well as reduction in suffering.

Not surprisingly, human rights workers look for violations of human rights and seek social changes that eliminate nonconformity to human rights principles. Humanitarian workers don't have the luxury of attending to violations or criticizing political parties; their goal tends to be constrained to reducing the suffering on all sides of a conflict (Fast 2014). Both humanitarian organizations and human rights groups contend with differences of opinion within their respective systems, however, the former tend to have the advantage of greater consensus on goals and strategies than does the human rights movement.

1.3.2   Humanitarianism

No single, universally accepted definition of humanitarianism exists, but the dominant view is that "humanitarian" refers to alleviating suffering and reducing loss of life, especially in emergency situations including armed conflict. The concept dates to the ancient Greeks and continues to expand in importance as International Humanitarian Law (IHL) increasingly serves as the basis for the accepted rules of warfare. In this narrow role of armed conflict, humanitarianism and IHL serve to define acceptable international boundaries of humane treatment, proportionality, and so on. These rules or laws serve as the legal basis for prosecution of war crimes (Barnett and Weiss 2008). Sznaider in Chap. 4 defines humanitarianism as the study and practice of "human benevolence, including compassion, love, and caring toward humanity." Hopefully, this will become a more commonly held definition because it emphasizes caring action.

In its broad sense, humanitarianism is the normative basis for philanthropy, widespread charity, desires to improve the human condition, and reduction of human suffering (Weiss 2007). Calhoun (2008) believes that humanitarian action is legitimized by three somewhat different value orientations or objectives: "to mitigate suffering wherever it occurs; to improve the condition of humanity in general; and to respond to sudden, unexpected and morally compelling crises." These three foundational platforms would merge as a single force, were it not for the instances when two or more of these platforms conflict. Calhoun documented such conflicts, which increasingly occur because violent conflicts seem less and less likely to have only one opposing side possessing all the moral high ground. Secondly, the mitigation of suffering has become more complex and difficult over time.

1.3.3 Humanitarian Aid

The organizational complex of global humanitarian aid has grown large and cumbersome. A report by the Active Learning Network for Accountability and Performance in Humanitarian Action (ALNAP), *The State of the Humanitarian System* (2012), estimated in 2010 a total of 274,000 humanitarian system fieldworkers, with half working for non-governmental organizations (NGOs) and a third working for the UN. The report estimates that at that time, there were 4,400 NGOs of which about 18 % were International NGOs. All these sectors spent USD $16 billion that year. Keep in mind that this does not include any direct governmental (national or local) spending for emergencies. Yet, the amount spent and the number of workers employed fell far short of that needed to address all of the disasters around the world. Nor does it allow them to ensure that full recovery occurs. The 2010 Haiti earthquake became a textbook example of how large expenditures for recovery make little difference without political and civic reform (Farmer 2013).

Growing tension in the past two decades between the intended neutrality of humanitarian assistance and the alignment of humanitarian projects and aid workers with specific conflicting parties arose because of government alliances (Bornstein and Redfield 2013; Weiss 2007). In addition, aid programs typically operate from Western countries and promote aid-related practices and lifestyles that make local aid recipients suspicious (Fast 2014; Kennedy 2011; Wilson and Brown 2009).

Another contextual complication, as noted by Calhoun (2008), stems from a trend toward greater sensibilities for civilian consequences of war. Humanitarian aid systems have become so widespread that they are seen as an element of globalization (Barnett and Weiss 2008). Emergencies in the wake of climate change are becoming the new normal, both in the media and by insurance companies and the very large budgets of relief organizations (Fast 2014). The expanding requirements and costs of the relief industry shift fund-raising toward government sources. Another rift in the humanitarian community emerges from the growing pressure for military action to curtail genocide and mass killings. Called "military humanitarianism," this pressure has been rejected by some aid organizations.

In such ways, the moral imperative to alleviate suffering became social action that could not be achieved without producing some suffering in the process. Thus, humanitarian causes become sidetracked by the demands of expanding and operating in contexts of greater complexity and interconnectedness (Wilson and Brown 2009). Fast (2014) proposes taking a more relational approach to humanitarian aid, the heart of which demands greater cultural appreciation and greater integration with the people who need help.

1.3.4   Overview of Part I: Chapters on Humanitarianism and Human Rights

A notable commonality of the authors in this section is that, while beginning with very different intellectual worlds, they agree that the foundational moral value for the survivability of humanity is the commitment to care, to act with compassion. The human rights movement, and the human interchange required by market capitalism and democratization, drove away the gross public cruelty of the nineteenth century, according to Sznaider (Chap. 4). While the causes of the reduction of cruelty in punishment may not be fully understood, the fact of major reduction in public cruelty makes plausible other social change in the direction of greater humanity in the near future. Ironically, while Sznaider may be correct that free markets helped reveal the desirability of compassionate relationships, uncontrolled capitalism carries the seeds of greed and power that could crush compassion and human rights.

Several authors in this first subset of chapters on the role of humanitarianism and human rights reveal the complexity of suffering and the need for better understanding and customization in the delivery of suffering relief. Upon examining the emergence of humanitarianism and human rights, it becomes obvious how globalization has helped shape these institutions. Some have come to rely on them for leadership in the assault on preventable suffering. This would not be a downfall, were humanitarian and human rights projects given the resources, both human and financial, needed to establish sustainable social arrangements and initiatives that would put a dent in world suffering.

Each of the chapters in Part I identifies ways in which world suffering, humanitarian action, and the human rights culture become entwined. Some authors identify ways in which the humanitarian and human rights communities morally promote the removal of specific types of suffering. Other authors found arenas within which suffering continues unabated because the humanitarian or human rights communities have not acknowledged the priority of specific types of suffering. It would appear that at present, the main resources to relieve suffering are the institutional networks of humanitarian and human rights activities, on one hand, and care delivery systems on the other.

Elise Feron (Chap. 2) pioneered a study of male rape victims during violent conflict, which could not have been done without ethnographic methods. Because sexual violence against men and boys in conflict zones had not yet been the focus of much research, Feron chose to conduct interviews in Burundi, Rwanda, and the Democratic Republic of Congo (DRC) of male victims during violent conflicts. In all three countries, she discovered that sexual violence of men against men and boys had been widespread and frequent during conflict times, though silenced and overlooked by political authorities and non-governmental organizations. Feron discovered that sexual assaults (rape, sexual mutilation, and forcing the victim to rape others) usually were accompanied by sexual torture, beatings, castration, starvation, and enslavement. After such unimaginable atrocities, the male victims often refused to report the event to officials or even to friends and family, because being raped like a woman, or being a victim of genital mutilation, was seen as the equivalent of losing one's status and identity as a man. Truly this type of suffering illustrates what I referred to earlier as *total suffering*, because these victims encountered every type of suffering in its extreme.

Iain Wilkinson in Chap. 3 provides a conceptual analysis, as do the two chapters following it, rather than a research report. He points out how some technical and critical approaches to the study of suffering are self-defeating unless they embrace the essence of humanitarianism and "the call to care." Having worked on social suffering so long and prolifically, he serves as the *de facto* leader of sociologists doing research on social suffering (Wilkinson 2005). He asserts that the essential goal of critical humanitarianism is to embrace the burden of those who care about threats to humanity; and those who study social suffering necessarily "examine relative conceptions and experiences of human rights." Building on the work of Chouliaraki (2013), he notes how she concluded that recent humanitarian campaigns unintentionally focus their audiences' attention and identity more on the celebrities than the plight of those actually suffering. He also notes that Calhoun (2004) concluded that campaigns of relief agencies often convey the social script that human suffering is an inevitable condition and that this state should not be targeted for political and social change. In the study of social suffering, Wilkinson claims that human suffering is viewed as "holding a mirror up to the moral and embodied experience of society." Not only does this raise awareness of the harms done to people by society, but it also sensitizes us to "social-structural oppression and cultural alienation." He argues that social researchers should be challenged to conduct research that shapes the character of our moral response toward others' suffering. In so doing, we will meet the needs of our audience as well. His concluding claim is that critical thought and research must not be an end unto itself, but "a call to care."

Natan Sznaider (Chap. 4) starts from the premise that the meaning of being human moved from acceptable cruelty toward compassion with the rise of democratization and capital markets. Pressure toward compassion, which is the concern for suffering others, including strangers, helped ignite the human rights movement and institutionalize humanitarianism. Public compassion in Sznaider's view is an organized, public response to the wrongdoing that results in unrelieved suffering. Despite those who demean and trivialize compassion, he views it as an affirmation of humanity, "the organized campaign to lessen the suffering of strangers," and a distinctly modern form of morality. The idea that the sight of suffering imposes a duty to ameliorate it "seems like a very old notion but it is largely a recent one."

Ruben Flores (Chap. 5) critiqued critical scholarship, specifically "critical social science," by contrasting it with Buddhism. Like Wilkinson's critique of critical scholarship, Flores focused upon the absence of an explicit ethics of care in critical social science, and on the need for researchers to gain understanding of the role that care can play, both in their own work and in addressing societal needs. Toward this end, he advocates using the language of human rights and the ethics of humanitarianism. As an alternative approach to the definition and relief of world suffering, Flores advocates examination of the Buddhist approach to suffering, specifically, a set of values and practices devoid of the religious and Eastern cultural traditions within Buddhism. Its value, he argues, arises from placing value in the self as freed by forming social commitments and to engage with compassion to all suffering human beings. In addition, Buddhism suggests that the source of most preventable personal suffering is the clinging to or craving of needless objects and aspirations. Flores principally admonishes us to compare, contrast, and combine different philosophical, theoretical, and methodological approaches so as to avoid paths that are self-defeating and unsympathetic to the suffering of the world.

Johannes von Engelhardt and Jeroen Jansz (Chap. 6) note that most of today's humanitarian catastrophes occur in countries of the so-called Global South. While the Global North plays the role of primary funder for the required humanitarian aid, few people in the Global North have firsthand knowledge of the cultures or calamities in the Southern Hemisphere. In this configuration, knowledge is acquired and funding decisions made through the lens and stories of the media. Scholars of media connections, while interested in this problem, have not made great progress in understanding the information and opinion flow. Engelhard and Jansz have developed a conceptual framework to assist in understanding the role of the media. They propose four key dimensions: *distance* from suffering persons; *actuality*, or believability of the suffering; *scale*, the number of persons affected; and *relievability* or resolvability. These draw attention to representations of distant suffering and create spaces that allow audiences to cultivate moral sensibilities and act out different forms of cosmopolitanism. It should be noted that the more intensive levels of cosmopolitanism overlap with universalism as promoted by the core of the human rights and humanitarian institutions.

1.4 Introduction to Part II Chapters on Caregiving

Studies of caregiving tend to use ethnographic and other qualitative methodologies to improve deep understandings of social life and the complex cultures associated with caregiving. The relationship between caregivers and care receivers is a complex one with idiosyncratic elements. Thus, full understanding depends to some extent upon understanding how the persons involved perceive and understand what is happening. It is not accidental that most of the caregiving studies in this volume use qualitative methods in collection of relevant data.

This first chapter underlines the concept of caring as "life's meaning and as the crucial facet of the social fabric of society." Effective caregiving depends upon understanding the individual sufferer and the nature of suffering. Thus, the aggregate relationships involving caregiving contribute in a major way toward the common good.

Care has been defined in many different ways, but the most comprehensive and practical definition can be found in Joan Tronto's (2013) *Caring Democracy*: "a species activity that includes everything that we do to maintain, continue, and repair our 'world' so that we can live in it as well as possible." Note how this goes beyond a person-centric definition and includes caring for elements of one's social and physical environments. Later she clarifies that such caring must be consistent with "commitments to justice, equality, and freedom for all." Caring, as opposed to power, popularity, happiness, and other candidates for life's purpose and meaning, has the motivational property of leading one into social relationships that have depth and reciprocity. Caring also leads to activities that promote the self-actualization of self and others. Philosopher Mayeroff (1971) described such caring roadmaps as:

> If my carings are inclusive enough, they involve me deeply and [they] fruitfully order all areas of my life. Caring then provides a center around which my activities and experiences are integrated (Mayeroff 1971).

Describing the choice of caring as one's goal or purpose offers a sense of meaning in life, which Mayeroff (1971) succinctly summarized as a *"deep-seated harmony of the self with the world that is neither passive nor manipulative."* The practice of this philosophy builds a lifestyle of caring or caregiving that can serve as a guide for decisions about suffering. Mayeroff wrote these insights more than four decades ago, but several chapters in this edited book propose the same philosophy. Chapters 3 and 4 by Wilkinson and Sznaider, respectively, support this same emphasis on care.

Several intellectual pillars support the idea that care and caring provide the most useful life purpose for alleviation of suffering. Kierkegaard (1941) and Frankl (1959) essentially designed the first pillar, the "will to meaning." Both intended to provide a deeper, truer purpose than Nietzsche's "will to power" (cf. Young 2010), and Freud's "will to pleasure" (Pruett 1987). The "will to" meaning implies that meaningful relationships that include mutual caring, or one-way caring for others, offer the most satisfying source of purpose, because living becomes more gratifying for both self and others. Those generous in alleviating suffering find new meaning in their lives, in the spirit of Frankl's (1959) characterization of humanity's search for meaning.

The second pillar of the notion of care as an exemplary basis of meaning comes from the tradition of care ethics. In the past 10 years, the ethics of caring has advanced rapidly, especially by Tronto (2013) who built a political theory on the notion of care in the context of democracy.

The third pillar of this position emanates from neuroscience research, mostly in the twenty-first century, which demonstrates that the human brain is structured to empathize with others and to engage cooperatively with other brains, as noted by Franks (Chap. 27). Finally, the fourth pillar relates to the deluge of research on positivity and happiness as the primary goal of human beings. Ironically, findings suggest that unhappiness and suffering more usefully clarify differences among social groups than do happiness and prosperity. These research findings imply that solidarity, social trust, mutual caring and suffering reduction serve as more meaningful bases of social differentiation than does aggregate happiness (Lelkes 2013).

The depth of human drive to care emerges from the socialization process throughout life. Those growing up in violent, aggressive families or communities may be less likely to enter a caregiving profession, but they still seek out the advantages of informal caregiving relationships. The stage of one's life course tends to shape one's purpose. E.g., in early adulthood the goals of learning social and work skills often have highest priority, but during later life, caregiving skills for those who suffer become much more highly valued. Clearly, the concepts of life purpose and meaning greatly enhance the analysis of caregiving in relation to suffering.

1.4.1 Synopsis of Part II Chapters

The chapters in Part II represent stories and perspectives on caregiving to victims of suffering. While some focus on the trauma and drudgery of caregiving, others concentrate on the potential gains. While several discuss the issues of informal or home-based caregivers, others discuss the stress of professional caregivers. The papers on loss and grief suggest that giving care to those mourning a major loss poses significantly different challenges than caregiving for those who remain alive but suffer.

Despite these contrasts, commonalities stand out. Caregivers of those suffering from grief and those living with chronic illnesses should be aware that both types of suffering lead to a struggle with aloneness. The sufferer may not need or want to be alone, but loneliness is a common feeling, perhaps a direct consequence of the bewilderment of a major loss. Caregivers who recognize this can probably be more effective in reducing the burden of the recovery process.

The depth of suffering cannot be seen and felt without the lens of culture. Caregiving must take this into account. Interpretations of the meaning of the loss or the suffering, as stressed by Neimeyer and by Johnston, make a large difference, but they are primarily shaped by local cultures. At the same time, suffering and effective caregiving are global in scope, and much can be learned from other societies and communities.

Cindy Cain, in Chap. 7, conducted exemplary ethnographic research while working as a volunteer hospice worker. She collected interview and participant observation data from 2009 to 2011 on the dynamics of hospices. Here she focuses on the ways in which the suffering, which was sometimes very extreme for the patients, affects the workers. She found that hospice workers suffered most when the patient's life brought out workers' greatest fears; when patients reminded them of their own personal loss; and when patients made ethical questions salient. While those unfamiliar with hospice often assume that it must be depressing and difficult work, some hospice workers in Cain's study adamantly refuted this assumption. They described work that was worthwhile, meaningful, and gave them new perspective on life. An important key to understanding this attitude, and how to maintain it, includes finding meaning in shared suffering or compassion.

Nancy Johnston (Chap. 8) in her chapter critiques aspects of the healthcare healing system, particularly medicalization and biological models, which minimize human interaction and empathy, rather than holistic approaches. The chapter's author does so with an enormous amount of empathy for care professionals and the sufferers they serve. As she notes, suffering raises deep questions about the meaning of our existence and the compassion of our relationships with those who suffer. She proposes new approaches to viewing self in commitment to others. She also proposes when to view suffering as a gift and a site for the cultivation of compassion and altruism. And she articulates how the societies committed to rapid economic growth at the expense of personal, social, and environmental values need a transformation of fundamental values to be successful in the alleviation of suffering. Johnston advocates hopeful views of the self as "hard-wired" for relationships, enlightened by suffering, attracted to altruism, and committed to social justice. She makes a strong case for restoration of the self as well as a more just society.

Robert Neimeyer (Chap. 9) has devoted his career to the study of grief, and here he portrays suffering following the death of a loved one from a "meaning systems perspective." This chapter explains this foundation and links secular and spiritual struggles finding human resilience in addressing suffering. He notes that research across a range of bereaved groups (e.g., young adults, older adults, parents, African American survivors of a loved one's homicide), has found complicated grief associated with an inability to find meaning in the aftermath of loss. The chapter reviews quantitative and qualitative measures that assess the degree of re-integration of meaning systems after a loss. He also reviews tools for identifying specific meanings made during the unwelcome life transition of bereavement. The overall intent of such work is "to pave the way for more nuanced research on the global suffering engendered by bereavement and on the effectiveness of interventions to ameliorate it." Given the burgeoning research in this area, many remain optimistic about the potential contributions of a meaning systems perspective as an integrative frame for studying suffering.

Pauline Boss (Chap. 10) writes how squeezed in between the sufferings of dying and normal living is a state called "ambiguous loss." The pioneer and expert on this subject, Boss summarizes here: the concept, a theory, and a set of interventions. In the interest of space in this volume, she limits her discussion to missing loved ones who are physically absent. The other type of ambiguous loss occurs when the loved one becomes psychologically absent as in cases of Alzheimer's disease. In the former case, when the loss is physical absence, ambiguity arises from not knowing what has happened to the loved one. A recent example of such losses is that of the families and loved ones of those traveling on Malaysian Airlines Flight 370, which disappeared in route to China on March 14, 2014, with 239 people aboard. As of this writing, no evidence of the plane or passengers had been found. Boss was called in to assist the grieving families. In many ways such loss of a family member causes greater suffering than deaths under known circumstances. Therefore, mourners often need special assistance in finding meanings, purposes, new hopes, reconstructing identities and revising attachments. What is particularly interesting is that Boss found that in Western cultures where people are socialized to greatly value achievement or mastery, they need help in reducing their need for control, whereas in Eastern cultures where people are socialized to live with little control, they need help establishing concrete steps to take, for example, creating a memorial to victims of their loss.

Graciela Tonon, Lía Rodríguez de la Vega and Inés Aristegui (Chap. 11) examined the stress of suffering from the perspectives of professional physicians, psychologists, and social workers in Buenos Aires, Argentina. The researchers were interested in not only their perceptions of their patients' suffering but the extent to which they suffered from "burnout," fatigue or any role-related distress. Rather than use an ethnographic approach, they gave each caring professional some questions and asked them to supply written answers. The questions were thought-provoking, for example, how do you define suffering? And does the suffering of those you work with affect your life? In general, they found most of their study subjects to be suffering from their work. The authors expressed their findings as follows: "They suffer alongside those they help, dealing with senses of injustice, loneliness, social stigma, vulnerability, and unhappiness. Care workers speak of helplessness and frustration, especially in those suffering situations that might have been avoided by suitable economic or public policy decisions." Because some healthcare workers did not have enough resources, they felt secondary social suffering due to their patients being stigmatized by illnesses, disabilities, and other ways in which they felt trapped. The researchers felt that existential or contemplative therapy such as yoga has the potential of helping to reduce this "secondary suffering."

Gloria Jacques (Chap. 12), as a researcher in Botswana, reviewed the research literature on the public health crises in southern Africa created by the HIV and AIDS pandemic, especially those studies of the home care system. Like the previous chapter, this study focuses on the distress of caregivers, but principally home-based caregivers. She gave special attention to Botswana because it has an exemplary African public health system, benefiting from partnerships with many Western institutions to try to reduce the devastation to the society from HIV/AIDS. The conclusion is that the well-being of home-based caregivers has been neglected and requires much greater support, given the enormous burden of suffering imposed upon them. New and improved caregiver support programs are needed in all countries with high HIV/AIDS prevalence. Adequate support for home caregivers is critical for the survival, as well as the quality of life, of southern Africa because it is afflicted by one of the most catastrophic health challenges of the modern era. As considerable strides have already been made in countries such as Botswana, there is reason to believe that the long-term prognosis could be a decline in the millions of casualties from HIV/AIDS in Africa. However, it is by no means certain.

Narelle Warren and Darshini Ayton in Chap. 13 sought to understand how the long-term suffering of a major stroke affected the lives of chronic stroke victims over age 70. Their ethnographic study of 20 stroke victims in Australia consisted of some observation time but mainly three co-interviews of the victim and informal caregiver at three points in time: at recruitment, 6 months later, and 9 months after the second interview. While lack of finances appeared to be a major problem curtailing the options and activities of many victims, social participation predominated their lifestyle difficulties. In general, their physical and mental limitations led to reduced social network size, lower levels of socializing and, perhaps most significantly, heightened social isolation. Those with a spouse-caregiver were most comforted and able to cope with their suffering. Disability victims had less and less social contact, because of two types of suffering. One type, social suffering, reduced social interaction because of the stigma of having both disabilities and a serious illness. The other type of suffering was labeled earlier as "interpersonal suffering," because the complexity and reduction of their interpersonal relations led to feelings of isolation and perceived rejection even by close friends. Warren and Ayton used capabilities theory, chronic illness concepts, grounded theory, and caregiving frameworks, each yielding strengths and limitations in pointing to the key traumatic consequences of suffering from major strokes.

1.5 Quality of Life and Part III Chapters

1.5.1 Introduction

When we suffer, our quality of life declines – it is an intuitive idea. What is not so obvious, however, is that by intertwining suffering and quality of life in our thinking, we can better understand and cope with suffering (whether our own or that of others). As a common phrase, "quality of life" (QOL) goes back only a few decades. However, in the twenty-first century, the concept has become rather popular, especially within research on health and economics (Land et al. 2012; Mukherjee 1989). A professional group called the International Society for Quality of Life Studies publishes several journals with "quality of life" in their titles. Many national and international policy reports also use the phrase, sometimes equating it with general well-being and/or happiness (Jordan 2012). The governments of several nations are now using the concept in attempting to construct new measures of national or human progress. Several research projects are working on indicators of "social progress."

QOL has two major roots, one psychological and the other social. From a psychological base, QOL tends to be equated with well-being, which may be measured as the balance of positive and negative experiences from moment to moment. From a social base, it may still be defined in terms of the balance of positive and negative experiences, but it is applied to a variety of social domains such as health, work, finance, productivity, sustainability, and so forth. Defining the relevant domains is a good place to start when one desires to apply the QOL concept to communities and societies.

From the standpoint of the individual, suffering fits easily with the notion of positive and negative experiences. But for purposes of defining the QOL of communities and societies, it may be more useful to associate suffering with crises, disasters, or other events that produce catastrophic changes to the community or larger system. Both suffering and social calamities are excellent indicators of negative quality of life. Unfortunately, the technical strategies for combining positive and negative elements in social measurement are not necessarily straightforward. This may explain why the measurement of QOL has largely ignored suffering as a component. Part of the purpose of this book is to rectify that omission.

1.5.2 Synopses of Chapters

The third part of the volume verifies that the incorporation of negative quality of life dimensions (such as suffering) into the assessment of QOL and well-being has moved slowly. One reason for the lack of major progress may be that the conceptual frameworks for suffering remain somewhat primitive. Greater clarity is needed in conceptualizing and distinguishing suffering as separate from causes of suffering like fear and anger. Multiple components or types of suffering add to the complexity. And a variety of outcomes or consequences of suffering add greatly to the challenge of measuring suffering and conceptually integrating it into the QOL construct.

Meanwhile, QOL has long been closely aligned with "standard of living" and even income. Given the many non-economic barriers of world suffering to human progress, the use of economic indicators as the primary measure of social progress would seem to be short-sighted at best. The increasing use of non-economic measures of human progress will put pressure on researchers to succeed in integrating suffering elements as negative components of QOL.

Ken Land, Vicki Lamb and Qiang Fu (Chap. 14) are well known for their work on the leading edge of research on child well-being. Not only does the chapter review the research literature on well-being and quality of life among children, but it also discusses progress on different types of measurement. The authors spend considerable time on the history of the UN's declarations on children's rights, especially the Convention of the Rights of the Child (CRC) and how it helped the United Nations establish the rights of children. Land and his associates make a strong case for the importance of investigating child suffering and measures of child suffering as routes to improving the measurement of the QOL of children around the globe. To illustrate the complexity and challenge of such work, they present several scatterplots showing the variety of distributions that different indicators of child suffering have with development as measured by the Human Development Index project. They propose the construction of an index of child suffering measures based upon systematic representation of the types of suffering outlined earlier in this chapter and methodologies that have been refined over the past few years to improve the quality of measures of cross-national development and well-being among children.

Yanjie Bian and Jing Shen in Chap. 15 report on their survey of two random samples of 10,000+ adults representing all one billion Chinese adults in each of 2 years, 2005 and 2010. Their scientific sample of Chinese adults in all provinces except Tibet, covering both urban and rural areas, asked each respondent if they had a *physical* ailment that "bothered their daily routine activities." If the person said "yes," they were considered to be "suffering physically." But if their response indicated its effect was only seldom or not at all, then the person was not considered to be physically suffering. The identical question set was asked about *mental* ailments too. Based upon these criteria in 2005, 23 % reported having physical suffering and 30 % reported having mental suffering. Five years later, those percentages had risen to 29 % and 34 % respectively. Similar levels of suffering and interactions with gender, age, and other such social factors have been found in highly developed Western nations (Anderson 2014; Johannes et al. 2010; Harstall and Ospina 2003; Tsang et al. 2008) but this is the first time that these patterns have been discovered to be an integral part of the social fabric of a major nation in Asia.

Mariano Rojas (Chap. 16) surveyed a sample representing all adults ages 17–70 in Mexico. But rather than asking the 10,000+ respondents about their suffering, he asked about the possible suffering of immediate family members. The "suffering" questions were asked in terms of the presence of any "grave ailments" or "addiction problems" among specific family members. Of the adults surveyed, 9 % reported a family member with an addiction problem and from 4 to 16 % reported a family member having a "grave ailment," the percent depending upon which type or role of family member was referenced. Rojas' remarkable finding was that the subjective well-being measures of the respondents were consistently lower when the person has a family member with a "grave ailment" or an addiction problem. The ailment language used in the survey clearly referenced a potentially suffering family member. Qualitative studies of suffering among family members have found it to degrade the well-being and quality of life of other family members, but this is the first time it has been established in a large-scale survey context.

Ferdi Botha (Chap. 17) of South Africa relied on data collected by the United Nations, World Health Organization, and a few NGOs. His subject matter was a vague, abstract concept generally called "Good Society," but which also is labeled

"Civil Society," and other terms that reflect a society devoted to the common good of all its members. Botha's research question was whether he could construct an index measuring national priorities for a "good society" in Africa. If so, he wanted to know if it would have any analytic value. Using what data he could find on most African countries, he built sub-indexes on nine factors. From these domains, he selected some indicators of suffering in societies and then examined the extent to which having a high standing on what he called the Good African Society Index (GASI) was associated with lower suffering. He found that higher GASI scores were likely to be associated with lower suffering, especially low child suffering. However, he also discovered that given that most African countries had relatively low outcomes associated with Good Societies compared to more developed countries, having a relatively high GASI score did not adequately protect a country from disasters and epidemics hindering future social progress.

Francisca Dussaillant and Pablo Gonzalez in Chap. 18 report the results of an important, large-scale survey that for the first time asked about *lifetime* suffering. In 2012, under the auspices of the UNDP–Chile project, they included in a survey a question asking: "Taking into account that all persons sometimes in their lives must face pain and suffering, could you tell me how much suffering you have experienced in your life?" Respondents gave their answers on a 10-point scale from 1 (no suffering) to 10 (a lot of suffering). Surprisingly, 75 % of the respondents responded with an answer from 5 to 10 (on a 10-point scale) indicating that upon reflection, most Chileans considered their suffering to be considerable. The survey was designed with the help and the vocabulary of the *capabilities approach* (Nussbaum 2011; Nussbaum and Sen 1993). On a theoretical basis, it distinguishes between *functionings*, which are enacted personal capabilities, and *evaluations*, which are self-perceived capabilities. The article explores the influence of capabilities and functionings on lifetime suffering beyond traditional controls such as personality traits, demographic characteristics and recent exposure to negative events. Those factors that significantly predict lifetime suffering include the following: being a woman, older age groups, lower income groups, social bonds, self-evaluated poor health, self-reported maltreatment, self-reported discrimination, exposure to recent negative events, and a high score on a "neurosis" scale.

China Mills and Diego Zavaleta (Chap. 19) asked questions in poverty surveys in Chile and Chad about loneliness and difficulties in finding companionship. Of the adults, 20 % reported they could never or could rarely find companionship when they wanted it. More than two-thirds of those unable to find companionship were women. And for both men and women, real companionship was considerably harder to find among the poor in contrast to the wealthiest in their society. The significance of both the discrimination against the poor and the social isolation of those in poverty is that it indicates substantial social suffering experienced by those struggling with poverty. Undoubtedly many of the poor experienced social suffering from specific types of violence and disability as well, but the survey was not designed to assess all forms of social suffering.

1.6   Part IV Chapters on Community and QOL

Community continues to be an amorphous entity but remains at the center of human social life and welfare. Communities guard the front lines of most disasters, even if the size of the emergency demands help from regional, national, or even international organizations. Tragically, in mega-disasters communities may be destroyed. The *community indicators* movement began several years ago largely because most communities, except the largest cities, felt demand for more information in planning and for building resilience to natural disasters and other calamities.

Reports in this part of the book include not only geographically located communities but also online communities of human interaction. While measuring quality of life in geographical communities adds obvious value to human and community progress, measuring it in online communities may not be useful to the participants themselves. The principal value of research within online communities likely derives from understanding basic human and social interaction. Thus, the three papers here about online communities address questions of emotional expression, identity formation, symbolism and expressed meaning.

Studies of suffering in the future will almost certainly continue to focus considerable attention on communities. Humans become more vulnerable to suffering from the lack of supportive social connections, and the harm of social isolation. Furthermore, communities provide the social context within which children first broaden their sources of social identity outside of their immediate family. It has been said that without community there can be no peace, which means ultimately, no life.

1.6.1   Synopses of Part IV Chapters

The chapters here implicitly, if not explicitly, try to answer the question as to what communities need to be more resilient or insulated from harm due to unexpected emergencies and a variety of obstacles. Sometimes they address the challenge of indicator priorities for a tracking system and how such indicators can be measured.

An attribute of communities that often receives attention in this context is social cohesion. While this is important, survival also depends on making good decisions and putting them into action. Karraker's (Chap. 23) community had enough of both attributes to survive two racial crises, but it might not survive another without vigilant attention to the social tensions and preparedness for additional crises. Larger communities pose greater challenges as revealed by *Jones and Murphy* (Chap. 21) in their case study of a community responding to a bureaucratic disaster that caused major injury or death to 150 children. The New Orleans community studied by *Harvey* (Chap. 20) appeared to have an unusual degree of resilience or at least toughness. Neither of these two communities appeared to have adequate community organization and leadership to keep them on track with common solutions. All three communities uncover many of the complexities of community functioning in the face of disaster and widespread suffering.

The last three chapters with the interactive web as a backdrop may provide a bit of a jolt for the reader upon discovering how deeply human feelings related to suffering can be expressed online with both words and visuals. Forty years ago, online communication was almost totally impersonal, so as the web evolves, much interaction may become indistinguishable from face-to-face emotional communication in natural social settings. As society moves in that direction, more and more research opportunities will be available as we attempt to understand suffering and the social dynamics associated with it.

What then, if anything, do the geographically located case studies offer the researcher and analyst of online communities and their suffering? Community members in an online forum could describe the physical characteristics of their neighborhood communities. However, it would take much longer for the researcher(s) to grasp and validate the role of the tangible environment in the survivability of the community. Secondly, while website discussion groups offer rapid response to opinion questions – without very costly creation of large databases of respondents – it is very difficult to collect data about communities needed in community indicator systems for planning and emergency response analysis. Finally, the major problems of disastrous emergencies tend to be physical, like finding food and shelter and creating a habitable space. Online services to provide assistance for these calamities are technically feasible, but as the Affordable Care Act in the United States has shown, building user-friendly systems requires lots of funding, time, and expertise.

Perhaps the most important finding to arise out of the online community studies was the discovery reported by *Döveling and Wasgien* (Chap. 24) of "virtual interaction chains." What they found was that in grief support relationships online, a caregiving posting very often followed a care-seeking post or message. Furthermore, over weeks or months, most online users gradually moved from care-seeking to care-giving. These types of interaction sequences may sometimes be easier to isolate online or in a laboratory rather than in natural field settings.

Daina Harvey (Chap. 20) conducted an ethnography of the Lower Ninth Ward of New Orleans in the aftermath of Katrina in 2005. His conclusion was that much like many developing countries with ongoing violence from warfare and other adversities, the Lower Ninth Ward's history can be characterized as a *culture of suffering*. In this geographical region, suffering is normative and the dominant basis for interacting with others. Their condition can also be appropriately labeled *social suffering* because discrimination, racism, and neglect by governmental agencies directly produced the trauma of the residents of the Lower Ninth Ward. In addition to extensive interviews, Harvey lived in the community for almost a year and helped them with all aspects of their community. In his interviews and conversations he discovered many victims felt deep empathy for others in parallel circumstances. Perhaps because of this empathy, a number of his interviewees in dire straits refused to acknowledge they had personally suffered. This distancing of suffering themselves from pain and distress, he concluded, served a kind of boundary-maintaining function, analogous to establishing the distinctiveness of their neighborhood from surrounding geographical areas.

Eric Jones and *Arthur Murphy* (Chap. 21) conducted an in-depth case study of a disaster in 2009 when a fire destroyed a day care center in Mexico killing 49 children and leaving 100 others with serious injuries. Behind the fire were a series of neglected safety measures, political stalemates, and failures to regulate. Jones, Murphy, and their research team carried out both structured and unstructured interviews with 226 parents and caretakers from 95 of the 134 families affected by the fire. Their primary interest was prolonged grief (defined as longer than 6 months) and the politics of grief. They completed two sets of interviews, one in early 2011 and the other in 2012. Jones and Murphy concluded "layers of diffuse responsibility created by the neo-liberal reforms with lax or absent regulations produce a system where blame cannot be assigned and laws are not enforced by the justice system." As the public interest was not served by the existing political system, the families who lost children had no clearly defined agency on which to focus their rage and grief. The Mexican day care disaster, like the Exxon and BP oil spills in the United States, revealed a legal context with entrenched political and economic interests that block attempts to deliver justice to those individuals directly affected by the breakdown of confidence in government.

Rhonda Phillips, in Chap. 22, explores what can be learned from community indicators of QOL related to community suffering and resilience. After tracing the history of *community indicators*, she describes cases of community disaster and tragedy to show how a community indicator system can greatly improve community resilience, which in turn minimizes suffering. Community indicators provide one type of community capacity and have the potential to bring out the benefits of a community's social capital. Community indicators, given that they are meant to represent the spectrum of the community's values and desires, as well as the resources citizens want to protect, can serve as a bridge between community-based planning and traditional disaster and risk assessment. Indicators can also be used to identify inequities and social suffering, independently or in tandem with a natural disaster.

Meg Wilkes Karraker (Chap. 23) emphasizes how racism engenders deep social suffering in communities, thereby depreciating QOL in profound ways. This chapter gives the history of a small city in Middle America toward the end of the twentieth century. *Small City*'s black citizens and their families suffered through cross-burnings and rocks thrown through the windows of their homes, as well as a rally organized by the Ku Klux Klan. Karraker used mixed methods to study the role of religious culture and caring capital in the mobilization of civic and religious leadership, to avoid additional suffering and improve the citizens' QOL. Many small cities face new challenges of immigration and racial discrimination, and Small City offers lessons for community resolve and action. Small City seems to have banked caring capital against future suffering; e.g., in 2012 a cross was, once again, burned in the front yard of a mixed-race family, but the mayor immediately issued a powerful statement to the media, condemning the action and committing law enforcement to stop such actions. Karraker's analysis of the community's civil history confirms that the nurturance of caring capital provides a foundation that transforms into community resilience when crises emerge.

Katrin Döveling and Katrin Wasgien (Chap. 24) sought to understand the attraction and interaction patterns of people using online communities intended to help those challenged personally by grief. More specifically, how does interaction related to *personal suffering* affect those who are sharing their grief and ultimately, how does it affect their quality of life? Three different bereavement platforms were examined in a qualitative content analysis. Emotional communication chains and their effects reveal that many care seekers in time become caregivers. The bereaved turn to social networking platforms largely because they don't feel adequate support from their face-to-face family members or friends. The authors' qualitative analysis discovered that privately shared emotions are now often expressed within these online communities. *Emoticons* as well as *ritualistic symbols* (such as candles) reinforce text messages. Without a doubt, many youth and older adults manage emotional distress and share emotional support through their online interactions.

Laura Robinson, in Chap. 25, illuminates the use of cosmopolitan identity frames in response to suffering caused by the 9/11 attacks in New York City in 2001. Drawing on empirical data from Brazilian, French, and American digital news forums shortly after the attacks, the analysis reveals the use of cosmopolitan and transnational frames to identify with those suffering. To do so, individuals redefine and expand identity boundaries to include those suffering through discourses bridging the distance between observer and sufferer. The most universalistic form of cosmopolitanism comes from those participants on the Brazilian forum. In the French forum, individuals were more likely to adopt more circumscribed versions of cosmopolitanism based on perceived transnational similarities. In the American forum, nationalism, transnational cosmopolitanism, and universalistic cosmopolitanism appeared side by side, albeit produced by different constituencies. While all cosmopolitans erase boundaries between themselves and those suffering, the Brazilian case offers the most vibrant example of cosmopolitan identification. The Brazilians show how empathy may be extended to those suffering as members of humanity regardless of any other identity category.

Anna Johansson and Hans Sternudd (Chap. 26) conducted a visual analysis, using words, of a common image found on the web of a girl sitting hunched over. Over and over, they found this dark image on websites devoted to self-cutting and other self-injury. They also discovered it on numerous video montages on YouTube. Johansson and Sternudd argue that the iconic images symbolize mental illness and depression elements of suffering. They conclude that the popularity of this icon stems from its generic character, making it easily remixed in new ways through social media. Furthermore, they argue that it both magnifies the suffering of depression and alleviates the dread of suffering by transmitting a sense of rebellion or opposition. Specifically, they suggest that the dramatization of shame, loneliness, and withdrawal from the world forms the basis for collective recognition, community-building, social support, and improved QOL by evoking unsuspected identification with the depicted, suffering girl.

1.7 Conclusions

An unintended outcome of this collection of eclectic chapters is that many of the authors have started using a similar language of suffering. Partly, this resulted from the definitions of suffering that I included in my recent book (Anderson 2014) and refined in this chapter. A common vocabulary takes time to emerge, and its direction cannot be predicted. In this instance, the words, phrases and definitions needed must encompass the relief of suffering as well as suffering itself.

The social contexts relevant to each instance of suffering vary from study to study. Some authors concentrate on the family, others on the community, and others on the society or societies as the principal social context that shapes the underlying suffering processes. Such questions as the degree of support from the social context determine for the most part the outcomes of the suffering,

Humanitarian actions and human rights protection play a critical role in the relief of suffering. In a parallel manner, the formal and informal caregiving systems play a critical function in ensuring adequate levels of quality in people's lives. Creative ideas will continually be needed to improve upon these systems, either separately or together. Helping crisis victims deal with adjustments in personal meaning may seem like a luxury, but several authors here argue that it often plays a critical role in successful recovery.

References

Alexander, J. C. (2012). *Trauma: A social theory*. Cambridge: Polity Press.

ALNP. (2012). *The state of the humanitarian system.* http://www.alnap.org/what-we-do/sohs. Accessed 25 May 2014.

Anderson, R. E. (2014). *Human suffering and quality of life – Conceptualizing stories and statistics*. New York: Springer.

Barnett, M., & Weiss, T. G. (Eds.). (2008). *Humanitarianism in question: Politics, power, ethics*. Syracuse: Cornell University Press.

Black, H. K. (2005). *Soul pain: The meaning of suffering in later life*. Amityville: Baywood Publishing Co. Inc.

Bornstein, E., & Redfield, P. (2013). *Forces of compassion: Humanitarianism between ethics and politics*. Santa Fe: SAR Press.

Borsook, D. (2012). *A future without chronic pain: Neuroscience and clinical research*. http://www.dana.org/news/cerebrum/detail.aspx?id=39160. Accessed 8 Mar 2013.

Bourdieu, P., et al. (2000). Understanding. In P. Bourdieu et al. (Eds.), *The weight of the world: Social suffering in contemporary society*. Stanford: Stanford University Press.

Calhoun, C. (2004). A world of emergencies: Fear, intervention and the limits of cosmopolitan order. *Canadian Review of Sociology, 41*(4), 373–395.

Calhoun, C. (2008). The imperative to reduce suffering: Charity, progress and emergencies in the field of humanitarian action. In M. Barnett & T. G. Weiss (Eds.), *Humanitarianism in question: Politics, power, ethics* (pp. 73–92). Syracuse: Cornell University Press.

Carr, D. B., Loeser, J. D., & Morris, D. B. (Eds.). (2005). *Narrative, pain and suffering* (Progress in pain research and management). Seattle: International Association for the Study of Pain Press.

Cassell, E. J. (1991). *Nature of suffering and the goals of medicine.* New York: Oxford University Press.

Chouliaraki, L. (2013). *The ironic spectator: Solidarity in the age of post-humanitarianism.* Cambridge: Polity Press.

Davidhizar, R., & Giger, J. N. (2004). A review of the literature on care of clients in pain who are culturally diverse. *International Nursing Review, 51*(1), 47–55.

Farmer, P. (2013). *To repair the world.* Berkeley: University of California Press.

Fast, L. (2014). *Aid in danger: The perils and promise of humanitarianism.* State College: University of Pennsylvania Press.

Francis, L. E. (2006). Emotions and health. In W. E. Stets & J. H. Turner (Eds.), *Handbook of the sociology of emotions* (pp. 591–610). New York: Springer.

Frankl, V. E. (1959). *Man's search for meaning.* Boston: Beacon Press. (Originally published in 1959)

Graaf, J., Wann, D., & Naylor, T. H. (2014). *Affluenza – How overconsumption is killing us and how to fight back* (1st ed.). New York: Berrett-Koehler Publishers.

Harstall, C., & Ospina, M. (2003). How prevalent is chronic pain? *Pain Clinical Updates. 11*(2), 1–4. Seattle: International Association for the Study of Pain.

Hemlow, J. (Ed.). (1975). *The journals and letters of Fanny Burney.* Oxford: Oxford University Press. http://www.segemi.de/files/kleinman_anthropology_cross-cultural_mental_health_6-2011_1_.pdf. Accessed 20 Jan 2013.

Johannes, C. B., Le, T. K., Zhou, X., Johnston, J. A., & Dworkinin, R. H. (2010). The prevalence of chronic pain in United States adults: Results of an internet-based survey. *Journal of Pain, 11*(11), 1230–1239.

Jordan, T. E. (2012). *Quality of life and mortality among children.* New York: SpringerBriefs.

Kennedy, D. (2011). *The dark sides of virtue: Reassessing international humanitarianism.* Princeton: Princeton University Press.

Kierkegaard, S. (1941). *The sickness unto death.* Princeton: Princeton University Press.

Kleinman, A., Das, V., & Lock, M. (Eds.). (1997). *Social suffering.* Berkeley: University of California Press.

Land, K. C., Michalos, A. C., & Sirgy, M. J. (2012). The development and evolution of research on social indicators and quality of life. In K. C. Land et al. (Eds.), *Handbook of social indicators and quality of life research* (pp. 1–22). New York: Springer.

Lelkes, O. (2013). Minimising misery: A new strategy for public policies instead of maximising happiness? *Social Indicators Research, 114*, 121–137.

Livingston, W. K. (1998). *Pain and suffering.* Seattle: International Association for the Study of Pain Press.

Mayeroff, M. (1971). *On caring.* New York: HarperCollins.

Morris, D. B. (2002). *The culture of pain.* Berkley: University of California Press.

Mukherjee, R. (1989). *The quality of life—Valuation in social research.* Newbury Park: Sage.

Nagappan, R. (2005). *Speaking havoc: Social suffering & South Asian narratives.* Seattle: University of Washington Press.

Narayan, M. C. (2010). Culture's effects on pain assessment and management. *American Journal of Nursing, 110*(4), 38–47.

Nussbaum, M. (2011). *Creating capabilities: The human development approach.* Cambridge: Harvard University Press.

Nussbaum, M., & Sen, A. (1993). *The quality of life.* Oxford: Clarendon.

Pruett, G. E. (1987). *The meaning and end of suffering for Freud and the Buddhist tradition.* Lanham: University Press of America.

Rummel, R. J. (1994). *Death by government.* Piscataway: Transaction.

Saunders, C. (2006). *Cicely Saunders: Selected writings 1958–2004.* New York: Oxford University Press USA.

Singer, M. (2006). *The face of social suffering – The life history of a street drug addict.* Long Grove: Waveland Press.

Thernstrom, M. (2010). *The pain chronicles: Cures, myths, mysteries, prayers, diaries, brain scans, healing, and the science of suffering.* New York: Farrar, Straus, and Giroux, LLC – MacMillan.

Trnka, S. (2008). *State of suffering: Political violence and community survival in Fiji.* Syracuse: Cornell University Press.

Tronto, J. C. (2013). *Caring democracy: Markets, equality and justice.* New York: NYU Press.

Tsang, A., Von Korff, M., Lee, S., Alonso, J., Karam, E., et al. (2008). Common chronic pain conditions in developed and developing countries: Gender and age differences and comorbidity with depression-anxiety disorders. *The Journal of Pain, 9*(10), 883–891.

Weiss, T. G. (2007). *Humanitarian intervention – Ideas in action.* Cambridge: Polity Press.

White, M. (2011). *Atrocities: The 100 deadliest episodes in human history.* New York: Norton.

Wilkinson, I. (2005). *Suffering: A sociological introduction.* Cambridge: Polity Press.

Wilkinson, I. (2012). *Social suffering and the problem of re-making sociology for caregiving.* http://www.academia.edu/1812508/Social_Suffering_and_the_Problem_of_Re-making_Sociology_for_Caregiving. Accessed 27 Jan 2013. (Published online at Academia.edu)

Wilkinson, I. (2013). The problem of suffering as a driving force of rationalization and social change. *The British Journal of Sociology, 64*(1), 123–141.

Wilson, R. A., & Brown, R. D. (Eds.). (2009). *Humanitarianism and suffering—The mobilization of empathy.* New York: Cambridge University Press.

Wilson, K. G., Chochinov, H. M., Allard, P., Chary, S., Gagnon, P. R., Macmillan, K., De Luca, M., O'Shea, F., Kuhl, D., & Fainsinger, R. L. (2009). Prevalence and correlates of pain in the Canadian National Palliative Care Survey. *Pain Research and Management, 14*(5), 366–379.

Wronka, J. (2008). *Human rights and social justice.* Los Angeles: Sage.

Young, J. (2010). *Friedrich Nietzsche: A philosophical biography.* Cambridge: Cambridge University Press.

Chapter 2
Suffering in Silence? The Silencing of Sexual Violence Against Men in War Torn Countries

Élise Féron

2.1 Introduction

Sexual violence against women within armies, or as a weapon of war in conflict zones such as in Syria, has recently attracted a large amount of media and academic attention. In the US for instance, a documentary film called "The Invisible War" was launched in 2012; it was widely acclaimed and has spurred various changes in how the US military deals with such crimes. However, much less has been said about the staggering figures published by the US Department of Defense about male soldiers as victims of sexual assault: of an estimated 26,000 soldiers who have been victim of sexual assault in 2012, 54 % were men (Department of Defense 2012). Similarly, a study conducted by Johnson et al. (2010) has reported that 23.6 % of men and boys living in Eastern DRC (39.7 % of women and girls) have experienced some form of sexual violence because of the conflict. This has not yet led to a major debate on how international funds for helping victims of sexual violence in that region were used. These examples highlight that victims of sexual violence, in its various forms such as rape, sexual torture, sexual mutilation, sexual humiliation and sexual slavery, can be both male and female. But why are we seemingly paying less attention to sexual violence perpetrated against men than when it is perpetrated against women? Is our understanding of sexual torture framed in such a way that it cannot be reconciled with situations in which men are the victims?

It is increasingly difficult to ignore a phenomenon that some researchers and NGOs have been describing and analyzing since the mid-1990s. As explained by Don Sabo, "whereas researchers and public health advocates began to recognize the sexual victimization of women in Western countries during the late 1960s, it was

É. Féron (✉)
Conflict Analysis Research Centre, University of Kent, Canterbury, UK
e-mail: E.Feron@kent.ac.uk

© Springer Science+Business Media Dordrecht 2015
R.E. Anderson (ed.), *World Suffering and Quality of Life*,
Social Indicators Research Series 56, DOI 10.1007/978-94-017-9670-5_2

not until the latter 1990s that the sexual abuse of men began to receive systematic scrutiny from human service professionals and gender researchers" (2005: 338). In the wake of research on sexual torture of male prisoners during civil wars in Chile, El Salvador and Greece, reports have begun to unveil how widespread sexual violence against boys and men is in military settings and conflict zones. It has been a constant feature of most conflicts and wars, though most of the time silenced by political and military authorities, if not by victims themselves (Nizich 1994; Schwartz 1994; Stener 1997; Oosterhoff et al. 2004; Carpenter 2006; Sivakumaran 2007).

These publications have also begun to shed light on the extent, features, and consequences of this phenomenon through exploring the destructive power of such violence on individuals and communities. It has been shown that sexual violence against men is not unlike that committed against women in that it is mostly perpetrated by men in arms who belong either to armed groups or to conventional armies. The combination of rape and sexual mutilation has been described as the most prevalent form of sexual violence against men and boys, especially in detention (Carpenter 2006: 94).

Beyond these scattered publications, no major international or national campaigns or funding have been set up in order to adequately respond to the suffering induced by these acts of violence. A few organizations in the humanitarian field have admittedly begun tackling the matter. The UNHCR has issued guidelines in July 2012 for UNHCR staff and other aid workers on how to identify and support male victims of rape and other sexual violence in conflict and displacement situations (2012). Such initiatives are so far isolated. The media and international community are capable of functioning as receptacles and amplifiers of testimonies in regards to suffering, but the case of sexual violence against male victims is being ignored. But what is exactly triggering such a downplay? This contribution, based on data collected in the Great Lakes Region (specifically in the Democratic Republic of Congo, Burundi and Rwanda), argues that gender roles and discourses hinder the acknowledgement of the various types of suffering faced by male victims of sexual violence. After a section presenting an overview of the phenomenon, we will discuss different types of suffering it entails for the victims. The chapter then explores what accounts for the silencing of this suffering, from representations of sexual violence where men stand as perpetrators, to patriarchal cultures associating masculinity to strength, protection and invulnerability.

2.2   Methodology

This paper builds on data collected mostly in the Great Lakes region of Africa, where I have been spending between 3 weeks and a month per year since 2009. I have collected data in the Kivu region of DRC (both North and South Kivu), which appears to be one of the regions in the world where sexual violence against both males and females is the most widespread, as well as in Burundi, where it is recognized as being one of the main features of the conflict that tore the country apart between 1993 and 2005. I have also used some data collected in Rwanda, and during interviews with Rwandan refugees settled elsewhere, on the issue of sexual violence during the genocide. All in all, my data includes more than 60 semi-structured as well as life-history interviews with combatants (former and still active) and refugees (both male and female), 30 semi-structured interviews with various local NGO leaders, doctors and surgeons, and numerous observation sessions. Some representatives of international organizations have also been interviewed.

Collecting data on the topic of suffering induced by sexual violence is far from being easy. Victims will rather talk about suffering inflicted upon others, than upon themselves. Similarly, perpetrators seldom acknowledge their direct participation and responsibility in these acts. They frequently use metaphors to speak about it, which is a good indication of the weight of the stigma surrounding these acts, but which also represents an obvious challenge when analyzing interviews. Moreover, fieldwork data on sexual violence perpetrated against men is difficult to gather because of the taboos surrounding that issue, but also because many people, including professionals in the field of gender, or in the medical field, are not familiar with the problem. I have often found, for instance, while trying to gather testimonies of doctors or of medical personnel, that many confused male on male rape with homosexuality. That was not the case of course in some highly specialized places such as the Panzi Hospital in South Kivu, well known for its expertise in dealing with the consequences of sexual violence, especially obstetric fistula. Public awareness on these issues seems to be a bit higher in DRC than in the rest of the sub-region (though still limited to hospitals and some specialized NGOs), but this is not a real surprise since over the past few years in DRC the issue has been brought up by some international NGOs such as Médecins Sans Frontières. In Rwanda, because of the numerous trials and cases involving sexual violence that have been examined by the traditional tribunals or gacaca, there is a growing awareness not only of the role played by women in violence (a fact which used to be taboo too), but also of the sexual violence perpetrated during the genocide on men, by both men and women. In Burundi, even those with a good awareness on issues pertaining to gender-based violence seemed to be totally unaware of the issue, and most people I spoke to even displayed surprise and dismay when I mentioned the matter and the cases or figures I had come across. This lack of awareness seems to be linked to the taboo existing around homosexuality, as well as to its penalization. (Homosexuality has been banned in Burundi since 2009. Those found guilty of engaging in consensual same-sex relations risk imprisonment of 2–3 years and a fine of 50,000–100,000 Burundian francs.)

Meeting perpetrators, and victims, has also been quite a challenge, since this is obviously not the kind of experience people would usually publicize and boast about. I have been quite lucky, though, since I first met several perpetrators and victims in 2009, while conducting several rounds of interview with former combatants (both male and female), on the issue of daily life within armed groups of the region. I subsequently decided to renew the experience, and, instead of conducting interviews on this issue of sexual violence only, met with combatants to speak more generally of their experience "in the bush". This was also a way for me to try to minimize as much as possible the risk of re-traumatizing my interviewees by asking questions that might have sounded intrusive or even offensive. In other words, a few spoke about it, most didn't, and in the latter case I did not push the matter.

Much could be said about my position, as a white, western and female researcher gathering data on such issues in one of the most unstable regions of Africa. Some local researchers have already told me that, as a Mzungu (a Swahili word meaning "someone with white skin"), local people were a lot more likely to speak to me, in the hope either of getting some money in return, or of having their situation somehow improved as a consequence of my research. I however have no way to say whether such dynamics were indeed at play when I investigated this specific issue. It is thus very difficult for me to have a precise idea of the proportion of my "sample" who has indeed been victim of such a type of violence; however I do not consider this a problem, since my research belongs unambiguously to the qualitative realm, and its objective is to unveil and explain processes rather than to come up with figures, which a few others have begun to gather (see in particular Johnson et al. 2010). I have also spoken to numerous NGOs workers dealing with sexual violence, and they have told me the stories of some of the victims, and sometimes put me in contact with them. Quite obviously, I have anonymized my data, and some dates/places have been changed in order to protect my interviewees. I have almost never recorded the interviews, and instead used a paper notebook, which I thought was less likely to destabilize the interviewees. Worth mentioning also is the fact that in some cases I have had to use the services of an interpreter, as some of my interviewees were not proficient in French or English. This might have caused misunderstandings, since the word "rape" for instance, especially when applied to men, doesn't have close equivalents in some local languages, for instance in Kirundi.

One of the main lessons I learned while working on this issue is that, when it comes to sexual violence against men in conflict situations, the usual clear-cut distinction between perpetrators and victims often doesn't stand. It appears that in the complex dynamics that characterize the situation in the Great Lakes region of Africa, some of the boys and men who had been, for instance, abducted, enslaved and raped by armed men (and, less often, by armed women), stayed in the group, and later became perpetrators themselves. The fact that a lot of authors who research sexual violence during conflicts tend to treat men as the obvious perpetrators has, in my view, veiled these interaction processes, and has prevented us from fully understanding these patterns of violence. This of course does not mean that I am trying to diminish or overlook the immense suffering induced by such practices.

2.3   Sexual Violence Against Men – An Overview

Reliable and precise figures on sexual violence against men are almost impossible to find. Some NGOs document an increase in such practices (Human Rights Watch 2005: 20), but it is difficult to say whether this is because such cases are indeed more numerous, or simply better reported. This phenomenon has been present in the great majority of contemporary conflicts, and during the last decade only it has been reported in 25 conflicts across the world (Russell 2007: 22). This type of violence often occurs in captivity, and marginalized groups, such as members of minority ethnic or religious groups, are particularly vulnerable. Many NGOs report such practices and underscore the fact that, even if there has been an improvement in reporting over the past few years, a large majority of cases are neither recorded nor reported. In Eastern DRC, Johnson et al. (2010) reports that 23.6 % of men and boys of that region (39.7 % of women and girls) have experienced some form of sexual violence; in 90 % of the cases, the perpetrators were male compared to 59.9 % in cases of sexual violence inflicted upon women. In some cases, perpetrators might have been prisoners, forced to rape or sexually assault others. These instances complicate the results. In any case, sexual violence against men during conflicts is not anecdotal, and deserves more political, medical and academic attention than it has been given.

My fieldwork compellingly shows that in all three countries covered by my study, sexual violence against men and boys has been widespread and frequent during conflict times, though silenced and overlooked by both political authorities and non-governmental organizations. Dionise,[1] a former combatant in the Burundian rebellion, explains that when he was abducted and forcefully integrated within the ranks of the combatants, he was first treated with great brutality. He was beaten and tortured, but as with many other men, he had to choose between the acceptance of "being treated as a nobody", "being used like a female slave", or being killed. He has stayed 2 years in the rebellion, and now feels broken, and incapable to "resume a normal life". Deo,[2] who used to be high in command in the Burundian rebellion, insisted that both men and women who had been kidnapped to be used as auxiliaries or as future combatants had "to be broken to be tamed."

At the Panzi hospital in Bukavu, Eastern DRC, the chief doctor reported[3] two cases that had been treated recently. The first involved a driver who had been stopped on his way to Bukavu by an armed group, and was forced to rape all the people, male and female, who were in his van. The members of the armed group then raped the driver. Interestingly, the doctor mentioned that none of the other male victims had come to the hospital, showing the low level of reporting of such acts. The second case included a young man who had been forced to help an armed group by carrying around goods they had stolen from various houses (including the young man's) and had been subsequently raped by the members of the gang. In both of these cases, there is a deliberate wish to instill terror, and to inflict pain and public humiliation. According to a person working for the International Rescue Committee in the Great Lakes Region of Africa,[4] sexual violence against men, and more

---

[1] Interview, Bujumbura, Burundi, 03 May 2011.

[2] Interview, Bujumbura, Burundi, 04 May 2011.

[3] Interview, Panzi Hospital, Bukavu, South Kivu, DRC, 30 April 2012.

[4] Interview, Bujumbura, Burundi, 12 May 2012.

specifically male on male rape, has become just another strategy of war for armed groups active in the region. Victims almost never report it, which makes this strategy increasingly successful. When this violence is perpetrated during raids on villages, males are often forced to rape their own family members (forced incest). This clearly entails humiliation, immense suffering and trauma for both the rapist and his victim, and family relations can never be fully mended. But in many instances, sexual violence happens during detention periods, or shortly after men and boys have been abducted by armed groups.

Combatants perpetrating such acts undoubtedly wish to emulate the hegemonic masculinity model (Connell and Messerschmidt 2005) embodied by their military leaders. In impoverished countries torn apart by decades of warfare, few men have the opportunity to attain the traditional model of masculinity promoted in their communities. In order to "be a man" in traditional cultures, one has to find a house (or build one), marry, have children and be able to feed and protect them. But conflict dynamics have complicated the fulfilling of such "simple" wishes. Parents often cannot help their children anymore, so young men have to find the money for building or buying a house, which is extremely difficult considering the tough economic conflict conditions. As a consequence, men marry and enter symbolic "manhood" later. Men also have trouble finding work, even in the sector of agriculture, and the lingering issue of land scarcity deprives them of a main source of power. Losing access to land implies a loss of control over economic and sometimes political resources. These difficulties explain why some men adopt a violent behavior as a way to gain or regain "respect". Men who do not comply with the conception of "hegemonic masculinity" are marginalized by the other men and face the harshest judgments, which in turn generate low self-esteem, sexual violence, and participation in armed groups. Getting involved in armed groups, and perpetrating atrocities, is seen as a way to reaffirm one's masculinity—even on individuals whose personal situation is very similar. Such processes might also explain why some male victims of sexual violence can turn into perpetrators, since this exercise of domination over both women and "weaker" men symbolically empowers the perpetrator and underscores his retrieved masculinity.

Strikingly, men who have been raped, forced to rape family members, or been mutilated, do not describe this as sexual violence. It is as though this concept is reserved to women only. Repeatedly, the men I talked to confused sexual violence against males with violence in general, or with homosexuality. According to a local source quoted in a report by OCHA (2011), "Men do not use the word rape, which is too hard. They prefer to talk about torture, abomination". My interviewees were no exception. In a sense, I had the feeling that it was less an attempt to euphemize what had happened, than an indication of their own incapacity to recognize that such a thing had happened to them. My interpretation of the metaphors and verbiage they used was made easier by the parallels they made between female prisoners and themselves. In that sense, it is clear that the main consequence of these acts – and probably also one of their main purposes – is to break their gendered male identity.

There are a few NGOs, like SERUKA in Bujumbura, that try to help both men and women of all ages who have been through such traumatic events. According to the person with whom I spoke,[5] only 5 % of the victims they receive are men and boys. In all of these cases, the major obstacle is that adult victims experience difficulty speaking about it and more so in sharing it with their wives: "How can I tell my wife than I have been turned into a woman?".[6] The taboo around homosexuality in extremely patriarchal societies partly explains their reluctance to ask for help, and some of their difficulties in coping with the suffering. Male victims of rape feel ashamed and mocked, and can be excluded from their local communities if the fact becomes public.

2.4 How the Suffering of Male Victims of Conflict-Induced Sexual Violence Is Silenced

As underscored by Ronald E. Anderson (2014: 8–27), suffering is not just physical, it often occurs with mental and social suffering. While many authors have highlighted such physical (e.g. fistula, HIV infection), mental (e.g. anxiety, humiliation) and social (e.g. social rejection, distrust) consequences for women who have been victim of sexual violence, including in conflict settings (see for instance Okot et al. 2005), research on what it entails for male victims is still lacking. For male survivors, suffering spans across these three dimensions too, with dire consequences.

First, as with female victims of sexual violence, male victims suffer from various types of physical pain, which can be related to castration, genital infections, ruptures of the rectum, and physical impotence. Because they are too ashamed to ask for help, many victims prefer to bear the suffering on their own with sometimes fatal consequences: "Aid workers here say the humiliation is often so severe that male rape victims come forward only if they have urgent health problems, like stomach swelling or continuous bleeding. Sometimes even that is not enough" (Gettleman 2009). The lack of training and of preparation of medical staff and health care professionals explains how these physical symptoms are often overlooked, and thus often not addressed in time. Communities in some regions where sexual violence against men is widespread, such as in the Great Lakes Region of Africa, do not view men as a possible victims of rape. In a rural hospital of South Kivu for instance, one of the doctors I spoke to did not understand when I was asking him about sexual violence against men. He thought that I was speaking about forced incest, or of cases where men have to watch other female family members being raped.[7] As a consequence, victims and sometimes health care professionals prefer to use more abstract categories for describing the abuse that veil its sexual nature, such as torture.

---

[5] Interview, Bujumbura, Burundi, 25 April 2012.

[6] Interview, Bujumbura, 25 April 2012.

[7] Interview, FOMULAC Hospital, Katana, South Kivu, DRC, 29 April 2012.

Most programs on sexual violence set up by international or national organizations in conflict areas specifically target female victims of sexual violence, and men may not be accepted in these facilities, thus impeding their access to adequate and indispensible medical care. As underscored by Chris Dolan, director of Uganda's Refugee Law Project: "There are indeed more raped women. But 100 % of raped men need medical help. It is not the case for women" (Dumas 2011).

Physical pain is often accompanied by mental and psychological suffering, which is similar to what female victims of sexual violence have to face; loss of appetite and sleep, exhaustion, anxiety, suicidal thoughts, and nightmares are the most commonly reported symptoms, all consistent with a post traumatic stress disorder syndrome (Christian et al. 2011: 236). While there are places where raped women can go and get some psychological help – though admittedly many of them don't or can't take advantage of these facilities – nothing of that sort exists for men. Even if there was, many of them would be too ashamed to ask for help. They struggle against a feeling of emasculation, of shame, of guilt, and they fear retaliation by perpetrators. Victims also often blame themselves for what happened and fear that they no longer will be able to function as men. In many patriarchal cultures of the developing world, a man is defined by his ability to cope with what befalls him. Male victims of sexual violence often think that they have to bear the mental and psychological suffering just as they have coped with the physical pain. Seeking help and speaking out would be another acknowledgement of the fact that they cannot act as men anymore. As a consequence, isolation, self-imposed exile, and flight often characterize the experience of survivors.

Suffering is also evident at the societal level. Social suffering, as defined by Ron Anderson (2014: 11), includes "suffering whose sources are social collectivities and/or social institutions. (…) Research on social suffering has uncovered that those affected by such dreadful events suffer in part from a devastating loss of their identity as human beings". Male victims may experience marital problems, alcohol and drug abuse, lack of trust, but also ostracism, segregation or even discrimination. When they speak out, they are often ridiculed by others, and many are left by their wives: "Not only do other adults mock survivors and their wives, children in the village will say to the children of male survivors, 'your father is a woman', stigmatizing the children of survivors" (Christian et al. 2011: 239). I have heard several stories of men being ostracized by their own families and wives after their "unfortunate experience" became known: "My wife and children thought it had happened because I was homosexual. I could not be their father anymore".[8] Since support mechanisms are almost non-existent for male victims of sexual violence, this societal suffering is not addressed either. Criminal justice systems are not taking the matter seriously because these cases of violence are not reported, so perpetrators are not prosecuted. This creates a climate in which sexual torture of men can become more widespread. Victims risk being accused of having engaged in illegal homosexual acts, making reporting and prosecution of sexual violence difficult.

---

[8] Jean-Claude, interviewed in Bujumbura, Burundi, 04 May 2011.

This would have both penal and social consequences for the survivor. He may be condemned to pay a heavy fine, or jailed, and he would also have to bear the stigma of being labeled homosexual in a homophobic society.

2.5 Men Are Assumed to Be Perpetrators, Not Victims

Research on sexual violence during conflicts, as well as international programs that address this type of violence, focus mainly on female victims. Girls and women indeed make up the great majority of victims of such type of violence, to the extent that "rape as a weapon of war" has almost become synonymous with sexual violence against girls and women during conflicts. The idea that the rape of women can be used as a weapon of war has become popular since the UN Resolution 1820 (2008) on Women and Peace and Security noted that "women and girls are particularly targeted by the use of sexual violence, including as a tactic of war to humiliate, dominate, instill fear in, disperse and/or forcibly relocate civilian members of a community or ethnic group." Although researchers and NGO workers have tried to raise awareness of male victims there is still no facility, clinic or hospital service specifically targeting men and boys.

Men are often viewed as the perpetrators of sexual violence and not the victims. Several factors can explain this myopia. First, no Human Rights instruments explicitly address sexual violence against men or male sexual abuse. Further, it seems that international law acknowledges men only insofar as their participation in preventing violence against women: "Men, like boys, are typically only included in language about violence in their instrumentalist capacity – as actors who are important to its reduction" (Stemple 2009: 623). The current international human rights framework is inadequate in addressing the problem and raising awareness about it. But international law is simply a mirror of national law. Many countries do not include male victims in their legal definitions of sexual violence, thus implicitly refusing to consider them as potential victims of that type of suffering. The only exception is sexual violence against boys in industrialized societies, whose suffering is fully acknowledged: "Where do male victims rank in the sexual violence hierarchy? Boys, with innocence still intact, certainly stand high above men, and arguably, very close to girls. But adult men are viewed as the aggressors" (Stemple 2009: 629).

Second, the understanding and framing of suffering induced by sexual violence in conflict areas is tightly related to how Third World masculinities (and related Third World femininities) are viewed. This is not to say that violent conflict only happens in developing countries, but rather that our understanding of sexual violence in conflict areas is shaped by accounts from Eastern DRC, Uganda or the Central African Republic. Women in developing countries are usually viewed as victims of a patriarchal order, in which men are preoccupied by struggles for power and domination: "How are we to understand "black men"? This is not a question that has received the attention it deserves, as the focus of gender work in underdeveloped world contexts and in terms of race has been insistently on women.

An ironic consequence has been to silence or to render black men invisible" (Morrell and Swart 2005: 96). When attention is drawn to men in conflict areas, they are usually seen as responsible for the very high levels of violence against women, as well as against other men. Such narratives explain that men are excluded from accounts on sexual violence in conflict areas; they also feed the assumption that sexual violence is a phenomenon only relevant to women and girls.

Third, it seems that speaking about sexual violence against men would undermine policies and programs designed to fight rape of women during wartime, through demonstrating that women are not the only victims – and might even also be perpetrators – of sexual violence. For instance, a UNHCR worker interviewed by Charli Carpenter argued: "I recognize our discourse is a bit outdated. But it's very difficult because as soon as you stop talking about women, women are forgotten. Men want to see what they will gain out of this gender business, so you have to be strategic" (Carpenter 2006: 99). It is true that the recognition of the plight of women during conflict times is relatively recent, and arguably still fragile. This feeds a competition between categories of victims, which is useless. Consequently, the suffering of men is almost completely invisible in the sexual and gender based violence narrative. Some authors even assert "health care workers have internalized stereotypical gender roles (men as aggressors, women as victims), to the extent that they are unable to recognize male victims of sexual violence who seek help, and may even dismiss them" (Oosterhoff et al. 2004: 68).

2.6   Men Should Be Strong and Able to Protect Themselves

Patriarchal cultures usually assign a role of protectors to men; they have to be strong and unyielding in order to protect themselves, their family, their community, but also their nation or State. Men who have been victim of sexual violence have failed to protect themselves and are thus less likely to be able to protect their family, provided that their family still accepts them. Male survivors have essentially failed to emulate the model of hegemonic masculinity that assigns to men the most important positions within the family, as backbones of their family and community. They are not "real men". Whether such sexual violence happens under the eyes of external witnesses or not is clearly important for understanding the victims' reaction and his ability to cope with the suffering – many male victims of rape flee their regions of origin or commit suicide.

The consequences on future gender relations, and society are severe. The figure of a glorified combatant is that of a cruel, fearless and extremely violent man, who intends to dominate physically but also psychologically all the individuals he is in contact with. In other words, this conception of masculinity gives birth to an extremely hierarchical social order, where "real" masculinity is defined by the ability to dominate others physically, men and women alike: "Yes, such things have happened, but not because we liked it, but because some combatants thought it was the only way to get local men to obey them".[9] The amount of frustration and resentment that is created by such practices is incommensurable; it also gives birth to a vicious circle by generating further episodes of symbolic and physical violence, either from the local communities on the victims themselves, or between spouses.

In this "exercise of power and humiliation" (Russell 2007: 22), one of the main goals seems to be the "feminization" of the victim and the "masculinization" of the perpetrator. Sexual violence against men and boys embodies the ultimate expression of hegemonic masculinity, as it has the power to symbolically turn male victims into women and to reinforce the masculinity of the perpetrator. The men with whom I spoke had the feeling of having been "homosexualized". Many of them find it impossible to report such acts, as complaining would symbolically reinforce their "feminization" by taking on the status of victim that is usually reserved to women: "They are treating only women over there. They do a good job, but this is not a place for me".[10] Most international programs dealing with sexual violence during conflicts focus on women and indeed tend to imply that only women can be victims. This leads to devastating consequences for male victims. They think that these programs are "made for women" and do not dare come forward. Male victims feel as if their own suffering was ignored, silenced, or too outrageous to even be spoken about. The equation that is made between women and victims further alienates them, because it confirms what most of them are already feeling—that having been raped or mutilated has "turned them into women", into "lesser men". The focus put on female victims of sexual violence furthers the suffering of male victims, by reinforcing the "de-masculinization" and "feminization" induced by what they went through.

2.7 A Collective Suffering

Some of my interviewees believe – and the existing literature tends to agree with them – that raping men stems from a similar strategy to that of raping women: an ethnic cleansing.[11] In societies where ethnicity is seen as being transmitted by males only, it is efficient to target specifically the bearer of ethnicity and hence destroy his own capacity to perpetuate his ethnic group. Sexual violence against men and boys can be considered as another weapon, both physical and psychological. It is thought to be more effective than sexually assaulting women as it targets the ones who are supposed to protect their community and to perpetuate the ethnic group (Zarkov in Moser and Clark 2011: 78). In that perspective, groups to which male victims of

---

[9] Jean-Baptiste, interviewed in Bujumbura, Burundi, 05 May 2011.

[10] Aimable, interviewed in Bubanza Province, Burundi, 18 April 2010.

[11] This was mentioned to me by an interviewee from the International Rescue Committee (Bujumbura, Burundi, 12 May 2012) as well as by another working for Caritas International (Goma, North Kivu, DRC, 03 May 2009).

sexual violence belong are also targeted through these practices, and they would rather silence these attacks that deeply undermine them.

This capacity of sexual violence against men to destroy family and community linkages is striking. In the Great Lakes Region of Africa, just like in most patriarchal societies (Sivakumaran 2007: 268), men are expected to protect their wives, their children, their aging parents, but also their whole community. If they cannot protect themselves, then their ability to protect the rest of the group can also be questioned. The suffering induced by sexual violence against men expands to include the whole community, which is left humiliated, unprotected and disempowered. As a result, the communities to which they belong lose their ethnicity. They symbolically become communities of women, of homosexuals, symbolically and psychologically deprived of any ability to regenerate and perpetuate themselves.

As I have discussed elsewhere (Féron and Hastings 2003), this type of violence is part of a repertoire where the perpetration of unforgivable and imprescriptible acts signals a rationale of a "definitive breach" of barbaric extravagance. In highly and traditional societies where sexuality remains extremely taboo, sexual violence against men and boys seems to embody the ultimate transgression. It will underline the omnipotence of the transgressor, while depriving the victim of the means and the will to revolt. It is a form of territorial domination that builds on the destruction of core political, cultural and social links. Sexual violence against men and boys, alongside that exerted against women and girls, thus illustrates the link underscored by Haugen and Boutros (2014) between the spread of violence and of other violations of human rights, as well as the deterioration of political and social orders. Communities and individuals alike are broken, more malleable, and less likely to revolt against the armed groups or armies that rob, loot, abduct, rape and seize precious natural resources.

2.8   Conclusions

Sexual violence against men and boys during conflicts is a tactic developed by armed groups in order to enforce domination on local men through a suffering that is symbolic, social, psychological, and physical. In many ways, it pushes the logic of gendered violence during conflicts to its utmost limits. Because this type of violence directly targets the ones who are considered to be the bearers of ethnicity and the protectors of their communities, it deeply breaks down the spirit of local populations by destroying core social links. It further deprives the victims and their families, and empowers the perpetrators, at the individual as well as at the collective level. It causes traumas that are almost impossible to overcome, and that may in turn feed the cycle of conflict. This type of violence is thus a product of the conflict as much as it produces it.

A series of assumption regarding "typical" masculine values and behavior however impede a wider recognition of, and response to, this suffering. Many also fear that acknowledging the suffering of men, or paying "too much" attention to it will distract attention from the suffering of women. However, this research highlights the multiple links and common characteristics existing between the suffering induced by sexual violence against women and girls, and that against men and boys. Just as sexual violence against both men and women has to be tackled jointly, an encompassing approach to the various categories of victims concerned has to be promoted, taking notice of the extreme complexity of such a phenomenon.

References

Anderson, R. E. (2014). *Human suffering and quality of life, conceptualizing stories and statistics.* New York: Springer.

Carpenter, C. R. (2006). Recognizing gender-based violence against civilian men and boys in conflict situations. *Security Dialogue, 37*(1), 83–103.

Christian, M., Safari, O., Ramazani, P., Burnham, G., & Glass, N. (2011). Sexual and gender based violence against men in the Democratic Republic of Congo: Effects on survivors, their families and the community. *Medicine, Conflict, and Survival, 27*(4), 227–246.

Connell, R. W., & Messerschmidt, J. W. (2005). Hegemonic masculinity: Rethinking the concept. *Gender and Society, 19*(6), 829–859.

Department of Defense. (2012). *Sexual assault prevention and response, department of defense annual report on sexual assault in the military* (Vol. 1). Washington. http://www.sapr.mil/public/docs/reports/FY12_DoD_SAPRO_Annual_Report_on_Sexual_Assault-VOLUME_ONE.pdf. Accessed 13 Mar 2014.

Dumas, M. (2011, August 2). Viols au Congo: Le jour où ils ont fait de moi une femme. *Rue 89.*

Féron, É., & Hastings, M. (2003). The new hundred years wars. *International Social Science Journal, 177*, 490–500.

Gettleman, J. (2009, August 5). Symbol of unhealed Congo: Male rape victims. *New York Times.*

Haugen, G. A., & Boutros, V. (2014). *The locust effect: Why the end of poverty requires the end of violence.* New York: Oxford University Press.

Human Rights Watch. (2005). *Seeking justice: The prosecution of sexual violence in the Congo War.* Human Rights Watch, New York. (Vol. 17(1(A))).

Johnson, K., et al. (2010). Association of sexual violence and human rights violations with physical and mental health in territories of the Eastern Democratic Republic of the Congo. *JAMA, 304*(5), 553–562.

Morrell, R., & Swart, S. (2005). Men in the third world. Post colonial perspectives on masculinity. In M. S. Kimmel, J. Hearn, & R. W. Connell (Eds.), *Handbook of studies on men and masculinities* (pp. 90–113). Thousands Oaks/London: Sage.

Moser, C. O. N., & Clark, F. C. (Eds.). (2011). *Victims, perpetrators or actors? Gender, armed conflict and political violence.* London: Zed Books.

Nizich, I. (1994). Violations of the rules of war by Bosnian Croat and Muslim forces in Bosnia-Herzegovina. *Hastings Women's Law Journal, 5*(1), 25–52.

OCHA. (2011). *DRC-Uganda: Male sexual abuse survivors living on the margins.* http://www.irinnews.org/Report/93399/DRC-UGANDA-Male-sexual-abuse-survivors-living-on-the-margins. Accessed 13 Mar 2014.

Okot, A. C., Amony, I., & Otim, G. (2005). *Suffering in silence: A study of Sexual and Gender Based Violence (SGBV) In Pabbo camp, Gulu district, Northern Uganda.* UNICEF, District Sub-Working Group on SGBV.

Oosterhoff, P., Zwanikken, P., & Ketting, E. (2004). Sexual torture of men in Croatia and other conflict situations: An open secret. *Reproductive Health Matters, 12*(23), 68–77.

Russell, W. (2007). Sexual violence against men and boys. *Forced Migration Review, 27*, 22–23.

Sabo, D. (2005). The studies of masculinities and men's health. An overview. In M. S. Kimmel, J. Hearn, & R. W. Connell (Eds.), *Handbook of studies on men and masculinities* (pp. 326–352). Thousands Oaks/London: Sage.

Schwartz, S. (1994). Rape as a weapon of war in the former Yugoslavia. *Hastings Women's Law Journal, 5*(1), 69–88.

Sivakumaran, S. (2007). Sexual violence against men in armed conflict. *The European Journal of International Law, 18*(2), 253–276.

Stemple, L. (2009). Male rape and human rights. *Hastings Law Journal, 60*, 605–645.

Stener, E. C. (1997). Sexual assault on men in war. *The Lancet, 349*, 129.

UNHCR. (2012). *Working with men and boy survivors of sexual and gender-based violence in forced displacement.* http://www.refworld.org/cgi-bin/texis/vtx/rwmain?docid=5006aa262. Accessed 13 Mar 2014.

Chapter 3
Social Suffering and Critical Humanitarianism

Iain Wilkinson

3.1 Introduction

In research and writing on social suffering, human suffering is viewed as holding a mirror up to the moral and embodied experience of society. The concept of social suffering is designed to draw a focus to the ways in which experiences of pain and misery are caused, constituted, and conditioned by the social circumstances in which people are made to live. Researchers operate with the understanding that social worlds are inscribed upon the bodily experience of suffering and that we should take such experience as a moral barometer of social life. This involves more than an attempt to have us recognize the harms done to people by society or the torments borne through culture; it also intends to make us critically oriented toward forces of social-structural oppression and cultural alienation. It aims to draw moral and political debate to both how social life takes place in lived experience and to people's social being. Here human suffering is taken as a social script and as a matter to awaken us to the imperative to care for the human-social condition as such.

Recent studies of social suffering share in the understanding that by documenting experiences of human affliction and providing spaces for individuals to voice their anguish and pain, scholars are also engaged in acts of social disclosure. They operate from the premise that, in having us attend to the brute facts of human suffering, readers are not only made open to a form of sociological/anthropological enlightenment, but are also equipped to think critically about human-social conditions. Seminal publications such as Arthur Kleinman's *Illness Narratives: Suffering, Healing and the Human Condition* (1988), Nancy Scheper-Hughes' *Death Without Weeping: The Violence of Everyday Life in Brazil* (1992), Pierre Bourdieu and colleagues'

I. Wilkinson (✉)
Faculty of Sociology, University of Kent, Cornwallis North East,
Canterbury, Kent CT2 7NF, UK
e-mail: I.M.Wilkinson@kent.ac.uk

© Springer Science+Business Media Dordrecht 2015   45
R.E. Anderson (ed.), *World Suffering and Quality of Life*,
Social Indicators Research Series 56, DOI 10.1007/978-94-017-9670-5_3

The Weight of the World: Social Suffering in Contemporary Society (1999), João Biehl's *Vita: Life in a Zone of Social Abandonment* (2005), and Philippe Bourgois's and Jeff Schonberg's *Righteous Dopefiend* (2009) ask readers to consider what suffering does to people in *experience* before embarking on the task of sociological and anthropological analysis. In this regard, social reality is understood to inhere in the welter of the individual, moral experience of life. Researchers take it as their sociological and anthropological task to trouble us in the recognition of this fact, foregrounding how social life is met in experience and focusing on social suffering so that we might root our analysis of societies in a concern for how this matters *for people*.

3.2   Social Suffering

In this chapter, I contend that a focus on social suffering leads social science not only in a humanitarian direction, but also traces back to the tradition of using the humanitarian appeal as a provocation to awaken social conscience. I aim to defend this practice against the arguments of contemporary critics. Writers such as Didier Fassin (2012) are inclined to cast the incorporation of "humanitarian reason" within projects of social science as an anathema to critical thinking and as a form of ideological corruption. By contrast, I maintain that it is a vital component of the pursuit of social understanding and the nurturing of social life. To be sure, I acknowledge the potential for humanitarian culture and its associated moral sentiments to be appropriated in the service of ideological agendas; nevertheless, I argue that a "critical humanitarianism" is essential in the attempt to understand social life in terms of the incidence and experience of social suffering.

First, I outline some of the arguments featured in recent sociological critiques of humanitarian culture and politics. I also review how these might be involved in a critical dismissal of research and writing on social suffering. In the second section, I contend that these critical standpoints lock us into an excessively narrow account of humanitarian political culture, when there is much more to uncover and explain in relation to the traditions of critical praxis developed within the history of campaigns for humanitarian social reform. In the third section, I locate recent developments in research and writing on social suffering as part of a critical tradition that courts moral and political controversies surrounding humanitarian motives and actions as a means to awaken social consciousness and action. In conclusion, I argue that insofar as problems of social suffering are brought to the heart of sociological and anthropological concern, they involve us not only in the attempt to apply tools of social analysis to conditions of human suffering, but also in a reconfiguration of the terms of social understanding. More directly, I argue that here we are challenged to have our thinking about society and our research conduct shaped by the character of our moral response toward the suffering others. In this setting, moreover, the value of social inquiry is to be sought not so much in its applications to critique, but in its service to the promotion of care.

3.3   The "Humanitarian Social Imaginary" and Its Reason

Charles Taylor argues that in any period of cultural history it is possible to identify distinct "social imaginaries" through which "people imagine their social existence, how they fit together with others, how things go on between them and their fellows, the expectations that are normally met, and the deeper normative notions and images that underlie these expectations" (Taylor 2003: 23). A social imaginary advances a conception of a presiding "moral order" and the appropriate behaviors that can and/ or should take place within this. While it operates as a social compass, the social imaginary also equips people with value orientations for determining how to live. On Taylor's account, as a social imaginary incorporates common apprehensions about "how the world works now," it also serves as a guide to the actions that are suited "to bring change to our world."

Recently this notion has been adopted to frame the cultural artifacts of humanitarian campaigns for analytical scrutiny. In this setting, however, it appears that commentators are chiefly occupied with casting humanitarian culture as a detriment to critical social understanding, creating a morally debased form of politics. For example, in studies of the ways in which celebrity ambassadors are used within the construction of "the humanitarian social imaginary" by organizations such as UNICEF, Lilie Chouliaraki (2013) contends, increasingly, publics encouraged to identify more with the feelings of celebrities than with the conditions of people in real life situations of adversity. Seizing upon the emotively laden performances of Angelina Jolie in her role as a UNICEF Goodwill Ambassador, Chouliaraki argues that audiences are encouraged to preoccupy themselves more with Jolie's feelings than with the plight of those actually in suffering (2013: 173). Insofar as celebrity-fronted media appeals are widely used to draw the human tragedy of large-scale disaster to public attention, Chouliaraki suggests that the humanitarian social imaginary encourages only the "low-intensity, fleeting sensibilities of a feel-good altruism," confining sympathizers to acting in "ironic solidarity" with distant sufferers rather than in any virtuous or authentic "solidarity of pity" (2013: 172–205).

In a similar vein, Luc Boltanski (1999) contends that modern humanitarian emergency appeals, such as those orchestrated by *Médecins Sans Frontières* (Doctors without Borders), ultimately undermine people's sense of political agency as well as their faith in the possibility of substantive social change (Boltanksi 1999). He contends that being a "detached observer" of human affliction creates a shared sense of powerlessness and moral inadequacy. On his account, the visibility brought to mass events of human suffering by modern communication media has created a cultural experience in which individuals are left feeling inadequate and impotent to respond to the imperative of action demanded by humanitarian appeal.

In a further development of this theme, Craig Calhoun (2004) argues that it may well be the case that people's apparent lack of concern and care for the suffering of others is connected to the fact that, in the context of humanitarian campaign work, the spectacle of human suffering is tethered to an "emergency imaginary" that normalizes a vision of the world as filled with frequent unforeseen crises.

Calhoun argues that "[a]pproaching conflicts as emergencies is, perhaps, the least unpalatable way of accepting their ubiquity, but it feeds unfocussed fear even as it reassures, and it encourages responses that may do good, but usually not deeply" (2004: 393). He worries over the extent to which the cultural artifacts of humanitarian appeals are involved in the creation of a social imaginary where global conditions of human suffering are seen as the result of "exceptional" and "unanticipated" disaster (Calhoun 2004, 2008). Suffering, then, is not an ongoing problem to be addressed on a global scale, but a series of short-term crises, each of which can be addressed individually. On this account, insofar as we are committed to the development of critical theories of our society, we should suspect a great deal of organized humanitarianism to "de-politicize" the public portrayal of large-scale events of human suffering. Calhoun contends that, consciously or otherwise, the social script that is offered discourages the privileged from a critical focus on the normalcy of human suffering in the conditions of global capitalism. Rather than applying our attention to the critical task of questioning the presiding order and ethos of society, we are more likely to be taken up with the task of marshalling resources in support of the efforts made by humanitarian organizations to "manage" its most damaging effects. Accordingly, Calhoun encourages us to associate modern humanitarianism with ideological discourses that not only provide tacit support for a status quo of grossly unequal power relations, but also prevent the arrangement from being taken up as a matter for critique.

This association is forcefully embraced by Didier Fassin, who, at the same time as he portrays humanitarianism as corruptive force within our politics, also casts it as an obstruction to the development of critical thinking within social science. In this regard, Fassin's critique of humanitarian culture is distinguished by an attempt to group it together with an angry dismissal of research and writing on social suffering so as to argue that social understanding is left skewed by "humanitarian reason" (Fassin 2012). On Fassin's account, research and writing on social suffering is part of a new development in modern culture that both fetishes the public spectacle of human suffering and is all too easily beguiled by moral sentiment. While such work might be portrayed as part of an effort to promote human rights and extend the bounds of social care, it is *really* a component of governmental discourses that police moral boundaries and impose categorizations of "victimhood" on the destitute, poor, and misfortunate (Fassin 2012: 252–57).

Singling out Pierre Bourdieu for particular criticism, Fassin claims that, in *The Weight of the World* (1999), Bourdieu was involved attempted to re-model sociology as a means to police the documentation of human experience. On Fassin's reading, this work served to advance the understanding that it is only insofar as we hear, see, and share in feeling for people's suffering that suffering should be recognized as a pressing social concern. Fassin writes:

> [O]n the basis of the sociologist's authority, social suffering acquired official status and empathetic listening became a legitimate tool, with the social sciences acting as a model for social work—and all the more because the book's success was partly due to the fact that unlike previous studies of exclusion, it showed that everyone was or potentially could be

affected by suffering. Rather than perpetuating the idea of a social world divided between excluded and included, as the sociologists of the second left asserted, Pierre Bourdieu, who can be seen as representative of the "first left" (neo-Marxist), revealed that everyone suffers, presenting a mirror in which all could recognise themselves. (2012: 32)

Bourdieu's promotion of social suffering as an issue for public concern served, to Fassin's mind, more to institute "a national policy of [only] listening." On these grounds, social suffering should be decried as a "mode of government" intent on making "precarious lives livable" by recognizing individual "misfortune" whilst leaving social conditions beyond critical scrutiny (Fassin 2012: 42). Fassin portrays Bourdieu not only as operating to diminish our social understanding of the world, but also as involved in the active creation of a cultural apparatus that serves to impose a sense of moral order on society rather than to hold it up for critical investigation.

More generally, Fassin regards the tendency for studies of social suffering to draw a particular focus to deprivations of health and embodied manifestations of suffering as representative of a movement to "reduce" people to problems of "biological life." Evoking arguments drawn from the works of Georgio Agamben (1995) and informed by Michel Foucault's later concern with issues of "biopower," Fassin declares an overwhelming disposition within humanitarian reason to only grant people social recognition insofar as they can be portrayed as "victims" of some form of detrimental health condition. Fassin argues that this focus on biological life operates to the exclusion of a concern for "biographical life" and that humanitarians intent on regulating bodily-health conditions operate with no concern for how the subjects of their interventions "give a meaning to their own existence" (Fassin 2012: 254). Accordingly, research and writing on social suffering within medical anthropology is held up as part of a culture that both obfuscates social analysis and diminishes our capacity for human recognition.

In all these studies, particularly the work of Didier Fassin, humanitarianism is cast as an enemy to social understanding—a force of political corruption and an obstacle to critique. In what follows, however, I aim to show that this casting relies on an excessively narrow conception of humanitarianism and draws a veil over the complex histories of humanitarian culture and politics. More directly, I contend that much of the incorporation of humanitarianism within works of social suffering is far more sophisticated and conscious of the political and moral risks inherent in its practice than critics are prepared to recognize or credit. I aim to defend the role of critical humanitarianism in the quest for social understanding and the promotion of human-social care.

3.4 Critical Humanitarianism as Praxis

Bartolomé de las Casas's *A Short Account of the Destruction of the Indies*, published in 1552, may well be the first document explicitly designed to illuminate human rights abuses in Western history (Las Casas 1992). Distinguished by his protest against the enslavement and violent persecution of the Amerindians, Las Casas points, above all, to the brute facts of suffering. In a series of graphic accounts of tortures, mass murders, and atrocities (in later editions, embellished by copper plate engravings of particularly gruesome acts of cruelty), Las Casas builds the vast majority of his case not so much on an appeal to matters of Christian conviction and theological principle, but on the evidence of human suffering. He repeatedly moves to bring moral recognition to the humanity of the Amerindians by describing the terrible details of their suffering. The public outrage and political controversies this account aroused across Europe were so destructive to the national reputation of Spain that considerable efforts were devoted to suppressing the details of his treatises. It was not until 1875 that Las Casas' full *History of the Indies* was finally published (Pagden 1992).

By this time, there was already a highly sophisticated politics of compassion within humanitarian campaign work. As Karen Halttunen records, by the mid-nineteenth century, humanitarian social reformers understood that graphic depictions of human suffering were liable to court public controversy, not least because it was widely understood that these accounts may be used for promiscuous pleasure rather than as prompts to civic virtue (Halttunen 1995). In this setting, the ongoing debates surrounding the motives behind Las Casas's documentation of atrocity (as most famously recorded in the dispute between Voltaire and Corneille de Pauw over the character of Las Casas's involvement in the conquest of the Americans) also helped cultivate a deep-seated awareness of the potential for people to be caught up in many morally conflicted states and actions by the force of sentimental feeling (Castro 2007; Arias and Merediz 2008). Particularly in the aftermath of the hostile literary and political condemnations of "sensibility" following the outbreak of revolution in France, it was widely feared that "the passion of compassion," as Hannah Arendt put it in a later reflections, might be deployed to erode commitments to rational public debate and to justify acts of violence (Arendt 1963).

Importantly, in this context, those who remained committed to the pursuit of humanitarian social reform via an appeal to the brute facts of human suffering did so in recognition of the fact that their campaign tactics risked public condemnation. They knew they were likely to fall under the moral condemnation of opponents committed to more rational-utilitarian approaches to managing social problems (Roberts 2002). There is now a literature devoted to detailing how anti-slavery campaigners, early feminist pamphleteer writers, and advocates of children's rights sought to broker with "the economy of attention to suffering" so as to craft texts that served the education of compassion (Abruzzo 2011; Spelman 1997). In the record of their diaries, letters, and public speeches, it appears that humanitarian campaigners such as Lydia Maria Child were all too aware that the graphic portrayal of human suffering might operate more as an erotic exploitation than as means to shock publics into supporting the cause of humanitarian social reform (Sorisio 2000).

Some of the more elaborate accounts of the politics of sentiment of the period are found in studies of the literary tactics of writers such as Charles Dickens and Harriet Beecher Stowe (Jaffe 2000; Ledger 2007; Roberts 2002: 258–331). Indeed, as far as the latter is concerned, Gregg Crane records that following the enormous public response to *Uncle Tom's Cabin* (1852)—the best selling novel of nineteenth century—Stowe actively attempted to clarify and defend the moral character and intention of her sentimental characterization of *Uncle Tom* in her next writing, *Dred: a Tale of the Great Dismal Swamp* (1856) (Crane 1996). Here, Crane records that not only did Stowe understand the rational culture of established law to operate in a conservative manner that set morally unacceptable limits on the issues that were taken up for public debate, she also understood that the strength of moral feeling than surpassed the processes of rational argumentation in moving people to act for the needs of others. Crane argues that while Stowe intended her depiction of Dred, the revolutionary leader of the slaves living on the swamp, to convey her misgivings over the potential for humanitarian sentiment to breed insurrectionary violence, she also sought to make clear her understanding that the struggle to imagine and realize better ways of living in the world was sustained more by passion than by point of principle. In this regard, Stowe's work might be taken as a manifestation of a critical praxis. Stowe regards the passion of compassion, whilst involving people in volatile feelings that might overwhelm their capacity to reason, each a necessary part of inspiring good reasons for involvement in the creation of humane forms of society.

3.5 The Return to Social Suffering

The origins of the concept of social suffering lie in the awakening of humanitarian social conscience in the second half of eighteenth century. The term conveys an early understanding of social life as mobilized and sustained by force of "fellow feeling," and it belongs to the "enlightenment of sympathy" (Frazer 2010). In this context, it was widely understood that, in the moral feelings aroused by the spectacle of human suffering, people were not only being made alert to their social ties to others, but also being challenged to care for their fellow humans' condition and needs (Mullan 1988). It is not merely the case that social suffering encourages us to understand that people's suffering as caused and conditioned by social circumstance; the perspective also invites us to recognize that, in what we feel for and how we respond to the suffering of others, we are *involved* in social experience and enactments of social value. Suffering is an incitement to social conscience and a spur to moral debate over the bounds of social responsibility and appropriate forms of humanitarian social action.

The more recent development of research and writing on social suffering marks a *return* to this tradition of social understanding. It ventures to rehabilitate a praxis that has been marginalized and/or denigrated within the institutionalization of social inquiry as a "science" within the academy. Once again, albeit through ethnography (the visualization of people's condition and circumstance through documentation of the ways people voice their experience of life), attempts are made to fashion social understanding through the arousal of moral feeling. In this regard, it is also vital to appreciate the extent to which such practices, embraced as a necessary component of the movement to awaken social consciousness and conscience, are also identified as inherently volatile risk-laden.

For example, Paul Farmer openly worries about the ways in which his graphic portrayals of human suffering serve to make his readers either 'habituated to horror' or outraged by the extent to which the stories might be taken as a form of voyeurism or pornography. Nevertheless, Farmer makes it his mission to court the provocation of a humanitarian social imaginary so as to shock readers into critical thinking and action. Following Susan Sontag (2003), he resolves "to locate our privilege on the same map as the suffering of our contemporaries," and, for this purpose, argues:

> …the road from unstable emotions to genuine entitlements—rights—is one we must travel if we are to transform human values into meaningful and effective programs that will serve precisely those who need our empathy and solidarity most (Farmer 2005: 152–6).

Similarly in their photo-ethnography of "dopefiends," Philippe Bourgois and Jeff Schonberg aim to make the moral disquiet aroused by images of bodies suffering the ravages of addiction a means to humanize the social perception of drug users (Bourgois and Schonberg 2009). Whilst anxiously concerned by the potential to encourage "a voyeuristic pornography of suffering," Bourgois and Schonberg hold it necessary to broker many moral tensions and unstable emotions so as to bring the human experience addiction to public attention: it is an issue for social conscience and political debate.

In both these examples, the acquisition of social understanding is taken to require a reconfiguration of moral feeling. Acknowledging the danger that their portrayals of human suffering might be culturally appropriated for ends that stand radically opposed to their humanitarian aims and objectives, nevertheless, these scholars still move to invoke the passion of compassion and, thus, social concern. They credit the most morally troubling, emotionally difficult, and semantically unstable passages of their work as those most capable of making the human-social condition a pressing matter for public debate.

A "critical humanitarianism" is at work here. At the same time these authors attend to concerns about sectional interests and even the possibility that their work might be fashioned as part of an arsenal of social abuse, they also see it as necessary for the cultivation of human-social understanding. In the struggle to make sense of difficult moral and intellectual tensions aroused through the witness of human suffering, readers might "see" the social situations occupied by others and become engaged in the challenge to care for all humans' social being.

3.6   Concluding Remarks

Pierre Bourdieu celebrated the potential for tools of critical social analysis to be directed towards privileged methods of social research and genres of writing about social life. Whilst he valued sociology and anthropology as disciplines that provided social enlightenment, he was wary of the ways in which they could be developed to eclipse the human-social condition. Reflecting on the motives that lay behind his documentation experiences of social suffering, Bordieu admitted that, in part, this was intended to draw debate toward the failure of social science to provide an adequate encounter with experiential suffering. Moreover, he was particularly worried by the potential for the language of social science to become a form of "symbolic violence" further contributing to the harms done to and suffered by people (Bourdieu 1999: 607–26). He sought to combat the conservativism of a critical counter-culture that critically denounced the world without venturing to involve itself in positive action.

The tendency toward technical, even clinical, writing in the social sciences risks obscuring more of the world than we bring to light. More troubling, sociologists and others risk a loss of social understanding in human terms. It is seems all too easy for social science to operate without human recognition, unintentionally renunciating care for the human as such. Under this conviction, research and writing on social suffering tries to enact a critical reflexivity that makes social science both consciously and conscientiously committed to exposing the moral experience of people in society (Kleinman 1999). We are encouraged to critically question our own values and to take up a critical stance with regard to how the culture of social science operates.

In the space of this chapter, I have sought to move beyond a mere review of how the concept of social suffering is featured and applied in contemporary social research. I hope to have emphasized how social suffering invites us to debate the character and conduct of our engagements with the task of social understanding. At various points, outlining its association to and involvement with the a critical praxis of humanitarianism, I have also noted that here there is a particular concern that we might see social inquiry fashioned not merely for purpose of critique, but also as a provocation to involve ourselves in real acts of care. A movement is at work here to have us recognize the quality of our social understanding to reside in the quality of our involvement in care for the suffering of people. Its 'critical humanitarianism' is far more an option taken up as an attachment to social inquiry, rather it is embraced as a necessarily troubling requirement for those who have any care for the human situation in social life. Critique must not be an end unto itself but a call to care.

References

Abruzzo, M. (2011). *Polemical pain: Slavery, cruelty and the rise of humanitarianism*. Baltimore: The John Hopkins Press.

Agamben, G. (1995). *Homo sacer: Sovereign power and bare life*. Stanford: Stanford University Press.

Arendt, H. (1963). *The social question in on revolution*. Harmondsworth: Penguin.

Arias, S., & Merediz, E. M. (Eds.). (2008). *Teaching the writings of Bartolomé de las Casas*. New York: The Modern Language Association.

Biehl, J. (2005). *Vita: Life in a zone of social abandonment*. Berkeley: University of California Press.

Boltanski, L. (1999). *Distant suffering: Morality, media and politics*. Cambridge: Cambridge University Press.

Bourdieu, P. (1999). Understanding. In P. Bourdieu et al. (Eds.), *The weight of the world: Social suffering and contemporary society* (pp. 607–26). Cambridge: Polity.

Bourdieu, P., et al. (1999). *The weight of the world: Social suffering in contemporary life*. Cambridge: Polity Press.

Bourgois, P., & Schonberg, J. (2009). *Righteous dopefiend*. Berkeley: University of California Press.

Calhoun, C. (2004). A world of emergencies: Fear, intervention and the limits of cosmopolitan order. *Canadian Review of Sociology, 41*(4), 373–395.

Calhoun, C. (2008). The imperative to reduce suffering: Charity, progress and emergencies in the field of humanitarian action. In M. Barnett & T. G. Weiss (Eds.), *Humanitarianism in question: Politics, power, ethics*. Ithaca: Cornell University Press.

Castro, D. (2007). *Another face of empire: Bartolomé de Las Casas, indigenous rights and ecclesiastical imperialism*. Durham: Duke University Press.

Chouliaraki, L. (2013). *The ironic spectator: Solidarity in the age of post-humanitarianism*. Cambridge: Polity Press.

Crane, G. (1996). Dangerous sentiments: Sympathy, rights and revolution in Stowe's anti-slavery novels. *Nineteenth-Century Literature, 51*(2), 176–204.

Farmer, P. (2005). *Pathologies of power: Health, human rights and the new war on the poor*. Berkeley: University of California Press.

Fassin, D. (2012). *Humanitarian reason: A moral history of the present*. Berkeley: University of California Press.

Frazer, M. L. (2010). *The enlightenment of sympathy: Justice and the moral sentiments in the eighteenth century and today*. Oxford: Oxford University Press.

Halttunen, K. (1995). Humanitarianism and the pornography of pain in Anglo-American culture. *The American Historical Review, 100*(2), 303–334.

Jaffe, A. (2000). *Scenes of sympathy: Identity and representation in Victorian literature*. Ithaca: Cornell University Press.

Kleinman, A. (1988). *The illness narratives: Suffering, healing and the human condition*. New York: Basic Books.

Kleinman, A. (1999). Experience and its moral modes: Culture, human conditions and disorder. In G. B. Peterson (Ed.), *The tanner lectures on human values*. Salt Lake City: University of Utah Press.

Las Casas, B. (1992). *A short account of the destruction of the Indies*. London: Penguin.

Ledger, S. (2007). *Dickens and the popular radical imagination*. Cambridge: Cambridge University Press.

Mullan, J. (1988). *Sentiment and sociability: The language of feeling in the eighteenth century*. London: Clarendon.

Pagden. (1992). 'Introduction' to Las Casas, B. In *A short account of the destruction of the Indies*. London: Penguin.

Roberts, F. D. (2002). *The social conscience of the early Victorians*. Stanford: Stanford University Press.

Scheper-Hughes, N. (1992). *Death without weeping: The violence of everyday life in Brazil*. Berkeley: University of California Press.

Sontag, S. (2003). *Regarding the pain of others*. London: Hamish Hamilton.

Sorisio, C. (2000). The spectacle of the body: Torture in the antislavery writing of Lydia Maria child and Frances E.W. Harper. *Modern Language Studies, 30*(1), 45–66.

Spelman, E. V. (1997). *Fruits of sorrow: Framing our attention to suffering*. Boston: Beacon.

Taylor, C. (2003). *Modern social imaginaries*. Durham: Duke University Press.

Chapter 4
Compassion, Cruelty, and Human Rights

Natan Sznaider

Say this city has ten million souls,
  Some are living in mansions, some are living in holes:
  Yet there's no place for us, my dear, yet there's no place for us (Auden 1967).

This poem, "Refuge Blues," was written by W. H. Auden just before the outbreak of World War II. It is a poet's outcry for a more humane world, for a world without cruelty. It is a poet's wish that his words and their display of compassion can make for a better world. Today, this outcry is couched in the language of human rights.

Rights and compassion mean much to many, and yet have no firm definition. Are we talking politics? If so, what are the political implications of human rights? Or are we talking aesthetics, a kind of "human rights experience" without great political consequence? Poets, politicians, and intellectuals seem only to agree that human rights matter.

In fact, contemporary societies are suffused with images making just this point. Imagine watching TV or browsing the Internet. Pictures of brutal beatings, forcible eviction, or military assaults on innocent civilians parade before your eyes. These are not movie clips; they are glimpses of reality near and far. Do we have a language that can make sense of these images and our reactions to them?

This essay is based on arguments developed in my jointly written book with Daniel Levy (Levy and Sznaider 2010) and my book *The Compassionate Temperament* (Sznaider 2000). I dedicate it to my former teacher Allan Silver, who introduced me first to the ideas of the Scottish Enlightenment and taught me to think sociologically.

N. Sznaider (✉)
Faculty, School of Behavioral Sciences, The Academic College of Tel Aviv Yaffo,
2 Rabeno Yeruham St, Tel Aviv Yaffo, Israel
e-mail: natan@mta.ac.il

© Springer Science+Business Media Dordrecht 2015
R.E. Anderson (ed.), *World Suffering and Quality of Life*,
Social Indicators Research Series 56, DOI 10.1007/978-94-017-9670-5_4

4.1 Human Rights

All human beings are born free and equal in dignity and rights. They are endowed with reason and conscience and should act towards one another in a spirit of brotherhood (UN 1948).

These noble words are Article 1 of the Universal Declaration of Human Rights. We must ask whether they have political meaning and, if so, consequential implications. The language of human rights provides a framework to begin to understand why pictures of strangers being beaten and tortured by other strangers concern us. Why do we care? Should we care? What is it about the power of human rights that makes the violation of them revolting? Is our passion for human rights historically contingent? At least rhetorically, human rights have become a kind of universal currency in politics; few politicians can afford to be *against* human rights. But rhetoric alone does not guarantee a world without violations.

Some believe the concept of human rights is nothing more than a Western ideological assertion, another sophisticated form of colonial imposition. Compassion and the public representation of suffering, too, have seen increasingly bad press among critical thinkers in the social sciences. These concepts are considered masks and screens covering up political realities (see Fassin 2012). Even if this may be the case, we still need to understand the phenomenon at hand.

There is a strong relationship between human rights consciousness and the emergence of a globalized cosmopolitan and liberal society, with its distinctive features of an expanded global awareness of the presence of others and the equal worth of human beings driven by memories of past human rights violations (Beck and Sznaider 2006; Levy and Sznaider 2005). Through these memories and their institutionalization in international conventions, the nature and sentiments of compassion have changed. Cruelty is now understood as the infliction of unwarranted suffering, and compassion is an organized, public response to this evil, as in human rights politics. With the lessening of profoundly categorical and corporate social distinctions triggered by the memories of barbarism, compassion can become more expansive, setting a politics of universal human rights into motion. The capacity to identify with others (in particular, with others' pain) is promoted by the profound belief in shared humanity, ontological equality. Compassion is also a revolt. It revolts against contempt, against torture, against humiliation, and against pain. It is more than "just" sentiment. It is the affirmation of humanity.

In addition, the globalization of media images plays a crucial role in society (Tester 2001). Compassion enters into current debates on foundations of ethics as depicted in the global media (Linklater 2007). Globalization has the potential to transform culture and through vocabulary influence meaning (Morley and Robins 1995). This transformation becomes most evident when the particularities that make up a culture are divorced from their original spatial (i.e., local and national) contexts. Transnational media and mass culture, such as film and music, loosen the national framework without abandoning it entirely (just note Sting's protest song 1987s "They Dance Alone," which was a symbolic gesture against Latin American dictatorships). Even those who never leave their hometown are challenged by the images on their televisions and computers to integrate global value systems that are produced elsewhere into their national frame of reference.

4.2 Compassion

Thus, my argument is that compassion – the organized campaign to lessen the suffering of strangers – is a distinctly modern form of morality that, itself, played an important role in the rise of modernity (Orwin 1980; Snow 1991; Sznaider 2000). And if we understand the nature of compassion and its connection to social structure, we can explain many social movements today that otherwise seem accidental, unprecedented, and post-modern. The idea that the sight of suffering imposes a duty to ameliorate it seems like it should be very old, but it is, in fact, a very recent one. There is a big distance between the duties that once bound (and even marked out) saints and that which is now considered incumbent upon all reasonable people. So little was suffering considered an evil before the nineteenth century that the guardians of morality paraded the spectacular suffering of evildoers before the public as a means of moral improvement (Gatrell 1994). Thus, for example, public hangings continued until the end of the eighteenth century. Even during the Reformation, often thought of as the first turn on the road toward modernity, people whose only crimes were doctrinal were routinely burned in the city squares of Europe's capitals. The movement to reform such cruelties reflected a change in the conception of human nature. No longer were public displays of cruelty thought to be salutary. They were thought brutalizing – to the people that watched them.

The moral sentiments that result from this process – what Norbert Elias (1978) called "The Civilizing Process" – constitute qualitatively new social bonds. I argue that the idea that we must remove "brutalizing" conditions in order to "civilize" people developed in tandem with capitalism and its "dark satanic mills." The result has been a qualitatively new outpouring of compassion (Haskell 1985).

I suggest two broad interpretations of the emergence and rise of public compassion. The *democratization* perspective suggests that with the lessening of profoundly categorical and corporate social distinctions, compassion becomes more extensive. A second perspective is linked to the emergence of *market society*. In this perspective, the market itself can be understood to extend the public scope of compassion. By defining a universal field of others with whom contracts and exchanges can be made, market perspectives extend the sphere of moral concern, however unintentionally.

In both perspectives, the nature and sentiment of compassion changed with the onset of civil society. As a "natural" moral sentiment, public compassion involves a revolution in sensibility and a new relationship to pain. Public compassion was initially the fight against cruelty, understood as the unjustifiable affliction of pain. Modern humanitarianism protests against a wider vision of suffering and pain. In its philanthropic version, it has tried to establish bonds of compassion among social groups and classes (for early formulations of this point, see Crane 1934). These modern humanitarian movements arose in the eighteenth and nineteenth centuries with fights to abolish slavery; cruelty to prisoners, animals, and children; and factory, sanitary, and prison reform. All of these movements continue today.

Humanitarian movements de-legitimized earlier values and practices as morally reprehensible. In the rhetoric of humanitarian reform, older practices were redefined as *cruelty*, the infliction of suffering, stripped of its outdated justifications. Compassion, in organized form, was framed as a public response to this evil. From that point on public executions, torture, and slavery all came under moral scrutiny (Peters 1985). Given the timing of these redefinitions and humanitarian sensibilities alongside the rise of market society and capitalism, it is no long stretch to see a connection (Haskell 1985).

I am aware that this is a counter-intuitive argument, particularly for sociologists. The more intuitive argument is that market behavior consists of the relentless pursuit of profit, so it is impossible to deduce a capitalist "moral cosmology." But the intuitive argument thinks of modernity as corrosive to moral sentiment. Sociologists see clearly the way in which modernity breaks down older social bonds, but they are much less attentive to the way in which it builds new ones. When waves of compassion break out into demands for political action, scholars searching for an explanation are forced to consider this humanitarianism exceptional – an atavism, an excuse, a subterfuge, or an irrelevancy.

To be sure, there are many ways to argue that modernization corrodes compassion. Hannah Arendt (1963), Michel Foucault (1965, 1977), Zygmunt Bauman (1989, 1993, 1995), and Giorgio Agamben (1998, 1999) are probably the most important and influential of these thinkers. Their indictments of modernity are the most original, as they are not simply a recycling of the Gemeinschaft/Gesellschaft distinction found at the base of so much other anti-modernism (Toennies 1965) or of critical theorists' accounts of the pitfalls of the Enlightenment (Horkheimer and Adorno 1971). Instead, these four scholars fasten on the most difficult empirical issues and carry their premises to logical conclusions. In so doing, they raise the most crucial objections to my own argument.

In the large outlines, I agree with those critics' characterization of the pre-modern era as one of "punishment" and exemplary cruelty. I also follow them in seeing an intellectual and experiential break between that era and our own. And I applaud them for putting the institutions of social control at the center of the analysis of society. But where we part company is in the characterization of the present. Where they see discipline, I see compassion. Where they see power, I see moral sentiments. And where they see social control as the state's control over society, I see social control as society's control over *itself*.

What critics of modernity ignore, on principle, is the experience of people. Under the first regime (pre-modernity), people are capable of taking their children to a public hanging as if it were family entertainment. Under the second (modernity), they feel queasy about violence on TV. The hypocrisy that, despite our queasiness, there is lots of violence on TV, should not obscure the sea change: real, physical violence – not the regulated violence of sports nor the stylized violence of the cinema – makes modern people shiver with disgust. To simply hear the details of torture produces, in most moderns, a physical revulsion. Sometimes it leads to outrage and clamoring that something must be done; sometimes merely to the desire to switch the channel. But what it does *not* lead to is laughter or a feeling of satisfaction. In the unusual cases in which we encounter people who enjoy killing or we come to believe a person must be put to death, it requires explaining. That is to say, we encounter real violence, cruelty, and unanswered suffering as an exception that needs to be reconciled with our worldview.

This shift – from people and societies that reveled in and prided themselves on killing and torture to societies that feel the pain of others so much that they have to hide it away or crusade against it – is essential. Many critics miss this, ironically, because they focus on continuities. It is true that there are still torturers in the world. But they are at the margins. They are hidden where they were once paraded. They are the exceptions where they used to rule (just note how popular culture has depicted the hero of a series "24" Jack Bauer as being in and outside the establishment of the security apparatus). This signifies a change in how we experience the world as well as how the world *is*.

I do not ignore this softening of manners as an epiphenomenon: I treat it as of central importance. The rise of modern compassion and human rights is not only the effect of structural changes, but also a contributing factor in its own acceleration. It is one of the keys to understanding the interaction between changing social structure and changing human nature. On my reading, the great critics of modernity share two main shortcomings when they argue that modernity has corrupted compassion. First, their concept of power seems to have neither actors nor responsible parties. Second, they rely on a State stretched so thin that it is in the end coextensive with the society over which it rules. I argue that the concept of society as constituted by moral sentiments overcomes both these problems in the best possible way – preserving their insights while resolving their contradictions.

4.3 Global Media

Another important criticism of the media portrayal of human suffering is known as "compassion fatigue" (Sontag 2003). That is, we are "becoming so used to the spectacle of dreadful events, misery or suffering that we stop noticing them. We are bored when we see one more tortured corpse on the television and we are left unmoved" (Tester 2001: 13). While it is perfectly reasonable to consider these negative features to be part of the global media, there is little question that a moral proposal is made to the viewer. It can be accepted or rejected, but hardly be ignored. Even the viewer whose compassion for others is *not* triggered by stories and images of the suffering of distant others must come to terms with those visions.

In global times the media are not only decisive in accelerating boundary-transcending processes but they also constantly remind us that the stories we tell ourselves are not the only sources of identification. It was Roger Silverstone (2007) who turned these insights into a complex media theory of moral and political space in which the new political space in which morality (and compassion for human rights) is negotiated is called "Mediapolis." Silverstone does not talk about a unified worldview, as we are constantly negotiating and moving between the universal and the particular. Instead, the Mediapolis is about plural experiences. Plurality, in turn, depends on the unique and the particular.

This is how the global media relates to the politics of human rights. It involves a moral minimalism that cannot be reduced to culture and nation. The moral space created by the media presupposes a universalistic minimum involving a number of substantive norms which must be upheld at all costs. The principle that women and children should not be sold or enslaved, the principle that people should be able speak freely about God or their government without being tortured or having their lives threatened – these are so self-evident that no violation is tolerated.

4.4 Moral Obligations

This is where contemporary human rights politics start: the highest principle is human well-being, and the greatest obligation is to prevent suffering wherever it occurs. This form of reasoning was embodied in the Scottish Enlightenment, specifically in the idea that there are duties imposed by sympathy and benevolence, motivated by exposure to heart wrenching stories (Silver 1990). The thinkers of the Scottish Enlightenment (like David Hume and Adam Smith) developed a theory of "moral sense", addressing the problem of compassion. They considered "natural compassion" both normative and descriptive of human nature (Hume 1751; Smith 1759). Human beings both have, and *ought* to have, fellow feelings for others. As an automatic mechanism for the common good, sympathy is thus seen to lie in the very nature of civil society. In this conception, imagination is key to compassion. Human beings are cruel when they cannot put themselves in the place of those who suffer.

Like the French Enlightenment, the Scottish Enlightenment also had a political program of reform. But unlike the French, its proponents did not place all their faith in reason and the wisdom of state officials. They instead argued that the social conditions that fostered sympathy were greater wealth, greater interaction, and greater equality, and that all of these conditions would be enhanced by the growth of the market. In other words, they argued that market cosmopolitanism and moral cosmopolitanism were mutually supportive. Thus it is perhaps not surprising that the Human Rights Regime began to take shape in hand with the spread of Neo-Liberalism after the end of the Cold War. That this mercantile outlook would produce a form of human rights activism targeting the market as a major source of social and economic human rights violations is only another manifestation of twists in the conditionality of human rights.

I am aware that to base human rights on sentiment rather than reason needs calls for justification. One view is that philosophy can become religion (Durkheim 1912). By embodying philosophy in rituals, such identities are created, reinforced, and integrated into communities. Richard Rorty (1989) makes the same argument in different terms. For Rorty, all moral philosophy an attempt to rationalize beliefs handed down as part of our religious heritage. We have been inculcated with them and believe them to be valid, but we do not believe the theology behind these beliefs. Hence moral philosophy – the attempt to provide a different foundation for ideas we already believe on faith. Secularized moralities, then, are moralities that are accepted on faith and anchored in identity. It matters very much to people if such things are questioned or if norms are flagrantly violated. Cruelty, violence, and breaches of the social contract make them feel personally injured, spur outrage, and connect those who feel similarly. And this provides the basis for political mobilization. A commitment to these values does not imply that moral cosmopolitans are rootless individuals preferring humanity to concrete human beings. Global values are *embedded* in concrete rituals such as war crime trials, with the extensive media and scholarly attention they garner (Turner 2006).

4.5   Relief of Suffering

Anderson (2014) offers some theoretical and philosophical suggestions as to how to ground ethical theories for a collective relief of suffering, claiming "human suffering is the greatest humanitarian challenge today" (p. 124). Compassion needs to be institutionalized and human rights are one important way of doing it.

I hope to complete some of Anderson's suggestions by providing some sociological underpinnings for such a task. It is not impossible and one's mind should not be clouded by the prevalent sociological discourse of suspicion around modern morality. Power and interests, of course, are important factors for understanding the social world, but they are not the *only* factors. Thus, I believe that a sociological study of compassion can and should clarify the historical processes through which compassion can shape the definition of "social problems" and investigate the means by which specialists in organizing moral sentiments strive to alleviate suffering. If we better understand the social and historical conditions that make this moral state possible, we can also move away from suspicion and look at morals as a social fact.

Compassion in liberal society involves not only action but also a strong belief in universal benevolence, optimism, and the idea that happiness can be achieved in this life on earth. That is, it requires humanitarianism. A nineteenth century humanitarian reformer concisely described the sentiment: "By humanitarianism I mean nothing more and nothing less than the study and practice of human principles – of compassion, love, gentleness, and universal benevolence" (Salt 1891, p. 3).

We need to distinguish public compassion from earlier models of compassion like religious charity, as well as models like the bureaucratic welfare state. Modern humanitarian movements are now venerable, the precursors to the current conception of human rights. Humanitarian movements de-legitimized earlier values and practices as morally reprehensible, even *cruel*. Compassion in this ethical system takes individualism and one's own experience of suffering as points of departure.

Emotional separateness and distance, essential to individualism, are constitutive of fellow feeling, as distinct from *agape* and *caritas*. Emotional separateness and distance, prevalent in market society, thus enables members of civil society to form a bond that shapes encounters with the suffering of others as in human rights consciousness.

Smith, in particular, emphasized the consistency between concern for the self and distance from others, on the one hand, and the emergence of moral conduct on the other. If sympathy grows out of the separate experiences of individuals, it is consistent with market society. Smith emphasizes the self-love of humankind in what he calls commercial society. People who were previously indifferent to each other can enter now into contractual market exchanges (Silver 1990). This reduction of structural distance between individuals makes it possible to bring them together in a common public realm (Boltanski 1993), and compassion arises as each recognizes the humanity of the other. This sort of compassion is an unheroic quality, unlike the absolute goodness of saints. Self-love and compassion are intrinsically linked and co-exist within individuals (Mizuta 1975).

Clearly, there is ambivalence about the concept of modernity and its moral sentiments. But just as clearly, there are more than two dichotomous answers for the relationships between modernity and barbarism or compassion. One view holds that the civilizing process is the principle of modern society. Modernity is characterized by the taming of aggression and the domestication of our psychic household. This view is now considered naïve by most social scientists. A second grand narrative came to answer the first: *barbarity* is an integral part of modernity. Moral sentiments like compassion become instruments of domination.

What of a potential third option: the project of modernity is being defined through a consciousness of the potential to barbarity and the attempt to overcome it though processes like compassion and human rights. If we are to see phenomena which are hostile, brutal, and violent as such, we need a moral baseline. Modernity is able to recognize barbarity in a self-reflexive process fostered by compassion and institutionalized through human rights.

Thus, one does one have to take the side of the deconstructionist, post-modernist. and other assaults on "foundationalism" in order to accept that human morality is historically contingent and a product of social relations? I have attempted, in this piece, to suggest a small alternative to these views by reconstructing the language of compassion from bourgeois discourse itself. We need to try to transcend idealistic or materialist theories concerning the origin of humanitarianism and maintain both aspects at the same time (see also Haskell 1985). There is indeed historical contingency with regard to the emergence of human rights consciousness which includes moral compassion. There are sociological forms of understanding that recognize the social origin of moral sentiments without reducing them to epiphenomena or ideological superstructures of the will to power or attempts by the ruling elements of society to control the masses or curb unrest.

Moral compassion is not merely epiphenomenal. It has arisen in a specific historical and social context – namely through the emergence of capitalism. The market, through its universal features, allows people participating in it to enter –

independently, of their will – into universal moral relationships. The market expands the horizons of people's moral responsibility, formerly limited by exclusivist bonds of memberships in corporate groups. Public passion emerges from market relationships and shows the possibility of compassion in a society of individuals. The rather common sense view found in the social sciences treats morality from a stance of skepticism, cynicism, even indifference. If at all, compassion is treated as an epiphenomenal, ideological superstructure, objectivizing practice, or method of carrying out symbolic violence. As useful as these approaches are in opening our eyes to hidden motives, they at same time obscure a tradition of modernity that *stimulates* this specific cultural value. Compassion and individuality are not mutually exclusive.

References

Agamben, G. (1998). *Homo sacer. Sovereign power and bare life*. Stanford: Stanford University Press.

Agamben, G. (1999). *Remnants of Auschwitz. The witness and the archive*. New York: Zone Books.

Anderson, R. E. (2014). *Human suffering and the quality of life*. New York: Springer Books.

Arendt, H. (1963). *On revolution*. New York: Viking.

Auden, W. H. (1967 [1939]). Refugee blues. In *Collected shorter poems, 1927–1957*. New York: Random House.

Bauman, Z. (1989). *Modernity and the Holocaust*. Cambridge: Polity Press.

Bauman, Z. (1993). *Postmodern ethics*. Oxford: Blackwell.

Bauman, Z. (1995). *Life in fragments: Essays in postmodern moralities*. Oxford: Blackwell.

Beck, U., & Sznaider, N. (2006). Unpacking cosmopolitanism for the social sciences: A research agenda. *British Journal of Sociology, 57*(1), 1–23.

Boltanski, L. (1993). *La Souffrance a distance*. Paris: Metaille.

Crane, S. R. (1934). Suggestions toward a genealogy of the 'man of feeling'. *ELH: A Journal of English Literary History, 1*, 205–230.

Durkheim, E. (1965 [1912]). *The elementary forms of the religious life*. New York: The Free Press.

Elias, N. (1978 [1938]). *The civilizing process, vol. 1: The history of manners*. New York: Pantheon.

Fassin, D. (2012). *Humanitarian reason. A moral history of the present*. Berkeley: University of California Press.

Foucault, M. (1965). *Madness and civilization*. New York: Random House.

Foucault, M. (1977). *Discipline and punish*. New York: Pantheon.

Gatrell, V. A. C. (1994). *The hanging tree: Execution and the English people 1770–1868*. Oxford: Oxford University Press.

Haskell, T. (1985). Capitalism and the origins of the humanitarian sensibility, parts 1&2. *American Historical Review, 9*, 339–361 and 547–566.

Horkheimer, M., & Adorno, T. (1971). *Juliette oder Aufklärung und Moral in Dialektik der Aufklärung*. Frankfurt: Fischer.

Hume, D. (1988 [1751]). *An enquiry concerning the principles of morals*. Indianapolis: Hackett.

Levy, D., & Sznaider, N. (2005). *The holocaust and memory in the global age*. Philadelphia: Temple University Press.

Levy, D., & Sznaider, N. (2010). *Human rights and memory*. University Park: Penn State University Press.

Linklater, A. (2007). Distant suffering and cosmopolitan obligations. *International Politics, 44*, 19–36.

Mizuta, H. (1975). Moral philosophy and civil society. In A. Skinner & T. Wilson (Eds.), *Essays on Adam Smith* (pp. 114–131). Oxford: Clarendon Press.

Morley, D., & Robins, K. (1995). *Space of identity: Global media electronic landscapes and cultural boundaries*. New York: Routledge.

Peters, E. (1985). *Torture*. New York: Blackwell.

Rorty, R. (1989). *Contingency, irony, and solidarity*. New York: Cambridge University Press.

Salt, H. (1891). *Humanitarianism: Its general principle and progress. Cruelties of civilization*. London: Humanitarian League's Publication.

Silver, A. (1990). Friendship in commercial society: Eighteenth century social theory and modern society. *American Journal of Sociology, 95*(6), 1474–1504.

Silverstone, R. (2007). *Media and morality: On the rise of the mediapolis*. Cambridge: Polity Press.

Smith, A. (1759). *The theory of moral sentiments*. Indianapolis: Liberty Classics.

Snow, N. (1991). Compassion. *American Philosophical Quarterly, 28*, 195–205.

Sontag, S. (2003). *Regarding the pain of others*. New York: Farrar, Straus and Giroux.

Sznaider, N. (2000). *The compassionate temperament*. Lanham: Rowman & Littlefield.

Tester, K. (2001). *Compassion, morality and the media*. Buckingham: Open University Press.

Toennies, F. (1965 [1887]). *Community and society*. New York: Harper.

Turner, B. S. (2006). *Vulnerability and human rights*. University Park: Penn State University Press.

UN. (1948). *Universal declaration of human rights*. New York: United Nations. Retrieved March 20, 2014, from http://www.un.org/en/documents/udhr/history.shtml

Chapter 5
Making Sense of Suffering: Insights from Buddhism and Critical Social Science

Ruben Flores

5.1 Introduction

Seeking to enrich our framework for studying and alleviating suffering, this chapter reflects upon the points of contact and tension between critical social science (CSS) and Buddhism—two traditions that have been compared at different times to the practice of medicine (Batchelor 1998; Bresnan 1999; Conze 1951; Eagleton 2011; Levine 2007) in that a key aspect of their *raison d'etre* concerns the alleviation of suffering. Both Buddhism and CSS offer causal understandings of suffering and recommendations for its alleviation. However, diagnoses and remedies differ in substantive ways, as it is to be expected from discourses developed in radically different historical contexts.

Part of my argument is that a dialogue between Buddhism and CSS is both necessary and useful. Necessary because, as Andrew Sayer has argued, CSS is bound to benefit from a constant engagement with different ethical perspectives (Sayer 2009); Buddhism, on the other hand, though strong on ethics, lacks a coherent understanding of societal suffering, which understanding CSS could provide. And useful because such debate could enrich the analytical perspectives of anyone interested in understanding and alleviating suffering.

Both Buddhism and CSS have long histories. I have attempted to avoid oversimplifications, especially regarding Buddhism, a tradition that, with over 25 centuries of reflection and practice, has given rise to a wide variety of schools and subtraditions spanning continents, languages, and times (Buswell and Lopez 2014; Bresnan 1999). My approach is best understood as drawing on Weberian "ideal

R. Flores (✉)
Faculty of Social Sciences, National Research University – Higher School of Economics,
20 Myasnitskaya Ulitsa, Moscow 101000, Russian Federation
e-mail: rflores@hse.ru

types," or conceptual constructions that seek to represent a given phenomenon, but that should not be confused with the varieties and nuances of its many manifestations.

5.2   Critical Social Science (CSS)

In a sense, all social research is critical. Varieties of CSS like Marxism or feminism can be clearly distinguished from mainstream social research in that they aim to dispel illusions not only in academic discourse, but also "in society itself" (Sayer 2009: 769). For example, "Marxism generally incorporates a critique of practices or social structures as contradictory and productive of unintended and destructive consequences (Callinicos 2006)," while feminism has criticized the incongruity of gender notions underpinning sexist/patriarchal practices (Sayer 2009: 769–770). Following Marx's celebrated eleventh thesis on Feuerbach, CSS has historically committed to understanding and criticizing social reality, as well as to transforming it through conscious individual and collective action (Feagin and Vera 2008).

In seeking to transform the world for the better, though, one is bound to benefit from taking a clear ethical standpoint. This is when CSS runs into trouble. Traditionally, CSS has implicitly aligned itself with notions like emancipation, thus effectively tending a bridge between "positive (explanatory/descriptive) social science and normative discourses such as those of moral and political philosophy" (Sayer 1997: 476). CSS has, however, tended to avoid spelling out the normative grounds on which it stands. While this uneasiness did not derail CSS at the time when criticism was fashionable, it has become a serious obstacle to its aspirations during more conservative times. The upshot is that, in the last three or four decades, critical researchers have been unable to go beyond shy demands for heightened reflexivity and "unsettling" discourses. Necessary though these activities may be, they can only amount to a "weak" version of critique (Sayer 2009).

Against this background, Sayer (2011) suggests CSS would be well advised to embark on a serious effort to make explicit and develop its normative dimension. This means defining what is taken to be human "good"—a task more difficult than it may at first appear. As Sayer argues, the categories of *suffering* and *flourishing* could offer a useful starting point. After all, an aspiration to combat social suffering has always been a powerful impetus not only for CSS but also for sociology more generally (Wilkinson 2005). CSS would be rendered intelligible if we were unable to understand that social practices that are typically the object of CSS's critique (capitalism, patriarchy, environmental destruction, compulsory heterosexuality, racism, or imperialism) bring about suffering and impede flourishing (Sayer 2009). CSS practitioners would be able to generate stronger versions of critique were they to recognize that one of their tasks concerns not only dispelling illusions about social life, but also unveiling the mechanisms through which human practices and structures bring about suffering. CSS could also free itself to explicitly search for social conditions that lead to individual and societal flourishing (Sayer 2009; Dussel 1998).

What we take to constitute suffering and well being is, of course, a function of our ethical framework. It is thus imperative for critical social scientists to engage in a permanent dialogue with ethical discourses, regardless of their provenance. The possibilities are as vast as the scope of humanity's ethical and political traditions, which include the religious and spiritual systems that have provided humanity with ethical guidance for thousands of years (Queen 2000).

5.3   Buddhism: Individual Suffering and Compassion for All Beings

Born around 500 BCE in the Indian sub-continent during what Karl Jaspers called the Axial Age (Bellah and Joas 2012), Buddhism remains one of the world's major spiritual traditions, as well as a visible "cultural institution" and "system of healing" (Safran 2003). As other such traditions, Buddhism provides an answer to the age-old question: "How do we find meaning in the midst of the pain, suffering and loss that are inevitably part of life?" (Safran 2003).

Buddhism is notoriously difficult to classify, with some interpretations highlighting its philosophical facet and others its more ritualistic and religious sides (Revel and Ricard 1998). In Western circles, Buddhism has been characterized as a "religion of no religion" (Watts 1999) and as a "religion without beliefs" (Batchelor 1998; cit. Safran 2003). In this account, "the goal in Buddhism thus becomes not one of transcending worldly experience [and suffering] but rather one of finding a wiser way of living within it" (Safran 2003: 461–462). Buddhism here is characterized as an agnostic, non-theistic and pragmatic way of life intent on addressing mental suffering through the letting go of attachments to ego, and the simultaneous cultivation of virtues like compassion, which in the Buddhist tradition is understood as "the wish that we may be free from suffering and the causes of suffering" (Wallace 2011: 137).

While there is truth in these descriptions, the history and practice of Buddhism is more complicated and not without numerous tensions. For one, like Christianity, many strands of Buddhism have sought to abolish the very realm where suffering and flourishing take place (Taylor 2011); for another, magic has historically played a very important role in Buddhist practice (Conze 1951). Buddhism thus inhabits a tension field that, far from undermining its credibility, has conferred it with vitality and dynamism throughout the centuries. Buddhist practitioners and schools have historically had to navigate their way between "the poles of agnosticism (or atheism) and faith (or commitment)" and "individualistic and communal orientations" (Safran 2003: 3). One of the reasons behind this diversity lies in Buddhism's remarkable ability to adapt to the different cultural contexts it has encountered (Conze 1951). It blended with Shamanic practices in Tibet, with the cult of the ancestors in Japan, and today is in dialogue with naturalistic discourses in the west (Flanagan 2011; Wallace 2006).

Common across the different schools of Buddhism is an understanding of suffering as stemming from the (wrong) view of self as a fixed, impermanent entity (as opposed to an ever changing construct) (Safran 2003), as well as an ethics system that stresses compassion, loving-kindness, equanimity, and sympathetic joy for all beings (Conze 1951; Flanagan 2011; Revel and Ricard 1998). These two features can be seen as standing in a productive tension with one another. On the one hand, the view of the self as non-substantial "leads to boundless contraction of the self—because everything is emptied out of it" (Conze 1951: 129). On the other hand, we are invited to identify with the suffering of ever wider circles of sentient beings and to strive for their liberation, a task leading to "a boundless expansion of the self—because one identifies oneself with more and more living beings. (…) The true task of the Buddhist is to carry on with both contradictory methods at the same time." (Conze 1951: 129; see also Wallace: 133).

In a very important sense, the interpretations outlined above hardly matter. For Buddhism, doctrine and theory are secondary to the question whether teachings/practices can be useful in overcoming suffering. Likewise, intellectual understanding of Buddhist teachings amounts to little, if anything, in the absence of the practice of virtues like compassion and loving-kindness for all beings and (in some sub-traditions) an utter detachment from the world, including our own bodies (Conze 1951). A multiplicity of methods is available to those aspiring to follow the Buddhist path, from lay rituals to the meditative practices traditionally associated with monastic life. Buddhist practitioners aim at cultivating a sense of serenity and inner peace that are independent of external conditions and the unavoidable ups and downs of life (Ricard 2003: 16–22).

Yet one can think of the basic condition of sitting in meditation as not adding much to the alleviation of the world's suffering or be as broad as helping to release all living beings from suffering. A key point to bear in mind is that scholars and practitioners of the Buddhist tradition have been much more interested in working with our minds in order to alleviate suffering via "world-denying love" (Bellah 2006) than in changing our social and natural environment (Wallace 2011). In other words, Buddhism has developed an avenue for overcoming suffering in which the stress is on changing our relationship to the world, rather than on changing the world. This has led a number of scholars to claim that drawing only on Buddhist teachings in order to understand and alleviate suffering under conditions of modernity leads to an aporia or irresolvable internal contradiction (Bellah 2006).

Buddhism's seeming inability to address modern social sources of suffering stems from its lacking a coherent understanding of political, economic, and social life (Smithers 2012; Van Arnam 2013; Flanagan 2011). As philosopher Owen Flanagan puts it: "Buddhism is a comprehensive philosophy that is very weak in the political philosophy department, overrating compassion and underrating the need for institutions that enact justice as fairness." (2011: xii). This shortcoming complicates the Buddhist response to the socially conditioned forms of suffering resulting from the dynamic of economic and political systems such as capitalism or authoritarianism. (See, however, Loy 2002). In fact, at some points during Buddhism's long history, rulers have found in Buddhist calls for compassion and non-violence an effective tool for pacification, conformism, and legitimation (Conze 1951). This is not to say that Buddhism is inherently "conservative"; there have been moments where social/resistance movements have adopted a Buddhist language in order to make sense of their struggles, the Chinese Boxer rebellion being a case in point (Conze 1951).

5.4 Healing Suffering

Though their approaches differ, some parallels are apparent between CSS and Buddhism. Both traditions share the conviction that we can avoid and overcome suffering, provided we are able to dispel delusions about its causes through an appreciation of the nature of reality (Ricard 2003: 22–24, 27; Wallace 2011). However, those aspects of reality to which they draw our attention differ: CSS bids us to pay heed to historical social processes while Buddhism advises refraining from giving undue attention to impermanent phenomena.

In spite of the aforementioned differences, or perhaps because of them, Buddhism and CSS are well placed for the tasks of dialogue, critique, and self-critique. Neither tradition exists, after all, for the sake of winning arguments; rather, just like medicine, each is intended to help us cope with the challenges of human existence and liberate humanity from suffering (see, however, Eagleton 2011, for a different take on Buddhism). The desirability of a dialogue has not been lost upon representatives of either "cultural institution", to use Safran's term (Safran 2003). Sayer has criticized CSS for its recent shyness and has encouraged a more active engagement with ethical traditions. And numerous Buddhist communities have come to the realization that addressing suffering in the contemporary world involves facing social problems (Malkin 2003; Van Arnam 2013; Queen 2000). Socially engaged Buddhism has emerged "in the context of a global conversation on human rights, distributive justice, and social progress" (Queen 2000). The same could be said about the 14th Dalai Lama's repeated statements on Marxism, which acknowledge the need to enrich Buddhism with other traditions in order to make sense of the socio-economic inequalities and political oppression found across the world, e.g., "I think of myself as half-Marxist, half-Buddhist" (Dalai Lama 1996: 110; see also Dalai Lama 1999) and "as far as sociopolitical beliefs are concerned, I consider myself a Marxist" (Dalai Lama as quoted by Namgyal 2011; see also Smithers 2012).

We could imagine the outcomes of the potential integration between the two traditions in concrete settings. Buddhism-inspired mindfulness interventions are already used to alleviate pain related to some medical conditions, like depression (Feldman and Kuyken 2011; Fraser 2013), as well as to combat compassion fatigue and stress among healthcare professionals (McClure 2013; Shapiro et al. 1998, 2005; Fraser 2013). In spite of their value, however, such interventions can do little to address the social inequalities that make such a big difference in the life expectancy and quality of life of people around the world. In order to challenge those inequalities, CSS speaks with a clearer voice than Buddhism.

Still, the salience of Buddhism in the spiritual landscape of contemporary societies can be interrogated as a possible symptom of the ideological problems of our time, and construed as a central piece in the ideological core of the twenty-first century capitalist "post-ideological era" (Žižek 2001; see also Smithers 2012). In this account, Buddhism allows people to search for salvation without having to confront the contradictions of capitalism and capitalist societies. Though this critique may be justified, its validity is limited. Reducing "Western Buddhism" to a form of escapism risks throwing out the baby with the bathwater. For the value of Buddhism and other achievements of the Axial Age arguably go well beyond the historical specificity of the capitalist age.

Dissonances should not be reasons for despair. Clashing notions can be fruitful grounds for the development of new ideas (Turner 2014), as the dialectical tradition teaches (Farr 2008; Jay 1996; Van Arnam 2013). Both sides require, however, the ability to listen attentively to the other (Barenboim 2010), a point worth mentioning because many strands of CSS have not been particularly good at listening. This flaw partly explains the charges of authoritarianism leveled against them in the past (Sayer 2009). How Buddhism fares on this count is an empirical question. We should note that, given its standing "in between" religion and philosophy, Buddhism is particularly well placed for building bridges between different traditions (Dalai Lama, cit. Revel and Ricard 1998: 25); that listening constitutes an important part of socially engaged Buddhism (Malkin 2003); and that some strands of Tibetan Buddhism in exile have shown a keen interest in encouraging a dialogue between science and religion (Wallace 2006). And yet, in spite of having anticipated many insights from sociology for thousands of years, in general Buddhism has arguably failed thus far to engage in a serious dialogue with social research (for an exception see Loy 2002).

5.5 Towards a Framework for the Study of Suffering

A process of active listening and dialogue could open up a "cycle of critique" (Abbott 2004), with both traditions addressing each other's weaknesses. A dialogue with Buddhist ethics could provide CSS the tools to counter its excessive emphasis on the individual self, which by the way is also common to much current social research (Anderson 2014; and personal communication). There is, of course, nothing wrong with individual emancipation and freedom. However, in taking the "free individual" as an implicit, ultimate goal when criticizing "undesirable social determinations," CSS has failed to grasp that flourishing requires not only liberation and "freedom from" undesirable social constraints, but also "freedom to" form social commitments (e.g., freedom to join communities and adopt responsibilities) (Sayer 2009).

In this context, Buddhism and traditions like care ethics (Tronto 1993) could help CSS gain clarity about the role of care as a positive social determination, and more generally on the social conditions that facilitate human flourishing for fragile yet resilient beings like us (Sayer 2011; see also Johnston [Chap. 8] and Wilkinson [Chap. 2]). For instance, engaging with Buddhism could help social researchers make sense of instances where suffering can be transformed into compassion (Johnston [Chap. 8]; Flores 2014). On a more applied level, CSS could benefit from Buddhist techniques for cultivating compassion and virtue in order to advance towards more humane forms of struggle against oppression; this is not a minor task given the cruelty committed in the name of the construction of revolutionary projects in the twentieth century (on compassion and politics, see Paz 1990). The ideals and actions of Mahatma Gandhi and the Rev. Dr. Martin Luther King, Jr. illustrate the potential for bringing together struggles for social emancipation with "world-denying love" (Bellah 2006).

As far as Buddhism is concerned, a dialogue with CSS could help make sense of suffering brought about by historical social practices and structures. As Conze writes, no major Buddhist school has developed in the last 1,000 years or so, but the conditions of the modern world may encourage a new creative impetus for Buddhism (Conze 1951: 68). Queen (2000) argues, similarly, that socially engaged Buddhism may be part of the formation of a new Buddhist stream—one more attuned to the needs of the modern world and the need to attain collective liberation and flourishing alongside personal liberation from suffering (see also Levine 2007).

But the more general point is this: in seeking to frame, explain, and alleviate suffering, we necessarily draw on the manifold intellectual, religious, and philosophical traditions that constitute humanity's heritage. Even when attempting to reject past understandings of the nature, causes, and solutions of suffering, human beings never start *ex nihilo*—they build on the stock of knowledge available to them (Berger and Luckmann 1966; Vera 2013). From these traditions, we have inherited some basic distinctions and intuitions leading to different conclusions as to the best courses of action individuals and whole societies might follow in their ethics, politics, and policies. Taking these traditions on their own terms and in dialogue could open new vistas for those interested in understanding and alleviating suffering. In seeking to illustrate this point focusing on Buddhism and critical social science, I have argued that both traditions could benefit from listening attentively to what the other has to say. This involves focusing on the harmonies between traditions as well as the points of dissonance. To the extent that these perspectives converge, they can enrich our toolkit to frame and heal suffering; to the extent that they collide, they call for dialogue, critique, self-critique, and reflexivity. This dialogue could also be useful to those who, without subscribing to either tradition, share a common goal to intellectually and practically address the challenges that suffering raises for human existence.

Acknowledgements The author wishes to thank Ron Anderson, Patrick Brown, Katja Bruisch, Ryan Burg, Letta Wren Page, Lili Di Puppo, and Sandy Ross for very useful comments and criticism. All the shortcomings of the text are entirely the author's responsibility.

References

Abbott, A. (2004). *Methods of discovery: Heuristics for the social sciences*. New York: Norton.

Anderson, R. E. (2014). *Human suffering and quality of life-conceptualizing stories and statistics*. New York: Springer.

Barenboim, D. (2010). *Everything is connected: The power of music*. London: Orion.

Batchelor, S. (1998). *Buddhism without beliefs: A contemporary guide to awakening*. New York: Riverhead Books.

Bellah, R. (2006). Max Weber and world-denying love: A look at the historical sociology of religion. In R. Bellah & S. M. Tipton (Eds.), *The Robert Bellah reader* (pp. 123–149). Durham/London: Duke University Press.

Bellah, R. N., & Joas, H. (2012). *The axial age and its consequences*. Cambridge/London: The Belknap Press of Harvard University Press.

Berger, P. L., & Luckmann, T. (1966). *The social construction of reality: A treatise in the sociology of knowledge*. Garden City: Doubleday.

Bresnan, P. S. (1999). *Awakenings: An introduction to the history of Eastern thought*. Upper Saddle River: Prentice Hall.

Buswell, R. E., Jr., & Lopez, D. S., Jr. (2014). *The Princeton dictionary of Buddhism*. Princeton: Princeton University Press.

Callinicos, A. (2006). *The resources of critique*. Cambridge: Polity.

Conze, E. (1951). *Buddhism: Its essence and development*. New York: Philosophical Library.

Dalai Lama. (1996). *Beyond dogma: Dialogues & discourses*. Berkeley: North Atlantic Books.

Dalai Lama. (1999, September 27). Long trek to exile for Tibet's apostle. *Time Magazine*. http://content.time.com/time/world/article/0,8599,2053819,00.html. Accessed 20 May 2014.

Dussel, E. (1998). *Ética de la liberación en la edad de la globalización y la exclusión*. Madrid: Trotta. English edition: Dussel, E. (2013). *Ethics of liberation: In the age of globalization and exclusion* (E. Mendieta, C. Pérez Bustillo, Y. Angulo, & N. Maldonado-Torres, Trans.). Durham: Duke University Press.

Eagleton, T. (2011). *Why Marx was right*. New Haven/London: Yale University Press.

Farr, A. (2008). The task of dialectical thinking in the age of one-dimensionality (book review). *Human Studies, 31*(2), 233–239.

Feagin, J. R., & Vera, H. (2008). *Liberation sociology*. Boulder/London: Paradigm.

Feldman, C., & Kuyken, W. (2011). Compassion in the landscape of suffering. *Contemporary Buddhism, 12*(1), 143–155.

Flanagan, O. (2011). *The Bodhisattva's brain*. Cambridge/London: The MIT Press.

Flores, R. (2014). From personal troubles to public compassion: Charity shop volunteering as a practice of care. *The Sociological Review, 62*(2), 383–399.

Fraser, A. (Ed.). (2013). *The healing power meditation: Leading experts on Buddhism, psychology, and medicine explore the health benefits of contemplative practice*. Boston/London: Shambhala Publications.

Jay, M. (1996). *The dialectical imagination: A history of the Frankfurt School and the Institute of Social Research, 1923–1950*. Berkeley/Los Angeles: University of California Press.

Levine, N. (2007). *Against the stream*. New York: HarperCollins.

Loy, D. R. (2002). *A Buddhist history of the west: Studies in lack*. Albany: State University of New York Press.

Malkin, J. (2003, July). In engaged Buddhism, peace begins with you. Shambhala Sun. http://www.shambhalasun.com. Accessed 21 Mar 2014.

McClure, R. (2013). *Sustaining compassion in health care, The Greater Good Science Center*.http://greatergood.berkeley.edu/article/item/sustaining_compassion_in_health_care. Accessed 4 Mar 2013.

Namgyal, T. (2011, June 8). Dalai Lama: "I Am a Marxist, But Not a Leninist". *Religion Dispatches*. University of Southern California.http://religiondispatches.org/dalai-lama-i-am-a-marxist-but-not-a-leninist/. Accessed 20 May 2014.

Paz, O. (1990). *Pequeña crónica de grandes días*. México: FCE.

Queen, C. S. (Ed.). (2000). *Engaged Buddhism in the west*. Somerville: Wisdom Publications.

Revel, J., & Ricard, M. (1998). *The monk and the philosopher: A father and son discuss the meaning of life*. London: Thorsons.

Ricard, M. (2003). *Plaidoyer pour le bonheur*. Paris: NiL éditions. English edition: Ricard, M. (2008). *Happiness: A guide to developing life's most important skill* (J. Browner, Trans.). New York: Hachette Digital.

Safran, J. D. (Ed.). (2003). *Psychoanalysis and Buddhism: An unfolding dialogue*. Sommerville: Wisdom Publications.

Sayer, A. (1997). Critical realism and the limits to critical social science. *Journal for the Theory of Social Behaviour, 27*(4), 473–488.

Sayer, A. (2009). Who's afraid of critical social science? *Current Sociology, 57*(6), 767–786.

Sayer, A. (2011). *Why things matter to people: Social science, values and ethical life*. Cambridge: Cambridge University Press.

Shapiro, S. L., Schwartz, G. E., & Bonner, G. (1998). Effects of mindfulness-based stress reduction on medical and premedical students. *Journal of Behavioral Medicine, 21*(6), 581–599.

Shapiro, S. L., Austin, J. A., Bishop, S. R., & Cordova, M. (2005). Mindfulness-based stress reduction for health care professionals: Results from a randomized trial. *International Journal of Stress Management, 12*(2), 164–176.

Smithers, S. (2012). Occupy Buddhism. Or why the Dalai Lama is a Marxist. *Tricycle*.http://www.tricycle.com/web-exclusive/occupy-buddhism/. Accessed 3 Feb 2014.

Taylor, C. (2011). What was the axial revolution? In R. Bellah & H. Joas (Eds.), *The axial age and its consequences* (pp. 30–46). Cambridge/London: The Belknap Press of Harvard University Press.

Tronto, J. C. (1993). *Moral boundaries: A political argument for an ethic of care*. London: Routledge.

Turner, M. (2014). Our blender brain: How mixing ideas made us human. *New Scientist*, Issue 2957.

Van Arnam, B. (2013, August 8). Buddhism and Marxism. *PaxMarxista: A radical forum for Marxist theory and revolutionary thought*.http://paxmarxista.org/buddhism-and-marxism

Vera, H. (2013). Norbert Elias and Émile Durkheim: Seeds of a historical sociology of knowledge. In F. Dépelteau & T. S. Landini (Eds.), *Norbert Elias and social theory* (pp. 127–142). New York: Palgrave Macmillan.

Wallace, B. A. (2006). *Contemplative science: Where Buddhism and neuroscience converge*. New York: Columbia University Press.

Wallace, B. A. (2011). *Minding closely: The four applications of mindfulness*. Boston and London: Snow Lion Publications.

Watts, A. (1999). *Buddhism the religion of no-religion*. Tokyo/Rutland/Singapore: Tuttle Publishing.

Wilkinson, I. (2005). *Suffering: A sociological introduction*. Indianapolis: Polity

Žižek, S. (2001, Spring). From Western Marxism to Western Buddhism. *Cabinet Magazine*, Issue 2. http://www.cabinetmagazine.org/issues/2/western.php. Accessed 29 Oct 2013.

Chapter 6
Distant Suffering and the Mediation of Humanitarian Disaster

Johannes von Engelhardt and Jeroen Jansz

6.1 Introduction

Many of the most extensively mediated events of the early twenty-first century have been instances of large-scale human suffering caused by violent conflict or natural disaster in countries belonging to the so-called Global South (World Bank 2010). What Western audiences know about victims of humanitarian disaster is therefore almost exclusively derived from various media. As Susan Sontag observed in her generative work *Regarding the Pain of Others*: "[B]eing a spectator of calamities taking place in another country is a quintessential modern experience" (2003: 16).

The first part of this chapter provides a brief overview of how Western media represent humanitarian disaster in the Global South. In the second part, we move our focus to Western audiences and the circumstances under which people tend to care and act. For this purpose, we propose four dimensions in the representation of distant suffering that can either open up or close down spaces in which audiences might engage with distant suffering: *Distance* encompasses the various ways representations render humanitarian crises distant or proximate to the spectator. *Scale* refers to the depiction of suffering as that of single, identifiable individuals as opposed to that of collectives. *Actuality* describes the extent in which stories of human suffering are told as real and consequential. And *Relievability* highlights the significance of representational practices that present distant suffering as something that can be mitigated in the present or prevented in the future.

We conclude with a brief reflection on the changing media landscape as social media and other online platforms challenge the dominant position of traditional

J. von Engelhardt (✉) • J. Jansz
Erasmus Research Centre for Media, Communication and Culture, Erasmus University
Rotterdam, 1738, 3000 DR Rotterdam, The Netherlands
e-mail: vonengelhardt@eshcc.eur.nl; jansz@eshcc.eur.nl

© Springer Science+Business Media Dordrecht 2015
R.E. Anderson (ed.), *World Suffering and Quality of Life*,
Social Indicators Research Series 56, DOI 10.1007/978-94-017-9670-5_6

mass media, in particular television. We present a number of pointers for future research that might contribute to a more balanced and engaging portrayal of distant suffering.

6.2   Representation of Distant Disaster

Through the mass media, we learn about and make sense of large-scale human suffering in distant countries. As simple and commonplace as this statement may appear, it offers a valuable entry point, as it forcefully draws our attention to the significance of two slightly more contentious observations: not all instances of mass human suffering receive the same amount of international media coverage; different types of human suffering are covered in different ways. Since this chapter focuses on audience engagement as manifested in emotional, cognitive, or behavioral responses vis-à-vis media coverage of humanitarian crisis, these two observations are key.

With respect to the first, research has repeatedly shown that contrary to a naïve window-to-the-world understanding of the media (McQuail 2010), the amount of media coverage received by a particular humanitarian disaster is only partly determined by its scope and severity. A number of quantitative studies have attempted to statistically model media attention as a function of both disaster- and country-specific attributes, revealing that the scope of human suffering typically explains merely a small proportion of the variance in media attention. What have repeatedly been identified as important predictors of Western disaster coverage are measures of cultural, economic and geographical proximity (Belle 2000; Adams 1986; Simon 1997; Singer et al. 1991; Joye 2010; CARMA 2006). For example, both Belle (2000) and Adams (1986) find that the level of popularity that a given country enjoys among U.S. tourists can serve as a significant predictor of the amount of disaster coverage.

Some of the world's largest humanitarian crises therefore hardly register with Western audiences (see Moeller 2006) or policy makers (Hawkins 2002). Specifically, devastating catastrophes such as the 1994 genocide in Rwanda and the second Congo War from 1998 to 2003 received little or belated coverage despite the fact that the latter was the most deadly conflict since World War II (IRC 2008). This partiality in coverage is often understood as a consequence of institutional, economic, and ideological structures that shape (and often constrain) the work of media professionals (Galtung and Ruge 1965; Harcup and O'Neil 2001).

These "forgotten crises" run the risk of remaining largely invisible to Western audiences. We observe the most direct and palpable effects in donation behavior. Not surprisingly, research has confirmed that the more coverage a disaster receives, the more people are willing to give money (Martin 2013; Simon 1997). For crises that are already ongoing, donations start pouring in only after media attention picks up (Waters and Tindall 2011). The sheer visibility of distant suffering is indisputably a necessary condition for any form of public engagement, but we will see that it is by no means a sufficient one. Our concern here is therefore not focused on *whether* but on *how* stories of suffering others are told.

Western publics are more likely to donate when a set of criteria regarding the disaster, its victims, and its media reporting are met. In an extensive literature review of studies on charitable giving, Bekkers and Wiepking (2010) identify a set of mechanisms that influence donation behavior. For example, they show that the perceived deservingness and helplessness of the beneficiary plays a decisive role. While there is some evidence that portraying victims as having a certain degree of agency (rather than as completely helpless) can increase willingness to give (Bennet and Kottasz 2000), findings from the same study also suggest representations should employ "unashamedly emotive advertising imagery" (p. 358) that shows beneficiaries as utterly destitute. At the same time, overly negative and offsetting depictions of suffering seem to work counter-productively in fundraising efforts (Dyck and Coldenvin 1992). Bekkers and Wiepking (2010) posit, "[i]t may well be that instead of the most needy, those with the best marketers receive the highest contributions" (24).

The high volume of research regarding media coverage of crises is, for the most part, critical towards representations of distant mass suffering for its frequent cultural stereotypes and imagined binaries of "us" and "them" (Joye 2009; Chouliaraki 2006; Konstantinidou 2007). For example, Joye's analysis of Belgian television's coverage of international disasters (2009) leads him to conclude that disaster reporting reproduces "a division of the world in zones of poverty and prosperity, danger and safety" (58). Contemporary discourses on distant disaster are also often said to deepen and reproduce historical chasms between colonial spectators and colonized sufferers by drawing on neo-colonial discursive repertoires and narratives of backward tribalism and pre-modernist irrationality (e.g., Bankoff 2001; Brookes 1995; Wall 1997; Franks 2005; Philo 2002). Additionally, mainstream Western media coverage of humanitarian disaster has been described as delivering little more than sensationalist sound bites, failing to provide audiences with sufficient context and meaningful explanations to inform action (e.g., Moeller 1999; Joye 2009; Franks 2005; CARMA 2006).

A related concern has been the degree to which victims are presented as *mere* victims, stripped of human agency, aspirations, self-sufficiency, or competence. In his analysis, Joye (2009) finds that distant victims are depicted as passive, vulnerable, and "part of the scenery" (Joye 2009: 52). The increasing focus on children in disaster reporting further serves to oversimplify complex tragedies: "Skeletal children personify innocence abused. They bring moral clarity to the complex story of a famine" (Moeller 2002: 36). In the case of famine in Africa, the eternal picture of the innocent, anonymous, starving child "reinforces the spectacle of an Africa full of passive, suffering victims" (Franks 2005: 134).

It should be noted, however, that while "the media" commonly is used as if referring to a coherent and homogeneous whole of outlets, this is a gross and precarious simplification. Relevant differences in coverage remain even within mainstream media. For example, with respect to the representation of Africa, Scott's study (2009) uncovers large differences among UK newspapers. This study is also one of the very few exceptions in the overwhelmingly critical body of literature as it concludes "coverage [of Africa] is not as marginalized, negative or trivial as it is often accused of being" (2009: 554). In short, Western coverage of humanitarian disasters in the Global South is neither all homogeneous nor all negatively skewed.

Futhermore, the literature is almost exclusively concerned with the study of Western media. Only recently, a handful of studies have attempted to also include analysis of non-Western media, often leading to valuable and unexpected findings (Scott 2009; de Beer 2010; Fingenschou 2011). For example Figenschou's (2011) study of the representation of distant suffering suggests a different kind of portrayal of victims on Al-Jazeera English.

6.3   The Audience: Reception & Responses

On the surface, media representations of humanitarian disaster provide audiences information about the scope and nature of an ongoing calamity. On a more essential level, these representations of suffering imply moral frameworks for how to relate to and care about the wider world (Chouliaraki 2006; Silverstone 2007; Tester 2001; Boltanski 1999): "teaching [us] how to feel and act 'right' – 'a sentimental education' – falls under the remit of journalistic work" (Pantti et al. 2012: 62). Moeller's (1999) *Compassion Fatigue* provides an in-depth analysis of the U.S. media's coverage of a range of humanitarian crises, such as the famines in Sudan and Somalia during the early 1990s and the genocide in Rwanda in 1994, arguing the U.S. television audience is oversaturated. Viewers have lost their ability to feel for those in misery due to an overflow of decontextualized stories and visuals. They feel powerless. For Moeller, compassion fatigue is "a consequence of rote journalism and looking-over-your shoulder reporting… sensationalism, formulaic coverage and perfunctory reference to American cultural icons" (1999: 32).

This thesis has received serious scholarly criticism and has been described as "an urban myth" (Cohen 2001: 191; also see Campbell 2012a). Compelling empirical evidence is lacking and a few studies seem to actually contradict its main argument. For example, a study by Höijer (2004) does not support the notion of an overall decline in compassion, but instead paints the picture of an audience that differently experiences and makes sense of distant suffering. Similarly, the results of Seu's focus group study (2010) also remind us that audiences actively re-interpret messages and respond in diverging ways.

Chouliaraki's (2006) work features this diversity in interpretations of and responses to "mediatized" distant suffering, contesting both overly pessimistic and optimistic generalities on the media's potential to facilitate moral engagement. In *Spectatorship of Suffering* (2006), she explores various modes of representation that may either invite or foreclose a spectator's position of cosmopolitanism—"a fundamental orientation to the stranger, a welcoming of differences" (Ong 2009: 450).

While Chouliaraki's work has inspired a number of recent studies (Joye 2009, 2010; Verdonschot and Von Engelhardt 2012), how and to what degree different forms of disaster reporting facilitate a cosmopolitan stance has not been sufficiently addressed empirically. Thus far, researchers have continued to concentrate on representation rather than on reception.

6.4   A Conceptual Framework for the Reception of Mediated Suffering

The framework discussed below is intended as a conceptual tool to think about and research the relation between mediated distant suffering and its interpretations and responses in Western audiences. The framework has four distinct yet interrelated dimensions: *distance*, *scale*, *actuality*, and *relievability*. These should be understood as ways through which media representations can create or close down spaces for audience engagement.

6.4.1   Distance

The extent to which we care about others in pain seems to be closely related with perceived cultural and geographical proximity. Loewenstein and Small (2007) have shown that proximity can play a potent role in fostering compassionate responses to suffering. The authors highlight what they call *sensory proximity*, suggesting that "one is more likely to care about other persons to the extent that one can... see them, feel them, touch them, or hear them" (117). Similarly, researchers have found a "here-and-now bias" when it comes to the arousal of empathy (Hoffman 2000).

Importantly, the positive sense of familiarity we experience towards those with whom we habitually interact face-to-face can be extended to distant others, provided the other is presented as not so different from us (Batson and Shaw 1991). The question of distance inevitably becomes an issue of representation. For example, Cialdini et al. (1997) developed the concept of "one-ness" to conceptualize how much of ourselves we see in a suffering other. In a series of experiments, one-ness was shown to be correlated with compassionate responses and was a significant predictor of a willingness to help. As Hoffman, a leading empathy scholar asserts, "[S]eeing that people in other cultures have similar worries and respond emotionally as we do to important life events ... should contribute to a sense of oneness and empathy across cultures" (Hoffman 2000: 294–295).

In addition, we posit another form of distance that carries implications for the way in which Western audiences make sense of mediat(iz)ed suffering. This distance stems from the audiences' limited capacity to imagine what it is like to be that other person. This limitation is not the result of a media-induced apathy, as the compassion fatigue thesis has it, but of the fact that the nature of the depicted suffering might remain truly *incomprehensible*. We must assume that few members of the Western public can empathetically relate to the lived experiences of constant food insecurity or famine, fleeing from civil war, or life in a refugee camp.

Psychological research has shown how a lack of shared experience restricts the capacity for empathetic responses. For example, experimental research on "empathy-gaps" has demonstrated that thirsty respondents are more likely than non-thirsty individuals to empathetically appreciate thirst-induced suffering (Van Boven and Loewenstein 2003). Correspondingly, research confirms that going through a traumatic experience, such as rape, increases the level of empathy for victims of the same type of suffering (Barnett et al. 1986).

We contend that this lack of first-hand experiential memory fundamentally shapes the Western experience of witnessing the suffering and dying in distant countries. This lack of "experiential overlap" is an obstacle to empathetic responses towards distant victims that is much greater than those created by geographical distance and perceived cultural or ethnic dissimilarity.

6.4.2   Scale

The suffering of individuals is perceived and processed differently from that of groups or masses. In an extensive review of studies on charitable giving, Bekkers and Wiepking (2010) show that awareness of need is a main mechanism affecting people's decision to make a contribution. As understood by the authors, this encompasses, but is not limited to, the scale of the humanitarian crisis. If the need is perceived as greater, overall willingness to donate tends to be higher.

Unfortunately, however, the mechanisms that underlie moral responses towards others have also been shown to not be 'well-tuned' to respond adequately to large-scale atrocity (Slovic 2007). Based on a review of a significant body of studies from cognitive and social psychology, Slovic (2007) explores what he refers to as "psychic numbing" in the face of mass atrocity. This is essentially different from a process of compassion fatigue; it does not point to an incremental emotional tiring of the audience, but instead emphasizes a fundamental human inability to "feel" for the masses. There is some evidence that this also applies to small groups. Participants in an experimental study (Kogut and Ritov 2005) showed significantly greater emotional response and willingness to help when shown a picture of a single child in need than when confronted with the suffering of a group of eight children. This "identified victim" effect, which leads people to respond more significantly to identified victims than to anonymous masses or small groups, corresponds to studies showing audiences respond more empathetically to news stories employing a human interest frame (e.g., Valkenburg et al. 1999).

Two explanatory vantage points emerge from the discussion on psychic numbing. In the first, researchers argue that people are simply less capable of being emotionally moved even by small groups than by the more psychologically coherent and concrete need of an individual (Slovic 2007). In the second explanatory model, the lack of empathetic reaction results from a mechanism of self-defense. People regulate their emotions to keep from becoming overwhelmed, leading to relative insensitivity towards the pain of groups (Cameron and Payne 2011). In either case, it needs to be stressed that whether a crisis is perceived and processed as the suffering of individuals or a mass is dependent on representation.

6.4.3 Actuality

The third dimension of *actuality* draws attention to the non-material nature of distant suffering. While related to *distance*, the dimension of *actuality* covers a more fundamental and radical detachment.

Witnessing suffering through the mass media differs from witnessing unmediated suffering: the sufferer and the spectator do not share a physical space. Tester (2001) speaks of "material solidity" and postulates that "the [suffering] other is, in a profound sense, not present in the world" of the spectator (79). Cohen (2001) states, similarly, that mediated distant suffering might be perceived as less real since "[t]elevised images of distant misery don't seem to belong to the same world as our familiar daily round" (17). The fact that large-scale human misery fails to become real for Western audiences reiterates the perceived chasm between the world of the spectator and that of the victim; the former is a world of order, predictable risks, familiarity, and safety. The latter is an unfathomable place of chaos, brutality, and inconceivable (seemingly inexplicable) human tragedy.

Audiences are also removed from distant human suffering in that any potential action to ease the other's pain is also mediated. Compassionate action never carries the promise of ending the mediated suffering that one is confronted with. Pantti et al. (2012) draw on Boltanski (1999) to postulate that "the distinction between reality and fiction may lose its relevance when the sufferer and the possibility of action are far away" (77). Similarly, Vestergaard (2008) argues that representations of suffering cannot enter the life world of the audience as real *unless* they result in meaningful action by the spectator. Actual suffering achieves realness mainly through the behavior that it triggers in audiences. Vestergaard pessimistically concludes that even in instances where members of an audience act by donating money, the moderate amounts they typically give do not even elicit a true feeling of sacrifice. Thus, the suffering of the other remains abstract, unable to elicit even mediated financial "pain".

6.4.4 Relievability

Reflecting on the implications of depicting suffering, the ever-quotable Sontag contends "[C]ompassion is an unstable emotion. It needs to be translated into action, or it withers" (2003: 90). In line with this, Moeller (1999) saw a widespread lack of audience efficacy as an integral element of what she observed as a general compassion fatigue in U.S. audiences.

Moral psychologists have provided empirical evidence that perceived self-efficacy can increase feelings of compassion towards others who are suffering (e.g., Goetz et al. 2010). Bekkers and Wiepking (2010) identify efficacy as one of eight mechanisms that affect decisions to donate. As their review shows, efficacy is primarily related to the amount and type of information potential donors have about how their contribution would be used to alleviate suffering. If this information is missing or unfavorable, the willingness to engage decreases.

Chouliaraki (2013) speaks of the *ironic spectator* who, rather than viewing a humanitarian crisis campaign from heart-felt compassion, views the suffering reports skeptically in light of persuasive techniques used previously by humanitarian organizations. An audience that increasingly consists of ironic spectators creates new challenges for humanitarian organizations, as recently illustrated by the massive critical backlash faced by the makers of the KONY2012 campaign video (see Madianou 2012; von Engelhardt and Jansz 2014; Nothias 2012).

We can also deduce that more public engagement can be expected for humanitarian disasters that appear more suitable for outside humanitarian intervention (e.g., a post-earthquake scenario) than crises that seem to have less straightforward remedies or even clear-cut victims (as in the case of a long-lasting civil war). When it comes to donation, experimental evidence provides support for this partiality, showing that donations for victims of "man-made" disaster are less likely than donations for victims of "natural" disasters (Zagefka et al. 2011).

At the same time, the perception of suffering as relievable is a matter of representation. How audiences understand suffering caused by poverty or complex humanitarian disasters is dependent, then, on the type of stories that are told. For example, it has been observed that famines – created by a combination of both man-made and natural factors – are routinely covered merely in terms of their "natural" causes, underexposing their social, political and historical genesis (Ploughman 1995; Campbell 2012b). While these reductionist accounts do not do justice to the realities on the ground, they might be more successful in rallying the public to donate money. Some encouraging evidence does show that more sustained engagement and interest in distant humanitarian disasters can be fostered by highlighting connections and interdependencies with the distant, suffering other (Philo 2002).

A tension may therefore exist between the agendas of different storytellers of suffering: humanitarian organizations and media organizations. In particular, when it comes to complex humanitarian disasters that typically also have a political dimension (such as famines and most refugee crises), the funding efforts of humanitarian organizations might be hampered by quality media coverage that foregrounds complexity. This tension becomes particularly visible and problematic whenever journalists in disaster zones must rely on humanitarian staff for access to local people and as primary news sources (Rothmyer 2011; Cottle and Nolan 2007; Franks 2008).

In addition, the effects of perceived relievability undoubtedly favor the plights of individuals (related to the dimension scale). Research shows that audiences are much less inclined to donate money when presented with statistical information about potential beneficiaries than when given descriptions of an individual victim.

One study even showed that when the description of an individual victim is *complemented* with general statistical information, average donations drop (Small et al. 2007).

6.5 Comments on New Technologies

When surveying the field, research on media and distant suffering has mostly focused on traditional mass media. It has had a slow start in reflecting on the consequences of contemporary information and communication technologies (ICTs). While a systematic discussion of potential implications of new ICTs is beyond the scope of this chapter, we conclude by briefly touching upon important aspects of these new forms of news gathering and reporting.

The ubiquity of the Internet in many countries affords the production and distribution of user generated content *during* crises. In some cases, this has resulted in an endless stream of pictures offering first-hand accounts of the disaster before international journalists even arrive. Some promising work has started to explore the implications of these trends in disaster coverage (see Cooper 2011), but if and to what extent these forms of amateur reporting might contribute to compassionate engagement deserves more empirical attention.

Furthermore, contemporary ICTs enable humanitarian organizations to engage new audiences, for example, by means of online petitions and persuasive "serious gaming," in which Internet users say, play a word game to trigger a donation (and are quietly exposed to a brand name) (Neys and Jansz 2010). Facilitating this form of online engagement is not without controversies, as forcefully demonstrated by the rise and fall of aforementioned KONY2012 campaign (Madianou 2012; von Engelhardt and Jansz 2014; Nothias 2012). Critics regard online activism "slacktivism"— a low-intensity, low-commitment, and low-impact form of political engagement. Authors such as Evgeny Morozov contend that it is not authentic engagement with a cause that makes people sign online petitions and join Facebook groups. Instead, "much of it happens for reasons that have nothing to do with one's commitment to ideas and politics in general, but rather to impress one's friends" (Morozov 2012: 186).

6.6 Looking Ahead: Avenues for Future Research

Future media and communication research will need to more fully address the question of how different forms of representation can cultivate a cosmopolitan position towards those who suffer. The four dimensions of our framework might serve to structure such research.

With respect to *distance*, research should explore what kind of imagery has the potential to increase the spectator's sense of proximity. This could be achieved by deliberately highlighting connections and interdependencies between the world of those who are watching and that of those who are being watched. Here, current practices of journalistic domestication (Clausen 2004) might provide a fruitful area of investigation. In their coverage of the 2010 Pakistan floods, Dutch public television news repeatedly linked the distant suffering to the devastating floods the Netherlands experienced in 1953 (Verdonschot and Von Engelhardt 2012). As trivial and far-fetched these attempts may appear, they might also be critical in connecting "us" with "them." As Pantti, Wahl-Jorgensen, and Cottle posit, "[s]stressing our common vulnerability can be a powerful tool for cosmopolitan education and encouraging cosmopolitan empathy that extends beyond the realm of the nation state." (2012: 136).

Research relating to *scale* has unveiled that feelings of compassion are most easily incited by individual cases. But that does not necessarily imply that human beings are insensitive to mass suffering. Research in collaboration with news reporters could help to develop the types of journalistic narrative and visualization that have the potential to counter a collapse of compassion and encourage audiences to feel and care even for large distant groups. In relation to *actuality*, empirical attention should be paid to the question to what extent and under which circumstances distant suffering runs the risk of being fictionalized – and what kind of representations can counter this. Also, on *relievability* more research is needed that investigates how different ways of representing humanitarian crisis affect perceived self-efficacy and the degree to which suffering is seen as inevitable, rather than relievable.

6.7   Conclusion

Coverage of distant suffering in Western media is generally described as decontextualized reporting that emphasizes the helplessness and passivity of local victims. The four dimensions we present above draw attention to specific characteristics of media representation that may allow or bar audiences from meaningful engagement with distant suffering. By no means do we argue that individuals will respond uniformly when faced with a particular representation of distant suffering. Rather, we follow Chouliaraki to contend that depictions of suffering carry frameworks that can allow audiences to cultivate and act out different forms of cosmopolitanism. The question of whether and how this actually happens is determined by factors outside representation.

References

Adams, W. (1986). Whose lives count? TV coverage of natural disasters. *Journal of Communication, 36*(2), 113–122.
Bankoff, G. (2001). Rendering the world unsafe: "Vulnerability" as Western discourse. *Disasters, 25*(1), 19–35.

Barnett, M. A., Tetreault, P. A., Esper, J. A., & Bristow, A. R. (1986). Similarity and empathy: The experience of rape. *The Journal of Social Psychology, 126*, 47–49.

Batson, C. D., & Shaw, L. L. (1991). Evidence for altruism: Toward a pluralism of prosocial motives. *Psychological Inquiry, 2*(2), 107–122.

Bekkers, R., & Wiepking, P. (2010). A literature review of empirical studies of philanthropy: Eight mechanisms that drive charitable giving. *Nonprofit and Voluntary Sector Quarterly, 40*, 924–973.

Belle, D. A. (2000). New York Times and network TV news coverage of foreign disaster: The significance of the insignificant variables. *Journalism and Mass Communication Quarterly, 77*(1), 50–70.

Bennett, R., & Kottasz, R. (2000). Emergency fund-raising for disaster relief. *Disaster Prevention and Management, 9*(5), 352–360.

Boltanski, L. (1999). *Distant suffering: Morality, media and politics*. Cambridge: Cambridge University Press.

Brookes, H. J. (1995). 'Suit, tie and a touch of Juju' – The ideological construction of Africa: A critical discourse analysis of news on Africa in the British press. *Discourse & Society, 6*(4), 461–494.

Cameron, C. D., & Payne, B. K. (2011). Escaping affect: How motivated emotion regulation creates insensitivity to mass suffering. *Journal of Personality and Social Psychology, 100*(1), 1–15.

Campbell, D. (2012a). *The myth of compassion fatigue*. Retrieved January, 2013, from http://www.david-campbell.org/wp-content/documents/DC_Myth_of_Compassion_Fatigue_Feb_2012.pdf

Campbell, D. (2012b). The iconography of famine. In G. Batchen, M. Gidley, N. K. Miller, & J. Prosser (Eds.), *Picturing atrocity: Photography in crisis* (pp. 79–91). London: Reaktion Books.

CARMA. (2006). *The CARMA report on Western media coverage of humanitarian disasters*. Retrieved February 20, 2011, from http://www.carma.com/research/

Chouliaraki, L. (2006). *The spectatorship of suffering*. London: Sage.

Chouliaraki, L. (2013). *The ironic spectator: Solidarity in the age of post-humanitarianism*. Cambridge: Polity Press.

Cialdini, R. B., Brown, S. L., Lewis, B. P., Luce, C., & Neuberg, S. L. (1997). Reinterpreting the empathy–altruism relationship: When one into one equals oneness. *Journal of Personality and Social Psychology, 73*(3), 481–494.

Clausen, L. (2004). Localizing the global: 'Domestication' processes in international news production. *Media, Culture & Society, 26*(1), 25–44.

Cohen, S. (2001). *States of denial: Knowing about atrocities and suffering*. Cambridge: Polity Press.

Cooper, G. (2011). *From their own correspondent? New media and the changes in disaster coverage: Lessons to be learnt*. Reuters Institute for the Study of Journalism. Retrieved February 13, 2014, from https://reutersinstitute.politics.ox.ac.uk/fileadmin/documents/Publications/Working_Papers/From_Their_Own_Correspondent.pdf

Cottle, S., & Nolan, D. (2007). Global humanitarianism and the changing aid-media field. *Journalism Studies, 8*(6), 862–878.

de Beer, A. S. (2010). News from and in the 'Dark Continent'. *Journalism Studies, 11*(4), 596–609.

Dyck, E. J., & Coldevin, G. (1992). Using positive vs. negative photographs for Third-World fund raising. *Journalism Quarterly, 69*(1), 572–572.

Figenschou, T. U. (2011). Suffering up close: The strategic construction of mediated suffering on Al Jazeera English. *International Journal of Communication, 5*, 233–253.

Franks, S. (2005). Reporting Africa: Problems and perspectives. *Westminster Papers in Communication and Culture*, (Special Issue), 129–134.

Franks, S. (2008). Getting into bed with charity. *British Journalism Review, 19*(3), 27–32.

Galtung, J., & Ruge, M. H. (1965). The structure of foreign news. *Journal of Peace Research, 2*(1), 64–91.

Goetz, J. L., Keltner, D., & Simon-Thomas, E. (2010). Compassion: An evolutionary analysis and empirical review. *Psychological Bulletin, 136*(3), 351–374.

Harcup, T., & Neill, D. O. (2001). What is news? Galtung and Ruge revisited. *Journalism, 2*(2), 261–280.

Hawkins, V. (2002). The other side of the CNN factor: The media and conflict. *Journalism Studies, 3*(2), 225–240.

Hoffman, M. L. (2000). *Empathy and moral development: Implications for caring and justice.* Cambridge: University Press.

Höijer, B. (2004). The discourse of global compassion: The audience and media reporting of human suffering. *Media, Culture & Society, 26*(4), 513–531.

International Rescue Committee. (2008). *Mortality in the Democratic Republic of Congo: An ongoing crisis.* Retrieved December 2, 2013, from http://www.theirc.org/resources/2007/2006-7_congomortalitysurvey.pdf

Joye, S. (2009). The hierarchy of global suffering. A critical discourse analysis of television news reporting on foreign natural disasters. *The Journal of International Communication, 15*(2), 45–61.

Joye, S. (2010). De media(de)constructie van rampen. *Tijdschrift voor Communicatiewetenschap, 38*(2), 139–154.

Kogut, T., & Ritov, I. (2005). The singularity effect of identified victims in separate and joint evaluations. *Organizational Behavior and Human Decision Processes, 97*(2), 106–116.

Konstantinidou, C. (2007). Death, lamentation and the photographic representation of the other during the Second Iraq War in Greek newspapers. *International Journal of Cultural Studies, 10*(2), 147–166.

Loewenstein, G., & Small, D. A. (2007). The Scarecrow and the Tin Man: The vicissitudes of human sympathy and caring. *Review of General Psychology, 11*(2), 112–126.

Madianou, M. (2012). Humanitarian campaigns in social media. *Journalism Studies, 14*(2), 1–18.

Martin, J. A. (2013). Disasters and donations: The conditional effects of news attention on charitable giving. *International Journal of Public Opinion Research, 25*(4), 547–560.

McQuail, D. (2010). *Mass communication theory* (6th ed.). London: Sage.

Moeller, S. (1999). *Compassion fatigue. How the media sell disease, famine, war and death.* New York: Routledge.

Moeller, S. (2002). A hierarchy of innocence: The media's use of children in the telling of international news. *The Harvard International Journal of Press/Politics, 7*(1), 36–56.

Moeller, S. (2006). "Regarding the pain of others": Media, bias and the coverage of international disasters. *Journal of International Affairs, 59*(2), 173–196.

Morozov, E. (2012). *The net delusion: How not to liberate the world.* London: Penguin.

Neys, J., & Jansz, J. (2010). Political internet games: Engaging an audience. *European Journal of Communication, 25*(3), 1–15.

Nothias, T. (2012). 'It's struck a chord we have never managed to strike': Frames, perspectives and remediation strategies in the international news coverage of Kony 2012. *Equid Novi: African Journalism Studies, 34*(1), 123–129.

Ong, J. C. (2009). The cosmopolitan continuum: Locating cosmopolitanism in media and cultural studies. *Media, Culture & Society, 31*(3), 449–466.

Pantti, M., Wahl-Jorgensen, K., & Cottle, S. (2012). *Disasters and the media.* New York: Peter Lang.

Philo, G. (2002). Television news and audience understanding of war, conflict and disaster. *Journalism Studies, 3*(2), 173–186.

Ploughman, P. (1995). The American print news media "construction" of five natural disasters. *Disasters, 19*(4), 308–326.

Rothmyer, K. (2011). *They wanted journalists to say "wow"* (Joan Shorenstein Center on the Press, politics and public policy discussion paper series). Retrieved March 15, 2011, from http://www.hks.harvard.edu/presspol/publications/papers/discussion_papers/d61_rothmyer.pdf

Scott, M. (2009). Marginalized, negative or trivial? Coverage of Africa in the UK press. *Media, Culture & Society, 31*(4), 533–557.

Seu, I. B. (2010). "Doing denial": Audience reaction to human rights appeals. *Discourse & Society, 21*(4), 438–457.

Silverstone, R. (2007). *Media and morality. On the rise of the mediapolis.* Cambridge: Polity Press.

Simon, A. (1997). Television news and international earthquake relief. *Journal of Communication, 47*(3), 82–93.

Singer, E., Endreny, P., & Glassman, M. B. (1991). Media coverage of disasters: Effect of geographic location. *Journalism & Mass Communication Quarterly, 68*(1), 48–58.

Slovic, P. (2007). If I look at the mass I will never act: Psychic numbing and genocide. *Judgment and Decision Making, 2*(2), 79–95.

Small, D. A., Loewenstein, G., & Slovic, P. (2007). Sympathy and callousness: Affect and deliberations in donation decisions. *Organizational Behavior and Human Decision Processes, 102*, 143–153.

Sontag, S. (2003). *Regarding the pain of others.* New York: Farrar, Straus and Giroux.

Tester, K. (2001). *Compassion, morality and the media.* Buckingham: Open University Press.

The World Bank. (2010). *Natural hazards, unNatural disasters: The economics of effective prevention.* Retrieved February 2, 2011, from http://publications.worldbank.org/index.php?main_page=product_info&products_id=23659

Valkenburg, P. M., Semetko, H. A., & de Vreese, C. H. (1999). The effects of news frames on readers' thoughts and recall. *Communication Research, 26*(5), 550–569.

Van Boven, L., & Loewenstein, G. (2003). Social projection of transient drive states. *Personality and Social Psychology Bulletin, 29*(9), 1159–1168.

Verdonschot, I. J. P. A., & von Engelhardt, J. (2012). Representaties van leed tussen "adventure" en "emergency". Een "critical discourse analysis" naar de representatie van de watersnoodramp in Pakistan (2010) in het NOS-journaal. *Tijdschrift voor Communicatiewetenschap, 41*(1), 62–81.

Vestergaard, A. (2008). Humanitarian branding and the media: The case of Amnesty International. *Journal of Language and Politics, 7*(3), 471–493.

von Engelhardt, J., & Jansz, J. (2014). Challenging humanitarian communication – An empirical exploration of Kony 2012. *International Communication Gazette, 76*(6), 464–484.

Wall, M. (1997). The Rwanda crisis: An analysis of news magazine coverage. *Gazette, 59*(2), 121–134.

Waters, R., & Tindall, N. (2011). Exploring the impact of American news coverage on crisis fundraising: Using media theory to explicate a new model of fundraising communication. *Journal of Nonprofit & Public Sector Marketing, 23*(1), 20–40.

Zagefka, H., Noor, M., Brown, R., de Moura, G. R., & Hopthrow, T. (2011). Donating to disaster victims: Responses to natural and humanly caused events. *European Journal of Social Psychology, 41*(3), 353–363.

Part II
Professional and Informal Caregiving

Chapter 7
Suffering and Identity: "Difficult Patients" in Hospice Care

Cindy L. Cain

7.1 Introduction

Hospice, an end-of-life care philosophy that emphasizes quality over quantity of life, takes many different forms worldwide. The first hospice opened in 1967 in the United Kingdom. Then, as now, U.K.-based hospice care primarily took place in small inpatient facilities, free to anyone in the end-stages of a progressive illness. In contrast, hospice in the United States has been more focused on home-based care, and has become institutionalized as part of the conventional care continuum. Hospice organizations have been slower to arrive in developing countries, but in the early twenty-first century, just under half of all countries worldwide offer hospice services (Lynch et al. 2013). Hospices in developing countries face shortages of pain medications and incomplete integration into the healthcare system (Twycross 2007), but as worldwide rates of HIV/AIDS and cancer remain steady, there is increasing need for hospice care (Clark 2007). Variation in organizational features of hospices by setting was an intentional decision. The original founders of hospice anticipated and encouraged variation, training new hospice leaders across the world to "adapt what you have seen to local circumstances, systems, needs, human and financial resources, and all of the other things that will make your programs distinctive and appropriate on the ground" (Corr 2007: 113).

Across organizational differences, the foundations of the hospice philosophy remain consistent. Summarizing the hospice approach 40 years after the first hospice opened, Twycross (2007) defined it as "the active total care of patients with life-limiting disease, and their families, by a multi-professional team when the disease is no longer responsive to curative or life-prolonging treatments" (9). For Twycross, the "essential task in palliative care is to help patients (and their families)

C.L. Cain (✉)
Division of Health Policy and Management, University of Minnesota,
C394 Mayo MMC 729 – 420 Delaware Ave SE, Minneapolis, MN 55455, USA
e-mail: clcain@umn.edu

© Springer Science+Business Media Dordrecht 2015   91
R.E. Anderson (ed.), *World Suffering and Quality of Life*,
Social Indicators Research Series 56, DOI 10.1007/978-94-017-9670-5_7

make the transition from fighting death to seeking peace" (9). Another scholar dubbed hospice "a safe place to suffer," emphasizing that relief of pain is one goal of hospice, but some suffering is inevitable (Stedeford 1987). More recently, hospice practitioners have argued that the goals of hospice should be to "companion" patients during their suffering, not necessarily try to end suffering (Yoder 2012).

Hospice workers argue that once they put aside their own agenda or inclination to "fix" the problem of suffering, they are able to "be there" with patients in a meaningful way. In this chapter, I use qualitative data gathered from U.S. hospice workers to show how this commitment to "being there" sometimes challenges hospice workers' sense of meaning about their jobs and identities.

7.2   The Work of Hospice

Hospice organizations in the U.S. approach the emotionality of caring for those at the end-of-life differently than other types of health care. In addition to emphasizing the value of "being there" with people during times of suffering, hospice organizations permit workers to express their emotions through two structural features of the work: the use of teams to provide care, and the administration of care in recipients' own residences. Working within a hospice team encourages hospice workers to form mutually beneficial connections with one another (Cain 2012). It also permits the sharing of emotions. Meanwhile, working in the homes of care recipients means that hospice workers are exposed to family life, personal items, and evidence of life beyond the illness, humanizing patients in the process (Cain 2014). Hospice organizations reconstruct workers' relationships to care for recipients and the emotional expressions surrounding those relationships, frequently accepting more emotional expression than is found in other care settings.

A source of meaning in hospice is the intentional reconstruction of ideas about death and dying. Hospice workers resist common understandings of death as scary or something to be avoided, reconstructing it as a beautiful, natural, and meaningful part of life. They emphasize that it is an honor to be present during this process. These reconstructed meanings about death can be helpful to workers as they try to make sense of loss. Ira Byock, an influential hospice physician and author wrote:

> I have learned from my patients and their families a surprising truth about dying: this stage of life holds remarkable possibilities. Despite the arduous nature of the experience, when people are relatively comfortable and know that they are not going to be abandoned, they frequently find ways to strengthen bonds with people they love and to create moments of profound meaning in their final passage (1998: XIV).

Another form of meaning is found in hospice workers' sense of self as care providers during difficult times. They see themselves as realistic about death and dying, while also sensitive to the needs of patients and their family members (Cain 2012). Because hospice has a long history of social movement action and advocacy, hospice workers in my study frequently adopted a mission to change others' ideas about death and dying. In this way, they also saw themselves as pioneering a much needed reform to American ideas.

These benefits (of accepting emotionality, reconstructing meaning about death, and forming identities around the work) do not completely mitigate the potential for suffering among hospice workers. Dealing with death and decline can be difficult, even when the hospice philosophy re-orients emotional responses.

7.3 Difficult Patients

Medical practitioners typically categorize difficult patients as those who are unwilling or unable to comply to orders. For example, a review of nursing literature found that patients whose illness or behavior made them difficult to work with were consistently considered "bad" or difficult by nurses (Kelly and May 1982). Non-compliance challenges the social order and makes it harder for practitioners to carry out normal routines of care. Non-compliance is certainly present in hospice, but the hospice philosophy seeks to redefine this struggle as an issue of patient autonomy. Ramon, a social worker, explained that he sometimes has to remind others on his team of this reframing:

> I will say, "Well, she's not going to do this because you have told her a thousand times, and she's not going to change her behavior. So, our only job is to change our behavior and our expectations to realize it's the client's right to lead their lives the way they want. They don't have to stop smoking; they don't have to stop drinking; they don't have to check their blood sugar four times a day; they don't have to go to a nursing home. You know?

This reframing puts patients in charge of their own lives, humanizing the medical encounter by encouraging hospice workers to see their patients as whole people, with complex needs, wishes, and desires (Gregory and English 1994).

The emphasis on seeing people as complex social entities is thought to improve care (Hutchinson 2011), but it also implicates another set of "difficult patients." I conceptualize difficult patients as those who challenge hospice workers' ability to continue to maintain a hospice approach of "being there." During 41 semi-structured interviews with hospice workers from all positions (physicians, nurses, social workers, counselors, chaplains, volunteers, and administrators), I asked workers about difficult patients and experiences as well as times they felt emotional about their work. Through the responses, I found that patients whose lives and experiences challenge workers' sense of meaning and identity create a diffused form of suffering that expands from the patients to the hospice workers.

7.3.1 Own Greatest Fears

Seeing patients at the end-of-life brought up workers' own fears about death. One of the greatest fears within this group was uncontrollable pain—physical or mental. Because controlling physical pain is so central to the hospice approach, unmanageable pain was sometimes taken as a signifier of failure, a challenge to the hospice identity. Ramon detailed one situation of uncontrollable pain: A typically tough, serious RN was overcome with emotion at a meeting and had to stop in the middle of her sentence in order to remain calm. She was discussing the corporeal state of the patient, who had ulcers and tumors all over his neck and face. Ramon said it seemed to be especially hard for her because "she is used to fixing the body and there was nothing she could do to make this better." The patient's condition brought out two fears: the fear of experiencing uncontrollable pain and the fear of not being able to offer relief. The latter is a powerful example of a threat to the hospice identity.

Another fear that contributed to workers' suffering was the fear of deaths that seemed to happen out of sequence. These deaths created what Boss (2007) calls "ambiguous loss" and were characterized as coming too soon, too suddenly, or without a sense of closure. In this context, an ambiguous loss can be either "leaving without good-bye," as is the case with sudden death, or "good-bye without leaving," as is often the case with Alzheimer patients. Ambiguous loss is difficult for families, but can also challenge workers. These processes of decline disrupt routines and force workers to relate the experience to their own lives. One administrator told a story about a patient whose experience caused a great deal of turmoil for workers in her hospice:

> We have a 45-year-old guy who's a quad, he's quadriplegic, and he decided—he's been a quadriplegic since 21, and he decided, "I'm done. I want the vent taken out. I'm done." So that was done, and he's still alive. What a freaking nightmare for everybody, the family, the staff. It's just—it's awful. It's sad. It's sad that he became quad at 21. It's sad that he—he was able to live for 24 years. I don't think I'd make it that long. I think I'd be insane. And then that he's still alive [after the removal of life support]… Well, sometimes it takes hours, sometimes it takes some days, but—and it's still—it's still looking like that's what will happen, but it hasn't happened yet. And the fear is that the 45-year-old heart and lungs are strong enough to keep him going, so that's sad.

Family and workers had prepared for the inevitability of the patient's death once the vent was removed, but because he was still young, it took some time. Additionally, he had suffered a great deal already, and his hospice team's knowledge of this suffering pushed the administrator to admit that she did not think she could have stayed sane if she were in his situation.

She went on to explain that the staff struggles in situations like these because they do not have a routine way to help the family through the process. Because the death is out of sequence, it is harder:

> [The staff are] having a hard time with it, they're having a really hard time with it. In other situations where a ventilator is pulled, the person is usually unconscious and pretty close to death already, and the family just says, "Come on. We're done." In this case, the guy's completely conscious and with it in decision-making. And he said, "I don't want to be conscious when you remove this, so please just give me something to sleep and then take it out." That didn't work. He didn't fall asleep. We had to go back the second day. So that is extremely hard on the staff, and then there's the poor family in the room finally having gotten to the place where they're in agreement and supportive with the brother or son—Mom's in the room—decision, and it's not happening.

In these situations, workers' own fears about decline and death are manifested in patients' experiences. For some, this was a matter of uncontrollable pain. For others, the most difficult patients were those who had already experienced hardship and were now dying out of sequence. These are both sets of problems with no immediate resolution, making it harder for hospice workers to reconstruct the experience as beautiful and meaningful. It also challenges their identities as hospice workers in that they are not able to produce "the good death" they see as their mandate and which is typically defined as a peaceful death, free of pain, and accepted by the decedent and the family members (Hart et al. 1998).

7.3.2   Reminders of Own Loss

Workers' selves become implicated again when patients or situations remind them of their own experiences of loss. When dealing with personal loss, many workers had a hard time "being there" with each individual patient. An administrator, formerly a nurse, explained how the loss of her dad colored her experience with a patient:

> So, I had a patient who not through any fault of his brought up lots of stuff about my relationship with my dad. And, at that time I hadn't completely explored all that to—it probably never would be but, you know, to a certain point. And, I had done enough of that that I was surprised at how emotional it was for me.

Even though her father's death had not been recent, this patient brought up residual feelings she was not prepared for.

The relationship between personal loss and ability to handle hospice work created a tension between caring for self and caring for others. Recent losses made the work of hospice difficult enough that some reported needing to take time away. When I asked one volunteer coordinator what made her work difficult, she said:

> Well, I guess the first thing that comes to mind is my own father died in April, and my 42-year-old niece died in September. And when you deal with your own personal loss, it's different. You can go sit with somebody. They die. You're sad. You were there for the family. It could have been a hard, a difficult, a stressful time, but when it's your own, it's completely different... I guess what really comes to mind is, in our staff meeting, we honor the patients that have died. And, right after my niece died, the chaplain read a poem, and I had to get up and leave because I started crying. I was just, you know, I had to get out of there. Because when she read it, she was reading it for a memory of the patients that we had served, but all I could hear is my own loss.

Hospice workers do not generally condemn crying in response to loss. In fact, crying to honor the patient who had died likely would have been seen as appropriate. Crying was a problem here because it was not about the patient and drew attention to the hospice provider.

Another form of personal loss is the imagined loss of self that accompanies watching others decline (Charmaz 1983). This came up most often when hospice workers discussed patients who were younger than they were. One nurse said:

> Well, I had a patient that was younger than I was and he had almost bottomed out four or five times when I'd been taking care of him for a year and a half and it does a real number on you when a patient's younger than you…. You're not supposed to think, "Well, you're going to get well." You're just not supposed to because it's a protection, but in so many ways I almost wish this person could have gotten well. And, it was emotional.

Because the patient was younger, this nurse had a hard time protecting herself from hoping for recovery. Part of the hospice identity includes accepting that all patients are going to die and supporting patients and family members as they move to greater acceptance as well.

Patients who had a hard time accepting their decline, especially when they were young, posed a challenge, too. A volunteer said,

> … it's a lot easier dealing with people who are older than I am than people who are younger. It really bothered me, because [the patient] wanted me to take him to get a computer, because he wanted to start a home business, and he wanted to get a new apartment, and he wanted all this stuff. And he admitted he knew, he talked about the fact that he was dying, and he probably didn't have much more time, but yet he wanted to do these things. And, inside, I was screaming at him in my own mind, "Why are you doing this? You're dying. Give it up." And obviously, fortunately, I knew that emotionally I couldn't tell him that, obviously. And that was very hard.

The volunteer knew his obligation was to "be there" with the patient and not try to change his thinking. However, he was upset that the patient did not seem to understand his condition. He wanted the patient to be in a place of acceptance, but the patient was young and unwilling to give up on dreams of starting a business or moving. The situation violated the norms of the hospice care relationship, and it threatened the identity of the hospice volunteer.

When workers were dealing with their own loss, it was all too easy to relate to the patients; it caused distress when care workers struggled to separate out the hospice reconstruction of death with their own feelings of senseless loss. Younger patients also sometimes challenged hospice meaning and identities as young patients did not always decline gracefully. This frustrated some workers who liked to imagine they would approach the situation more realistically.

7.3.3   Ethical Questions

Envisioning one's self in patients' situations makes ethical questions salient. Because of the ethic of "being there," hospice workers sometimes find it difficult to determine appropriate lines of action. This frequently came up in cases of suspected neglect. While overt physical abuse in nursing and assisted living facilities is rare, workers told me neglect was more common. Several hospice workers expressed how this posed a dilemma: if they reported the neglect, they harmed their relationships with care home staff and it was unlikely that anything would change. But if they did not report the neglect, they feared patients would not get the care they deserved—the care hospice workers wanted for themselves and their loved ones. Volunteers were more privy to neglect than other types of hospice workers, because they made regular, unannounced visits to care facilities. One volunteer said:

> I had another client that I felt in the home that she was in that she wasn't really being treated well. And again, I reported that to [the volunteer coordinator]. And this is just my interpretation of what I was seeing. And, she was kind of a cantankerous woman. She and I hit it off

right from the start. So, we had no trouble at all. And, I'd see her every single week. But, I felt that the staff there—it was another adult care home—I felt that the staff was not being very nice to her the way they were treating her and the way they were talking to her and the way they would ignore her. And so, again those were just emotional things for me because the more they were doing that, the more I was trying to overcompensate on the other side.

The volunteer reports trying to "overcompensate" because of the suspected neglect, but felt uneasy because she could not imagine letting her patient be ignored.

Workers also felt ethical difficulties when patients revealed information that could be reported, but patients expressed a desire to keep it private. This frequently came up in terms of some patients' desires to hasten death. A chaplain tells the following story:

> I'll say a situation where a patient indicated that she wanted to take her own life. And we're dealing with psychological stability in addition. But personally, philosophically I'm not opposed to the right to die for people, but that's not what our system and the laws allow. And so, I have to separate some of that out. And, in one case she was really confiding in me confidentially about a way in which she was going to attempt suicide and I was pretty fearful about what I should do about that in the sense of the extent to which I need to be informing people and so on… But I was kind of fearful about what was my obligation to her, how much I should be keeping confidential as opposed—you know, in other words there is, in the training that a priest receives, the idea of the seal of confession, which is legally and in other ways you're not supposed to—you are not to share anything that someone tells you under the seal of confession. Now legally that's being challenged these days so you can be called into court on it.

The irony in this situation is that, because the chaplain related to the patient as another person, not as a medical worker, she felt comfortable sharing this information. The chaplain had to consider his dueling ethical obligations. He describes the situation's resolution:

> Actually here's how it sort of plays out: because of the fact that she was confident and trusting me that she wouldn't—that I wouldn't go and call the police and tell other people, then she went into it in more depth than she did with other people. Now that also then opened the door for me to have conversations with her about, "Now how will your granddaughter respond to that when she comes and finds you? Is that what you want to leave with her?" and so on. I mean, kind of, "Let's play this out," and able to talk about some dimensions of it that she may not have talked about with other people otherwise.

Because of this in-depth conversation, the chaplain felt confident that the patient was not a threat to herself, but the experience still made him feel very uneasy. It brought out many of his own thoughts about death with dignity and one's right to end their own life, while also complicating his sense of responsibility to patients and his profession.

Lines of action are not always clear within caring work, especially in settings like hospice where people are facing complex issues and workers are encouraged to relate to patients. These ethical issues were difficult for hospice workers to handle, and remained with them as they tried to think through the appropriate response. They felt two pains through this process: one that was in response to the pain of the patient, and another as they tried to make sense of their own identity in relation to patients' life and care.

7.4 Discussion

Hospice workers' experiences show that suffering can be reframed and directly confronted as part of the work of caring for the dying. For instance, hospice's reframing of death as a meaningful, beautiful part of the life cycle provides hospice workers with cultural tools that allow them to build relationships with patients, construct meaning from suffering, and establish an identity around their work. But, some patient experiences are more difficult than others. Patients who challenge workers by making fears salient, reminding them of their own loss, and bringing up ethical dilemmas pose a problem for the hospice approach of "being there."

Social scientists have expanded perspectives on pain by theorizing suffering. Suffering is a subjective state goes beyond physical pain: it can include psychological, spiritual, family, and mental anguish. In fact, Charmaz (1983) refers to suffering as a "loss of self," providing a definition that encompasses all arenas of social life. Suffering might also be a product of loss of identity or a challenge to one's sense of self (Anderson 2014). Loss that seems to be without meaning is much more difficult to recover from than loss that fits meaning (Boss 2007; Neimeyer 2014). From these perspectives, we can see how experiencing the suffering of others can disrupt hospice workers' sense of meaning and identity, causing the diffusion of suffering beyond the initial patient and their family members.

Other researchers have tried to capture the same phenomenon. For instance, some scholars have used the term "compassion" to mean suffering that is shared: "compassion is defined as a sense of shared suffering, combined with a desire to alleviate or reduce such suffering" (Schulz et al. 2007: 6). However, compassion does not completely capture the processes described in hospice. First, "being there" and "companioning" are explicitly premised on not trying to solve the problem of suffering. In fact, Byock, wrote:

> Most fundamentally, clinicians can serve the dying person by being present. We may not have answers for the existential questions of life and death any more than the person dying. We may not be able to assuage all feelings of regret or fears of the unknown. But it is not our solutions that matter. The role of the clinical team is to stand by the patient, steadfastly providing meticulous physical care and psychosocial support, while people strive to discover their own answers (1996: 250).

By acknowledging suffering that diffuses between people, but not seeking to fix the problem, hospice workers' experiences of suffering extend beyond the common definition of compassion.

Reciprocal suffering is a concept that seeks to explain why one person may feel suffering in response to the pain of another. Some research has found that team-based care may mitigate suffering if team members support one another and feel empowered to call upon mental health experts (Swetenham et al. 2011). While the application of this concept does help to understand the social nature of workers' experience of suffering, it does not theorize how workers' identities and larger constructions of death and dying condition suffering. In fact, by looking at how identity intersects with suffering, this chapter is able to make sense of how difficult experiences become integrated into workers' general responses to the work.

In particular, some of these instances of suffering later became some of the most meaningful parts of hospice work. A chaplain explained:

> But I really was drawn to it because I recognized, especially in the retirement activities and conversations with people when I left parish ministry, that it was these kinds of times when people were facing significant change in their lives, and certainly including death and dying, experiences within their families that we have made bonds that were really significant, that it seemed like the most meaningful ministry I was doing, so I wanted to focus on that.

Like many other hospice workers I interviewed, this chaplain came to realize that his work was most meaningful when he was able to intervene in critical life moments—like death. Others described end-of-life care as "where the juice [of life] is" or "when the bullshit is over and there is honesty." Working as a volunteer, I realized that the imminent end to the relationship made many of my encounters with patients intimate quickly. Many hospice workers in this study reported that this level of intimacy was what made the work worthwhile, especially when they contrasted it to other types of medical work that was always too hurried.

While meaning is possible in these difficult situations, hospice workers are not equally prepared for the process of making meaning. Handling emotional aspects of the work is a learned skill, and professional training differentially prepares hospice workers. Those with counseling backgrounds had a refined language for discussing how to "be present" while still recognizing problems with becoming too involved with another's pain. For instance, one counselor said,

> Young parent—parents with small children are very poignant and very deeply touching. Or sometimes somebody's whose child is dying that's the same age as my kids or somebody who's my age and I deal with their children who are the age of my children. And there are similarities in my personal life that are reflected in the cases I work in. Those can be—those are emotional if I start to over-identify with them, I feel I can get pulled too far, and I need to kind of do whatever work I need to do to get my perspective back and remember that they too need to do their suffering. They need to do their grief and have their hurt so that they can experience the healing that awaits them on the other side of their hurt.

Another counselor describes this as "knowing where [we] end and they begin." Those without counseling backgrounds, especially nurses, were often thought of as unprepared to walk the line of sharing suffering without moving attention off the patient. Nurses' sense of self was sometimes seen as too bound up with the experiences of patients.

7.5 Conclusion

Those unfamiliar with hospice may assume that it must be depressing, difficult work, but hospice workers in this study adamantly refuted this assumption. They described work that was worthwhile, meaningful, and gave them new perspective on life. Reconstructed meanings about death, openness to emotional expression, and strong hospice identities allow hospice workers to find meaning in their work, even as it is sometimes emotionally difficult. However, there are limits to these approaches. Some patients or experiences are nearly impossible to find meaning within and sustain one's identity. Those patients who brought out workers' great fears, who reminded workers of their own loss, and who made ethical questions salient were frequently described as the most difficult patients. Each demonstrates the ways that difficult patients challenge hospice meanings and workers' identities, causing a diffusion of suffering from the patient to the worker.

References

Anderson, R. E. (2014). *Human suffering and quality of life: Conceptualizing stories and statistics*. New York: Springer.

Boss, P. (2007). Ambiguous loss theory: Challenges for scholars and practitioners. *Family Relations, 56*(2), 105–111.

Byock, I. (1996). The nature of suffering and the nature of opportunity at the end of life. *Clinics in Geriatric Medicine, 12*(2), 237–252.

Byock, I. (1998). *Dying well: Peace and possibilities at the end of life*. New York: Riverhead Books.

Cain, C. L. (2012). Integrating dark humor and compassion: Identities and presentations of self in the front and back regions of hospice. *Journal of Contemporary Ethnography, 41*(6), 668–694.

Cain, C. L. (2014). Orienting end-of-life care: The hidden value of hospice home visits. In M. Duffy, C. L. Stacey, & A. Armenia (Eds.), *Caring on the clock: The complexities and contradictions of paid care work*. New Brunswick: Rutgers University Press.

Charmaz, K. (1983). Loss of self: A fundamental form of suffering in the chronically ill. *Sociology of Health & Illness, 5*(2), 168–195.

Clark, D. (2007). End-of-life care around the world: Achievements to date and challenges remaining. *Omega, 56*(1), 101–110.

Corr, C. A. (2007). Hospice: Achievements, legacies, and challenges. *Omega, 56*(1), 111–120.

Gregory, D., & English, J. C. B. (1994). The myth of control: Suffering in palliative care. *Journal of Palliative Care, 10*(2), 18–22.

Hart, B., Sainsbury, P., & Short, S. (1998). Whose dying? A sociological critique of the 'good death'. *Mortality, 3*(1), 65–77.

Hutchinson, T. A. (Ed.). (2011). *Whole person care: A new paradigm for the 21st century*. New York: Springer.

Kelly, M. P., & May, D. (1982). Good and bad patients: A review of the literature and a theoretical critique. *Journal of Advanced Nursing, 7*(2), 147–156.

Lynch, T., Connor, S., & Clark, D. (2013). Mapping levels of palliative care development: A global update. *Journal of Pain and Symptom Management, 45*(6), 1094–1106.

Neimeyer, R. A. (2014). Meaning in bereavement. In R. E. Anderson (Ed.), *World suffering and the quality of life*. New York: Springer.

Schulz, R., Hebert, R. S., Dew, M. A., Brown, S. L., Scheier, M. F., Beach, S. R., & Nichols, L. (2007). Patient suffering and caregiving compassion: New opportunities for research, practice, and policy. *The Gerontologist, 47*(1), 4–13.

Stedeford, A. (1987). Hospice: A safe place to suffer? *Palliative Medicine, 1*, 73–74.

Swetenham, K., Hegarty, M., Breaden, K., & Grbich, C. (2011). Refractory suffering: The impact of team dynamics on the interdisciplinary palliative care team. *Palliative and Supportive Care, 9*, 55–62.

Twycross, R. (2007). Patient care: Past, present, and future. *Omega, 56*(1), 7–19.

Yoder, G. (2012). *Companioning the dying: A soulful guide for caregivers*. Fort Collins: Companion Press.

Chapter 8
Healing Suffering: The Evolution of Caring Practices

Nancy E. Johnston

8.1 Technology and the Biologic Model: At a Crossroads

Considering that our modern era has been distinguished by nothing so much as its conquest of nature through scientific methods, it is ironic that our scientific and technical achievements have precipitated many new forms of the perplexities they were designed to diminish. While it is evident that suffering at the global level cannot be considered apart from technological, economic, and political factors, there is also clear evidence that suffering at the level of individual human beings has been influenced by the incursions of science, technology, and economic markets. Up until recent times suffering has been understood as part of the human condition; the unsought misfortune that sooner or later comes to us all. Explanatory frameworks that privilege biological models have changed the way we think about suffering and provided the footing for the development of lucrative Western business enterprises; consider for example, that the sale of antidepressants in the US alone has reached 12 billion dollars in total sales annually (Hirsch 2010). Particularly in Western, developed nations, suffering is now understood as medical illness, diagnosed by psychiatrists and general practitioners, managed by classification (e.g. depression, anxiety, and post traumatic stress disorder), and treated as biochemical imbalance to be corrected by psychotropic medication (Horwitz and Wakefield 2007; Mehl-Madrona 2010).

Positive recovery rates and symptomatic relief have been lauded. Indeed, psychotropic medication can play an important role in relieving some suffering of a psychological, persistent, and life-threatening nature. However, there are questions about the legitimacy of many of the medical claims. Critiques point to the unreasonably wide range of criteria used to diagnose, as well as flaws in the process of

N.E. Johnston (✉)
Faculty of Health, School of Nursing, York University,
4700 Keele St, Toronto, ON M3J 1P3, Canada
e-mail: johnston@yorku.ca

© Springer Science+Business Media Dordrecht 2015   101
R.E. Anderson (ed.), *World Suffering and Quality of Life*,
Social Indicators Research Series 56, DOI 10.1007/978-94-017-9670-5_8

choosing which studies come to be cited in professional journals, given the many potential conflicts of interest among clinical medicine, biomedical sciences, journal publishing, and scientific advisory panels (Horwitz and Wakefield 2007). In one striking example, a meta-analysis on the effectiveness of antidepressants reported directly to the Food and Drug Administration (as opposed to those published in professional journals), showed no difference from placebo when all trials were reported (Hirsch 2010).

Responding to increasing concern about conflicts of interest, Cosgrove et al. (2006) investigated the financial ties between the pharmaceutical industry and 170 panel members who contributed to the diagnostic criteria produced for the revised DSM-IV and the DSM-IV-TR. A full 56 % of the panel had one or more financial associations with pharmaceutical companies. Connections were especially strong in those diagnostic areas where drugs are the first line of treatment for mental disorders.

Recent literature adds to the criticism of the biological model by showing that, after diagnosis, some individuals report a loss of a sense of personal agency and freedom. They have come to see their behavior and choices as primarily influenced by a disease beyond their personal control. Kaiser, cited in Mehl-Madrona (2010), documents this erosion of personal agency and the effort required for patients to regain sustaining relationships, commitments to meaningful causes, and, ultimately, self-healing. In 2007 Horwitz and Wakefield drew attention to an "epidemic" of depression in North American society. Pointing to statistics that one in ten people suffer from depression every year and 25 % are diagnosed with the "disease" at some point in their lives, the researchers delved into the etiology of the epidemic. They found that the diagnosis of depression had now come to include transient and completely reasonable responses to life events such as loss of financial security and death of a spouse. They argued persuasively that the DSM-IV criteria professionals (and, indeed, the public) used to diagnose depression did not sufficiently distinguish between "normal sadness" and depression. By showing how normal, transient feelings had become diagnosed as pathologies and treated with medications, these authors argued that normal emotional response has been almost completely medicalized.

A revised version of the diagnostic manual, now titled DSM-V, was published in 2013, 6 years after Horwitz and Wakefield criticized the previous volume's depression criteria. Unfortunately, much of their critique still stands. Diagnostic criteria continue to lack the power to differentiate between normal sadness and depression. It can even be argued that the emotional territory represented by the DSM-V actually *expands* the territory claimed by the medical profession. Dowrick and Frances (2013), in their incisive critique of the DSM-V, point out the problems of assuming depression in cross-cultural consultations with patients who have experienced loss and are seeking asylum. They further express concern about replacing distress and loss with psychiatric diagnosis. Such an approach individualizes and conceals issues that were previously seen as social problems. Diagnosing *grief* within the category of major depressive disorder adds unnecessary medication, increases the risk of side effects, and adds significantly to the cost of care for those who may suffer painfully, but for good reason and for relatively short periods of time.

Joel Paris, a prominent psychiatrist in Canada, was asked in a leading newspaper (Kirkey 2014) what he thought about Canada having "achieved" the third highest level of consumption of antidepressants among 23 member nations surveyed by the Organization for Economic Co-operation and Development. Paris said:

> We're not always happy, and there are often good reasons for unhappiness. But there's this idea that we should all have high self-esteem, fantastic relationships and tremendous jobs. It's like cosmetic psychopharmacology: If you don't like the way you look, you go to a plastic surgeon and get it fixed. If you're not happy enough, go to a doctor and go on antidepressants.

Somber reflection on the mutually-influencing relationship of heightened, unrealistic life expectations and the legitimization of pharmaceutical agents to manage emotional life raises questions of great consequence: Is the medicalization of emotional life weakening our capacity for resilience? Has the time come to retrieve the notion that suffering may offer opportunities to gain wisdom, empathy, and compassion? Is it possible to recover humanism and work with it in a way that is complementary rather than hostile to the materialist, biologic paradigm, which *has* assembled a prodigious body of knowledge about how our brains work?

Fricchione (2011) believes in the value of humanist approaches, empirical science, *and* principles and practices drawn from the wisdom traditions—traditions which represent mankind's deepest source of knowledge regarding harmony, sustainable existence, developing the inner self, and the realization of enlightenment (Chodron 1997, 2010; Miller 2006). Using insights, concepts, and findings drawn from all three spheres, Fricchione (2011) advances a theory and new philosophy of medicine that empowers the re-integration of love and compassion into the science of medicine. Drawing on Bowlby's (1973) seminal "attachment theory," evolutionary/complexity theory, and cutting-edge neuroscientific research, Fricchione's theory shows potential for overcoming the materialist/humanist divide, deepening our respect for the wisdom traditions, and furthering our understanding of how suffering can be healed. He shows that positive neurochemical and neurobiological states occur in humans when just, fitting, attuned, and compassionate responses are experienced. These positive states can be perpetuated, even when threatened. Strategies to call forth and perpetuate positive states are labeled "attachment solutions", while the situations that activate fear and the loss of integrity, meaning, and connection constitute "separation challenges". When we return to suffering, it is clear the separation challenges lie at the very heart of human suffering. Attachment solutions, which involve restoring meaning, then, lie at the heart of caring and healing.

8.2 What It Means to Be Human: The Self and Social Justice

Newer understandings of what it means to be human that have emerged in the past two decades offer a crucial dimension: they advance our knowledge of our relational nature as humans and give *centrality* to this understanding, which is backed up by empirical science. Asserting emphatically that humans are self-interpreting entities, new scholars recognize that humans build humanity within relationships. What is truly significant and meaningful to us happens within and between us *as humans* (Jordan et al. 1991; Jordan 1997, 2004; Miller and Stiver 1997; Fricchione 2011). Johnston (2007) writes bluntly that the self is not a thing. It is not an intrinsic substance or entity, but is assembled from the stories we tell ourselves *about* ourselves in making sense of our relationships with other people. Neibuhr (cited in Harland 1960) asserts that there are certain conditions that attend the relational self, with its endless internal conversations and its external dialogues with other people. These include acknowledgement of the following:

> The self faces the other self as a mystery which can never be fully penetrated; the self sees the other as an instrument for its purposes and as a completion for its incompleteness; the self cannot be truly fulfilled if it is not drawn out of itself into the life of another; the self recognizes the other as the limit of its expansiveness… there must therefore be an element of reservation and reverence for the other in even the most mutual relations; the uniqueness of the individuals which enter into any dialogic relation makes each one of these relations highly unique, and finally while the self is a unique center of life it is indeterminately 'open' to other selves. (p. 61)

Reflection on the conditions that attend the self raises important implications for healing practices. The self is shifting, changing; we can never get to the bottom of who we or others *are*. The changeability of self-identity is both an irremediable problem for "objective" science and a cause for hope. This is because our human nature, essentially open, liberates us from determinate causes and effects. The flexibility of self places us in novel situations, unlocks an infinite number of contextual analyses, invites new self-interpretations, and perpetuates an ongoing range of possibilities. Standing before others and ourselves as a mystery not only inspires awe and reverence, but also ignites the expectation of surprise. It promotes the exciting prospect of continual transformation and the transcendence of the past (Johnston 2005).

Research based on observation of mothers and infants reveals just how essential connections are to well-being. Stern (1985) writes that human connections are permanent, healthy parts of mental growth and that forming relationships is the primary task of infancy. Schore (cited in Robb 2007), commenting on the neurobiology of connection in infants and children, asserts that we are hard-wired to develop in tandem with an "other," even before words are spoken. Miller and Stiver (1997), eschewing an understanding of the self as isolated and greedy, write that "The goal of development is not forming a separated self or finding gratification but something else altogether—the ability to participate actively in relationships that foster the well-being of everyone involved" (p. 2). Suggesting implications for the healing (and healers) of suffering, relational-cultural theorists assert that only a good relationship can teach a person to limit the damage from bad relationships. To the relief of most, such good relationships can be built even by adults who have experienced disappointing or disruptive early bonds. New possibilities arise when these same adults are able to experience the pain of another person and stay engaged. Robb (2007) writes that it occurs for both the sufferer and the caregiver: "It is apparent that we cannot touch without being touched" (p. 189). Staying engaged when we feel averse or terrified requires altruism (a subject to be taken up in more detail later in this chapter); altruism dilutes aversion, domesticates fear, and points in the direction of self-respect and personal fulfillment Johnston 2002. It also points the way for concrete action toward ameliorating suffering at the societal level. The notion is only beginning to dawn on conventional, mainstream psychotherapy.

Comas-Diaz (2012) writes,

> Currently mainstream psychotherapy addresses the individual, family, group and community. However, the next developmental step in psychotherapy will be to address the societal realm… and will involve the promotion of societal change under the rubric of social justice. (p. 474)

Personal authenticity involves speaking the truth, ending abuse, and resisting oppression. For many who are healing from various forms of trauma, the final stage of healing involves a commitment to the kind of social and political action that is meaningful to the individual's own particular form of suffering. Herman (cited in Robb 2007) writes this approach to healing trauma: "while there is no way to compensate for an atrocity, there is a way to transcend it, by making it a gift to others. The trauma is redeemed when it becomes the source of a survivor mission" (p. 412). Evolutionary progression in healing practices demands that counselors, therapists, and other health-care practitioners not only understand the potential redemptive role in healing of their client's "survivor missions," but that they facilitate and actively play such roles themselves.

Urging practitioners to end uncritical acceptance of injustice, Comas-Diaz stresses the importance of revealing the gap between the special privileges of dominant groups and the misery of marginalized and radicalized groups. Gilbert (2002, 2009, 2010) also writes about the necessity of reform at the societal level. Hypothesizing a link between western, materialist values and psychiatric illness, Gilbert finds the roots of psychological disorders in the self-rejection of individuals who cannot live up to the demands and values those values. Coulehan (2003) asserts that nothing short of a radical reevaluation and rebalancing of North American society is required: emphases on individual rights, personal entitlement, and self-determination (to the exclusion of social duty, sharing, and communal responsibility) have perpetuated suffering and hindered healing by concealing our hard-wired need for empathetic connection. Since human beings are seen to be self-interpreting, intensely relational entities with the capacity for compassion and self-transcendence, it seems reasonable that the call to address the root causes of social injustice will be key to the next wave of caring practices. Getting there, however, necessitates a more finely nuanced understanding of the paradox of suffering.

8.3   Can Suffering Be a Gift?

With an increasing awareness of the social and political causes of suffering and our obligation to address them, the notion that suffering includes gifts can seem outrageous. Many believe that suffering and loss—especially among the poor and the ill and the oppressed—are simply irredeemable (Young-Eisendrath 1996, p. 2). They understandably argue that some forms of suffering—genocide, the death of children, and catastrophes visited by natural disaster, industrial accident, or war, to name but a few—defy any possibility of acceptability. Some authors (Anderson 2004) go further to warn that the acceptance and valorization of suffering, let alone the idea that it may hold benefits for the sufferer, risks the perpetuation of suffering: it may allow for acquiescence rather than resistance to social oppression.

These compelling perspectives require an unambiguous position: inviting or conceding to suffering in order to experience and expand the self is neither reasonable nor defensible. Without exception, suffering introduces great risks and painful uncertainties and gifts are never guaranteed.

That being said, the possibility of receiving or being able to convey benefits to others in the wake of suffering cannot be refuted. Johnston (2007, pp. 128–130) illuminates this paradox of suffering by providing numerous vignettes drawn from her qualitative research. How is does the process of experiencing suffering as gift unfold? What conditions and ways of dwelling amidst suffering influence the probability of meaningful versus meaningless suffering?

Johnston (2007) and Young-Eisendrath (1996) write of the jolt that can accompany suffering. Illusions of personal control are shattered and people come to question "who" they are and their very purpose in life. The scholars' research reveals how the unavoidable mysteries of pain and suffering inaugurate prolonged and unrelieved despair, but their work also shows evidence that such suffering can be gradually transformed into hidden resources of compassion, courage, and solidarity with others. The self expands. Those who suffer see that they are not alone in their struggles and that new resources are needed to address their own and others' needs. When the illusion of self-sufficiency breaks down, habitual barriers are destroyed and new intersubjective fields are built, which bring pain to expression, overcome isolation, and join the sufferer to others.

When the vitality of suffering is not dulled and obscured, when it is not viewed as disease or dysfunction and rationalized away, suffering can teach. It offers an opportunity to mine the inevitable losses of life to enrich notions of ourselves and the nature of being human. Thus, suffering can be a useful and helpful—indeed, a transformative—gift when it reveals the truth; enables self-awareness awakens responsibility for our own attitudes, thoughts, and actions; reveals what is truly important in life; and promotes compassion (Young-Eisendrath, pp. 6, 33, 42; Johnston 2002, pp. 114–128).

Suffering, then, can be (but will not *necessarily* be) much more than anguish, misery, and travail. For care practitioners working in systems increasingly driven by the demand for "efficiency" the challenge, indeed the obligation, is to resist the pressure to privilege efficiency over caring approaches. When efficiency is valued over the human imperative to care for and connect with others, visible signs of suffering are ignored, and the sufferer agonizes in silence and isolation. Meaning can break down for client and practitioner alike. When patients cannot trust that their emotional needs will be responded to, hospitals lack hospitality and agencies are emptied of the sense of devotion to meaningful causes. Social service providers become spawning grounds for burnout and despair among their workers (Pask 2005).

Instead, when the notion that suffering could bring gifts rather than just misery is, in itself, cause for hope. Hope, in turn, enables alertness to new possibilities for alternate sources of meaning and purpose. This empathy-centered approach has the power to transform suffering.

8.4 The Wound as the Locus of Compassion

Next, I must turn to the means by which suffering becomes transformative and redemptive by appreciating how the psychological and spiritual wounds inflicted by suffering can become a locus for compassion and a vital impetus for healing of the self and others.

The word compassion derives from the Latin *com patior*, to suffer with. Compassion involves feeling another's suffering as keenly as one's own, and being moved to succor. *Pity*, the emotion of tenderness aroused by the suffering of another, and *mercy* toward the powerless, are subsumed in compassion and intertwined with *empathy*—the ability to understand and enter into another's feelings—a twentieth-century coinage from the German *Einfühlung* (Gregory 2004). Current views accept compassion as a form of humanitarian benevolence that includes the interrelatedness of all life and the welfare of the planet itself. In tracing our unfolding understanding of compassion, Gregory characterizes it as a

> tender-mindedness outraged at the deliberate infliction of pain; it extends across national boundaries to the distant and unknown victims of persecution, to all social classes and ethnic groups, to domestic and wild animals, and in the past twenty years to the planet itself. (2004)

Olthuis (2001) deconstructs the word compassion, pointing out that *com* "with" and *patior* "to feel" mean more together than resistance evil and suffering. Compassion transforms them. Suffering may befriend pain in a way that is neither coercive nor dominating, but is rather inviting, congenial, mutual. Rather than preventing or removing pain, compassion lets pain be shared, shouldered by many and thus lightened. Practicing compassion involves "connecting with one's self and owning one's own woundedness" (Olthuis 2001, p. 46). Younger (1995) shares the view that one's own wounds and flaws (aspects of the self she calls the "shadow side") must be confronted and accepted. Instead of accepting our negative traits, however, we tend to project them on others rather than ourselves. In their most extreme form they become the impulse for scapegoating others. Compassion may be a hallmark of humanity, but it is still no easy feat.

Based on Buddhist teachings, Chodron (2010) offers an understanding of the roots of suffering, the wounds that arise from it, and the practices that ameliorate it. She shows how our natural inclination is to avoid unpleasantness, holding tenaciously to all that we experience as pleasant and striving to get things on our own terms (that is, we bend to ego). But, according to Buddhist thought, everything is impermanent and pain is inevitable. When we avoid facing the ephemeral nature of all things and insist on doggedly clinging to that which has and must pass, when life satisfaction is judged by the extent to which our cravings are satisfied, we turn ephemeral pain into intense and lasting suffering. Chodron says the reason we behave in ways that intensify our suffering is easily explained: our actions and thoughts are protective. There is, in each of us a soft spot—what she calls "the tender, warm vulnerable heart of *bodhichitta*, which we instinctively protect so that nothing will touch it" (Chodron 2010; 88). Likening the "protected" ego to an imprisoning room, Chodron urges a gradual opening of the door, not through judging our actions toward others or toward ourselves, nor through clinging to comfort, but by cultivating and acting upon a courageous intent to gather humor, curiosity, openness, and knowledge (p. 89).

Chodron offers the view that compassion for another arises because we all share the basic experience of raw, painful vulnerability. We "have been there." Opening up to, rather than resisting, the pain of our own wounds enables us to get past the identification of self as victim. Yes, others have injured us, but a singular focus on how we have been hurt leads to more and more protective maneuvers; more anger, more bitterness, more withdrawal, more closing off of life. A willingness to experience pain while cultivating kindness and compassion (to others and the self), on the other hand, results in a gradual opening up to life. Greeting pain in this way shifts the focus from "me" to "we"—the Buddhist statement "the light that is within me bows to the light within you" also creates its companion, "the pain that is in me is within you." Embrace of pain enables a sense of solidarity and agency.

Feldman and Kuyken (2011) also affirm the importance of altering the "story line." They write that those who suffer from anxiety and depression must reframe their personal narrative in order to develop self-compassion. The story that the self is inadequate or a failure shifts to one in which the self is suffering—in need of and *deserving* of compassion.

The idea that healing requires *explicitly* non-judgmental and compassionate approaches to the self is not new; in fact, it is one of the central tenets of Buddhism, which has been around since 520 BCE. Only within the last 10–15 years, however, has this notion found its way into western therapies. New approaches integrate traditional cognitive behavioral approaches with fresh strategies influenced by Buddhist teachings and spiritual practices. One example of such an approach is Mindfulness Based Cognitive Therapy (MBCT) (Segal et al. 2012). The goal of MBCT is to teach clients to interrupt automatic processes of negative and depressive thinking, focus less on reacting to incoming stimuli, and accept and observe such stimuli without judgment. This mindfulness practice enables a reflective, curious approach to difficulties and the fostering of resilience. Research supports the effects of MBCT in people who have been depressed three or more times; it has been demonstrated to reduce relapse rates by 50 % (Hougaard 2011).

Compassion Focused Therapy (CFT) (Gilbert 2009), another example of this genre of therapies, is specifically directed toward individuals for whom "woundedness" takes the form of heightened sensitivity and overactivity of the threat-protection and/or drive systems. Such sensitivity and overactivity results in constant vigilance, a tendency toward protective stances, creates confusion and conflict, and a high drive to constantly search for resources. Readers may note that this sounds rather like popular depictions of Post-Traumatic Stress Disorder (PTSD). As cited earlier in this chapter, Gilbert associates this preoccupation with the values of western culture, which emphasizes amassing material possessions, status, and power. Accordingly, when extreme levels of vigilance are activated, when the drive to acquire is unleashed, and when intense needs for self-protection result in unremitting demands on the self, severe levels of shame and self-criticism can be experienced. People who suffer in this way are unable to generate feelings of contentment and warmth in their relationships with themselves and other people. Sharing some similar theoretical underpinnings with MBCT and drawing upon Buddhist thought and conceptual viewpoints similar to Fricchione (2011), Gilbert (2009) stresses the importance of early patterns of attachment in protecting against such later difficulties. These early patterns, he writes, either lay down (or fail to lay down) the neurochemical substrates responsible for self-soothing capabilities. The role of CFT is to help clients develop an internal compassionate, appreciative relationship that replaces their aggressive, blaming, bullying, cold, condemning, and self-critical inner tone. Once such a relationship is formed, thought patterns and behaviors can change.

The understanding of the wound as the locus of compassion has significant implications for the evolution of healing practices. As a place of painful vulnerability *and* the motivating force that ignites and motivates empathy, understanding, warmth, and acceptance, the wound carries great risks and opportunities. The risks are that, when suffering is extreme, meaning breaks down. Fear, projection, and estrangement ensue. The goal of caring practices is not to take the pain away, but to render the suffering bearable, and a site of insight (Feldman and Kuyken 2011). Helpful, empathic, and stabilizing relationships, both professional and personal—what Johnston (2007) calls "skilled accompaniment" and Fricchione (2011) labels an "attachment solution," can bring about that enormous change. In a climate of warmth, compassionate acceptance, and safety, mute suffering finds a voice, self-rejection is transformed, isolation is overcome, and healing begins.

8.5 Self-Transcendence and Healing Through Altruism

Interspersed throughout this chapter have been fleeting allusions to self-transcendence and the attraction to altruism as a natural consequence of experiencing compassion born of suffering. In this section, some of these assertions are revisited alongside emerging research that supports the proposition that altruism can be as much a route to healing as a manifestation or outcome of healing. In fact, this is what characterizes the fourth evolutionary development in caring practices related to suffering.

In further support of the idea that suffering may be transformed into a redemptive gift, I offer the personal story of Abraham, gathered as part of a qualitative research study (Johnston 2007). In the Israeli/Palestinian conflict, Abraham's son was killed by a suicide bomber on a bus. In discussing the initial impact of his son's death and his subsequent attempts to make meaning of this loss, Abraham told Johnston:

> I felt that life had stopped completely, that everything was over for me…. I became terribly depressed; I couldn't do anything. I couldn't eat; I couldn't sleep. I couldn't make any sense of it at all. I wanted to die just to be with my son again…. Then one day I am watching TV. I see Palestinian people weeping and wailing because Israeli soldiers have killed their sons. Their coffins are being carried through the streets and suddenly it just hits me. They feel just as bad as I do. Their hearts are breaking just like mine, and I feel so close to them. They are not my enemies they are by brothers and sisters. And then I know what I have to do. I go to a Palestinian family and I say to them that I am so, so sorry and I tell them that I lost my son too and then we just all sit down and we weep together… We are family… and then the idea takes root that we have to do more…. Now we have formed an organization for Palestinian and Israeli families who have lost children and want the war to stop. Today I am a different man, and some people don't want anything to do with me. They want to keep up the barriers that I want to tear down. Still I know what is important and I realize that it is my pain that connects me with the suffering of other people and [that] has made me a better person. (pp. 128–129).

In this story, two "great evils" of suffering (Cushing 2010)—the loss of relationship and the loss of hope—are redeemed. The self is transcended and intense suffering becomes the impetus for profound identification with others who suffer. Enabling the rejection of the categorization of others as enemies, Abraham's experience reinforces a sense of common humanity and propels an intense desire to reach out to others who suffer. A renewed sense of purpose and personal growth evidence community benefit in the wake of extreme suffering.

Staub and Volhardt (2008) affirm that altruism born of suffering (ABS) is different than resilience or even posttraumatic growth (PTG). This is because "altruism requires a focus beyond the self…. [T]o develop altruism in the context or aftermath of suffering experiences beyond those that foster resilience are necessary" (p. 269). While it can result in positive self-regard for the actor, altruism involves action that is primarily driven by caring and the unselfish desire to benefit others (Staub and Volhardt 2008, p. 276). Understanding the kind of experiences that call forth altruism is extremely important: it sheds light on how suffering can be translated into social justice and expressed in actions that benefit individuals *and* communities. While research on ABS is still in its infancy, findings do show positive, significant correlations between the severity of suffering, commonality with victims, and involvement in pro-social activities that extend to outgroups in activities like, for example, volunteer work with victims of disasters, the elderly, and the homeless (Staub and Volhardt 2008).

Placed in perspective with the understandings that have influenced the evolution of healing practices, such findings should not be surprising. Newer philosophic understandings supported by empirical research reveal the self to be a self-in-relation. Since this is a self which is hard-wired for and inseparable from relationships, healing from suffering for sufferer and personal growth for healer (or altruistic giver) occur simultaneously. This is because as Robb (2007, p. 189) reminds us, we "cannot touch without being touched."

Accordingly, a circular and continuous relationship can be proposed among: healing by learning to care for, be compassionate toward, and have positive regard for the self; healing by developing and maintaining a cohesive self by way of experiencing oneself compassion and caring from others (Fricchione 2011; Gilbert 2009); and healing by engaging in altruistic acts that involve extending compassion and social justice to others (Staub and Volhardt 2008; Volhardt and Staub 2011; Comas-Diaz 2012). The circularity of the feedback loops inherent in this circuit of compassion can be expected to enhance healthy regard for the self.

8.6 Conclusion

Evolutionary developments in caring practices for suffering hinge on conceptual breakthroughs in the understanding of self and society. They also depend on new, catalyzing influences arising from confluences of thought in areas that have been quite separate. Buttressed by scientific evidence, we now understand the self to be much more flexible and relational than ever before. Confronted with the precarious nature of western society, committed as it is to rapid economic growth at the expense of social and environmental health and security, we have begun to appreciate the need for a transformation of fundamental values if we are to reduce suffering.

In a manner that will likely characterize the ongoing evolution of caring practices, an exciting new trend can be observed: the converging conversation about the interaction of spiritual traditions and science. By describing the integration of ancient spiritual, contemplative, wisdom traditions, and practices with recent developments in evolutionary biology and neuroscience, this chapter has shown that outmoded perceptions of the self and suffering have been upended. The self is not isolated and alone. The wound is not a flaw. Suffering is not irreparable loss. More hopeful views reveal a self that is "hard-wired" for connection, fulfilled in relationship, enlightened by suffering, attracted to altruism, and committed to social justice. These understandings guide and will, in the future, provide vital momentum for caring practices aimed at not only the restoration of the self, but also development of a more just society.

References

Anderson, J. M. (2004). Lessons from a postcolonial-feminist perspective: Suffering and a path to healing. *Nursing Inquiry, 11*(4), 238–246.

Bowlby, J. (1973). *Attachment Vol. 1: Attachment and loss*. London: Hogarth Press.

Chodron, P. (1997). *When things fall apart. Heart advice for difficult times*. Boston: Shambhala Publications Inc.

Chodron, P. (2010). *Taking the leap: Freeing ourselves from old habits and fears*. Boston: Shambhala Publications Inc.

Comas-Diaz, L. (2012). Psychotherapy as a healing practice, scientific endeavor, and social justice action. *Psychotherapy, 49*(4), 473–474.

Cosgrove, L., Krimsby, S., Vijayaraghaven, M., & Schneider, L. (2006). Financial ties between DSM-IV panel members and the pharmaceutical industry. *Psychotherapy and Psychosomatics, 75*(3), 154–160.

Coulehan, J. (2003). Metaphor and medicine: Narrative in clinical practice. *Yale Journal of Biology and Medicine, 76*, 87–95.

Cushing, S. (2010). Evil, freedom and the heaven dilemma. In J. Schlegel & B. Hansen (Eds.), *Challenging evil: Time, society and changing concepts of the meaning of evil*. Inter- Disciplinary Research retrieved from: http://www.svri.org/evil.pdf#page=72 on 8 Feb 2014.

Dowrick, C., & Frances, A. (2013). Medicalising and medicating unhappiness. *British Journal of Medicine International Edition, 347*(7937), 20–27.

Feldman, C., & Kuyken, W. (2011). Compassion in the landscape of suffering. *Contemporary Buddhism, 12*(1), 143–155.

Fricchione, G. L. (2011). *Compassion and healing in medicine and society: On the nature and use of attachment solutions to separation challenges*. Baltimore: Johns Hopkins University.

Gilbert, P. (2002). Evolutionary approaches to psychopathology and cognitive therapy. *Journal of Cognitive Psychotherapy, 16*(3), 263–294.

Gilbert, P. (2009). Introducing compassion-focused therapy. *Advances in Psychiatric Treatment, 15*, 199–208.

Gilbert, P. (2010). *Compassion-focused therapy (CBT distinctive features)*. New York: Routledge.

Gregory, R. L. (Print publication date 2004, online version published 2006). *The Oxford companion to the mind* (2nd ed). Oxford/New York: Oxford University Press. eiSBN 9780191727559.

Harland, G. (1960). *The thought of Reinhold Neibuhr*. New York: Oxford University Press.

Hirsch, I. (2010). *The emperor's new drugs: Exploding the antidepressant myth*. New York: Basic Books.

Horwitz, A. V., & Wakefield, J. C. (2007). *The loss of sadness: How psychiatry transformed normal sorrow into depressive disorder*. New York: Oxford Press.

Hougaard, J. P. (2011). The effect of mindfulness-based cognitive therapy for prevention of relapse in recurrent in recurrent major depressive disorder: A systematic review and meta-analysis. *Clinical Psychology Review, 13*(6), 1032–1040.

Johnston, N. E. (2002). *Finding meaning in adversity*. Doctoral dissertation. Retrieved from: http://www.collectionscanada.gc.ca/obj/thesescanada/vol2/001/nq86530.pdf. 8 Apr 2014.

Johnston, N. E. (2005). Beyond method: Toward embodied ways of knowing. In N. Diekelmann & P. Ironside (Eds.), *Beyond method: Interpretive studies in health care and the human sciences*. Madison: University of Wisconsin Press.

Johnston, N. E. (2007). Finding meaning in adversity. In N. E. Johnston & A. Scholler-Jaquish (Eds.), *Meaning in suffering: Caring practices in the health professions* (pp. 98–139). Madison: University of Wisconsin Press.

Jordan, J. V. (Ed.). (1997). *Women's growth in diversity: More writings from the Stone Center*. New York: Guilford Press.

Jordan, J. V. (2004). Relational learning in psychotherapy consultation. In M. Walker & W. Rosen (Eds.), *How connections heal: Stories from relational-cultural therapy* (pp. 22–30). New York: Guilford Press.

Jordan, J. V., Kaplan, A. G., Baker Miller, J., Stiver, I. P., & Surrey, J. L. (1991). *Writings from the Stone Center*. New York: Guilford Press.

Kirkey, S. (2014). *Drugging unhappiness: Canadians now among world's biggest consumers of antidepressants*. Ottawa Citizen retrieved from: http://www.ottawacitizen.com/health/Drugging+unhappiness+Canadians+among+world+biggest+consumers+antidepressants/9405515/story.html. 21 Jan 2014.

Mehl-Madrona, L. (2010). *Healing the mind through the power of story: The promise of narrative psychiatry*. Rochester: Bear & Company.

Miller, J. P. (2006). *Educating for wisdom and compassion: Creating conditions for timeless learning*. Thousand Oaks: Corwin Press.

Miller, J. B., & Stiver, I. P. (1997). *The healing connection: How women form relationships in therapy and in life*. Boston: Beacon Press.

Olthuis, J. H. (2001). *The beautiful risk: A new psychology of loving and being loved*. Grand Rapids: Zondervan.

Pask, E. (2005). Self sacrifice, self transcendence and nurses' professional self. *Nursing Philosophy, 6*(4), 247–254.

Robb, C. (2007). *This changes everything: The relational revolution in psychotherapy*. New York: Picador, Farrar & Giroux.

Segal, Z. V., Williams, J. M. G., & Teasdale, J. D. (2012). *Mindfulness-based cognitive therapy for depression* (2nd ed.). New York: Guilford Press.

Staub, E., & Volhardt, J. (2008). Altruism born of suffering: The roots of caring and helping after victimization and other trauma. *American Journal of Orthopsychiatry, 78*(1), 257–280.

Stern, D. N. (1985). *The interpersonal world of the infant*. New York: Basic Books.

Volhardt, J., & Staub, E. (2011). Inclusive altruism born of suffering: The relationship between adversity and prosocial attitudes and behavior toward disadvantaged outgroups. *American Journal of Orthopsychiatry, 81*(3), 307–315.

Young-Eisendrath, P. (1996). *The gifts of suffering: Finding insights, compassion and renewal*. Boston: Addison-Wesley.

Younger, J. D. (1995). The alienation of the sufferer. *Advances in Nursing Science, 17*(4), 53–72.

Chapter 9
Meaning in Bereavement

Robert A. Neimeyer

9.1 Introduction

If suffering is universal, so too is one of its most profound causes: death and loss as an ineluctable reality of the human condition. When we pause to think of it—as we rarely choose to do—we recognize that every person, every project, every place, and every possession we hold dear will one day be lost to us (at least in an earthly sense). Indeed, most readers of this volume, whatever their culture or geography, will already have already lost many and much. How we live with this intimate knowledge of impermanence shapes who we become, as individuals, families, communities, and nations.

Working as a psychologist engaged with loss and transition in both research and applied contexts, my interest in this phenomenon is one part theoretical, one part practical. In both domains I have found that viewing human suffering through the lens of the *meaning systems* people use to orient to loss is clarifying. This is true whether I am focused on the molar secular and religious discourses with which different cultures and traditions shroud the human encounter with death or concentrated on the more molecular meanings individuals place on the intimate losses of family members.

In a similar vein, discussing the psychology of spirituality, Paloutzian and Park write:

> religion should be conceived in terms of religious meaning systems, that is, as a subset of meaning systems in general. Meaning systems, as we understand them psychologically, comprise mental processes that function together to enable a person… to live consciously and nonconsciously with a sense of relative continuity, evaluate incoming information relative to his or her guidelines, and regulate beliefs, affects and actions accordingly. (2013: 6–7)

R.A. Neimeyer, Ph.D. (✉)
Department of Psychology, Faculty of Psychology, University of Memphis,
400 Innovation Drive, Rm 202, Memphis, TN 38152-6400, USA
e-mail: neimeyer@memphis.edu

© Springer Science+Business Media Dordrecht 2015
R.E. Anderson (ed.), *World Suffering and Quality of Life*,
Social Indicators Research Series 56, DOI 10.1007/978-94-017-9670-5_9

Nowhere are such meaning systems—whether secular or spiritual—more relevant than in conferring significance on the end of life and offering perspective, understanding, and consolation to survivors.

Working within the specific field of bereavement studies, my colleagues and I find this perspective both congenial and comprehensive, comfortably conjoining with the constructivist conceptualization (Kelly 1955; Neimeyer 2009) that undergirds our research. In the present chapter, I hope to illustrate the utility of a meaning systems perspective in addressing the effort to (re)establish meaning in the wake of the loss of a loved one, with special attention to the significant struggles that arise for some mourners. Briefly reviewing our longstanding program of research on the quest for meaning in loss, I hope to illustrate its relevance to understanding and even ameliorating human suffering, touching not only on our chief findings to date, but also on several new methods we hope will prove useful to other researchers.

9.2   Loss and the Quest for Meaning

Framing our study of secular and spiritual sense making in the wake of loss is a *meaning reconstruction* model of bereavement (Neimeyer 2001, 2006). In this perspective, a central feature of grieving is *the attempt to reaffirm or reconstruct a world of meaning that has been challenged by loss* (Neimeyer 2002). In distinction from highly "cognitive" theories in psychology, such meanings are understood here in terms of the sometimes explicit but often implicit ways that we human beings seek "replicative themes" (Kelly 1955), discerning and imposing regularity and significance on the unfolding patterns of our lives (Neimeyer 2000). When these lives are relatively unproblematic, the prereflective meaning and coherence of experience go largely unnoticed; this forms a tacit ground for an orderly perception of the world and our actions within it (Merleau-Ponty 1962).

But there are times when the conscious need to find meaning in experience stubbornly or even agonizingly asserts itself. Deeply unwelcome life transitions such as the death of a beloved other, especially under tragic circumstances, are among these moments when the taken-for-granted coherence of life is disrupted. The simplest routines of daily living require painful review and revision, as when we no longer need to wake to nurse a baby that has died, or in our widowhood, go to bed alone. These and a hundred other violations of the "micro-narratives" of our lives can ultimately vitiate our capacity to make sense of the larger "macro-narrative" of loss and our existence in its wake. The disjuncture launches a search for meaning that may find few simple answers (Neimeyer 2004, 2011).

In summarizing our research program on grief and the quest for meaning, I should acknowledge at the outset that I will adopt primarily a clinical psychological approach in view of my active concern with the lives of those challenged and changed by tragic transition. I recognize—and indeed demonstrate—that many mourners negotiate their losses with surprising resilience, such that even in their bereavement, the meaning of life (and death) remains secure and unproblematic

(Bonanno 2004; Bonanno et al. 2004). When it does not, however, grief can be complicated by a profound struggle to integrate loss in both secular and spiritual terms, sometimes to a point that professional assistance is warranted (Neimeyer 2012). This focus on life vitiating losses of a sort that often leads people to seek psychotherapy situates our work at a mid-level of Paloutzian and Park's (2013) multi-level model of meaning systems (MS). It is concerned primarily with the personal resources (and vulnerabilities) that individuals bring to bereavement, though these of course both presuppose basic neurological processes (Gundel et al. 2003) and are in turn nested within broader family interactions (Hooghe and Neimeyer 2012) and social/cultural structures (Neimeyer et al. 2013) involved in processing and integrating the loss.

One of the clearest and best researched implications of the MS model concerns just interface where abiding meanings meet with apparent challenge and invalidation. As Park notes:

> [W]hen individuals encounter potentially stressful or traumatic events, they assign a meaning to them… and trauma is thought to occur when appraised meanings "shatter" or violate aspects of one's global meaning system. (2013: 360)

The death of a loved one certainly ranks high on the list of potentially traumatic events, and can carry serious consequences for survivors at the levels of both symptomatology and life significance. The struggles that can attend bereavement are painfully apparent in our research on African Americans who have lost a loved one to homicide. Studying a group of 54 survivors on average less than 2 years from the death, we discovered that more than half struggled with intensely complicated grief marked by preoccupation with the death, the sense that a part of *themselves* had died, and an inability to function in the spheres of family, work, and the social world. Nearly as many suffered clinically significant depression, and almost 20 % met criteria for a diagnosis of posttraumatic stress disorder (PTSD), whether or not they were present when their loved one was killed. Importantly, the majority contended with more than one of these syndromes; nearly all of those with PTSD, for example, also tested positive for depression and complicated grief. However, it is worth noting that even in the wake of this horrific loss, a resilient 37 % somehow emerged with none of these diagnoses (McDevitt-Murphy et al. 2012).

What role does the search for meaning play in accommodation to such horrific loss? Evidence from our research on general meaning making suggests that the answer is "a great deal." For example, one study of over 1,000 ethnically diverse young adults confirmed the significantly greater complication that followed the shattering impact of violent death (by homicide, suicide, or fatal accident) than of natural death losses, even when the latter were sudden and unanticipated. Consistent with our rationale, however, meaning making emerged as an explanatory mechanism for the difference in outcome following these forms of loss, as an inability to make sense of the loss functioned as a nearly perfect mediator of this relationship (Currier et al. 2006). Even in the case of the loss of a partner to natural causes in late life, an anguished search for meaning that extended 6 or more months prospectively predicted exacerbated grief and depression several months or years later (Coleman and Neimeyer 2010).

Fortunately, whether in the context of formal psychotherapy or simply in the course of living, most survivors ultimately accommodate the unwelcome transitions introduced by many kinds of losses (Currier et al. 2008; Neimeyer and Currier 2009). Here too, current research from a meaning-based perspective is beginning to illuminate some of the underlying processes in accommodation. For example, a study of bereaved parents demonstrates that the ability to make sense of the loss is a potent predictor of grief symptomatology, accounting for five times the variance in normative grief symptoms (e.g., missing the loved one, crying) and 15 times the variance in complicated grief responses (e.g., feeling that the future is bleached of purpose, being unable to function in one's work) as other factors, such as the passage of time or whether the death was violent or natural (Keesee et al. 2008).

Particular patterns of meaning making triggered by different causes of death (e.g., violent vs. natural) also have been reported (Lichtenthal et al. 2013). The salutary effect of sense making is further supported in longitudinal research on older widows and widowers; those who are better able to find significance in the loss by 6 months report higher levels of positive emotion and wellbeing as much as 4 years into the future (Coleman and Neimeyer 2010). These and several other studies by our group (see Neimeyer and Sands 2011, for review) comport with Park's argument that

> the meaning making process helps people reduce their sense of discrepancy between appraised and global meanings and restore a sense that the world is comprehensible and that their lives are worthwhile. (2013: 360)

9.3   Religion and Meaning Making in the Context of Loss

In many communities and cultures, as Park (2013) also recognizes, meaning making in the wake of loss naturally involves recourse to religious and spiritual beliefs. These provide a sense of divine purpose in or consolation for the death of a loved one. This was certainly the case in our sample of parents struggling with the death of a child. Beyond the general relation between sense making and improved adjustment, our systematic coding of parents' narrative responses suggested patterns of meaning that were especially associated with better outcomes, including viewing the death as congruent with God's will, endorsing the prospect for reunion in an afterlife, and the (potentially more secular) belief that the child was no longer suffering. Likewise, better accommodation of the loss was reported by parents who found unsought spiritual benefits in the tragedy (e.g., deepened faith, the prospect of reunion in an afterlife), who realigned life priorities, or who dedicated themselves to needed lifestyle changes (Lichtenthal et al. 2010).

When such meaning making proves elusive, evidence suggests the impact can be severe in terms of survivors' spiritual and psychological wellbeing. For a substantial subset of the predominantly Christian, African American homicide survivors we studied, the murder of their loved one not only ushered in depression, PTSD, and complicated grief, but it also gave rise to *complicated spiritual grief*, understood as an intense form of spiritual struggle precipitated by the death. When it occurred, complicated spiritual grief often suggested a disruption in the mourner's relationship to God, as illustrated by the comments of one 69-year-old woman grieving her grandson's murder:

> I felt that God had allowed the capriciousness of life to invade our world. I wondered aloud if our entire family and our belief system were merely a cosmic joke. I questioned why God permitted such a painful and horrendous act when he had the power to stop it.

For others, the complication arose from changed relationships with fellow church members. Another 59-year-old woman spoke of the aftermath of her husband's homicide:

> I thought I could rely on my church community, but they grew tired of trying to console me and took advantage of my vulnerability. They said they would be there for me, but I didn't know there would be a time limit.

For many survivors, the two forms of struggle were conjoined, becoming a constellation of "negative religious coping" (Koenig et al. 1998) that compounded the literal loss with a symbolic and social one. We have subsequently documented the association between such spiritual struggle and poor grief outcomes in ethnically diverse, but predominantly Christian, samples grieving a variety of natural and violent deaths (Burke and Neimeyer 2014).

Longitudinal study of the relation between attempts at religious meaning making and distress has also begun to suggest some interesting overlap. For example, tracing the adaptation of the African American homicide survivors across 6 months, we discovered that complicated grief at Time 1 prospectively predicted complicated *spiritual* grief at Time 2, suggesting that the violent sundering of attachment associated with this horrific loss also undermined a sense of meaning and relationship with God and the spiritual community in the months that followed. Interestingly, the reverse was not the case. Spiritual struggle earlier in bereavement did not portend later complicated grief. Nor, to our surprise, was "positive religious coping" in the form of grounding oneself in one's beliefs or turning to God or coreligionists for consolation predictive of less complicated grief (Burke et al. 2011), a finding we have replicated in other samples (Burke and Neimeyer 2014). Further study has demonstrated that neither Time 1 depression nor PTSD forecasts spiritual struggles at Time 2; instead, intense grief uniquely seemed to provide the instigating context for such crisis (Neimeyer and Burke 2011).

The absence of a clear link between positive religious coping and attenuated grief notwithstanding, a strong spiritual orientation may nonetheless predispose to positive bereavement outcomes in another sense: those who self-identify as religious and who practice their tradition tend to report greater post-loss growth in our studies, as do those who mourn a violent death as opposed to a natural death (Currier et al. 2012). Thus, while religiousness might not mitigate the pain of loss, it may nevertheless set the stage for greater growth through the experience.

9.4   Methodological Contributions

If research is to do more than document the existence of global suffering, and even hope to illuminate the mechanisms that exacerbate or ameliorate suffering, then appropriate methods are required to render these visible and open to analysis. From a psychological standpoint, the concept of meaning systems holds promise, but only if psychometrically valid and existentially relevant methods are devised to do so. Here, I summarize some of our own attempts to construct such methods, several of which are currently being translated to permit their application and adaptation to other cultural settings.

Park and Paloutzian (2013), too, argue for a "multilevel methodology," rightly recognizing that methodologically distinctive studies—such as those using quantitative questionnaires, qualitative interviews, and experimental research—when converging on similar conclusions, contribute to the identification of more robust principles than do those relying on a single methodological base. In keeping with this principle, and to augment the fairly narrow range of measures currently available to advance the MS research agenda in bereavement studies, we have constructed a number of quantitative and qualitative assessments of relevant constructs to which I will briefly orient the reader.

9.4.1   Assessing General Meaning Systems

Because my colleagues and I have been interested in the role of meaning systems in general in helping people accommodate unwelcome life transitions and losses, we have developed both quantitative and qualitative approaches to the assessment of meaning amenable to both secular and spiritual contexts.

9.4.2   Inventory of Stressful Life Experiences Scale

One such measure is the 16-item *Inventory of Stressful Life Experiences Scale*, or ISLES (Holland et al. 2010). This is an easy-to-use, multidimensional, and well-validated measure of the meaning made after a stressful life event. In two samples of young Americans—178 who experienced a variety of stressors and 150 who experienced a recent bereavement—ISLES scores were shown to have strong internal consistency and, among a subsample of participants, to exhibit moderate test–retest reliability. In both samples, support was also found for a 2-factor structure, with one factor assessing one's sense of *Footing in the World* (e.g., "This event made me feel less purposeful") and a second measuring the *Comprehensibility* of the event (e.g., "I am perplexed by what happened"). Convergent validity analyses revealed that ISLES scores are also strongly associated with other theoretically related measures and with mental and physical health outcomes, offering support for the potential utility of this measure in research and clinical settings. Subsequent research on a large sample of 741 bereaved adults confirmed the factor structure of the scale in both its original and in an abbreviated 6-item form and demonstrated the incremental validity of both formats in predicting health and mental health outcomes even after such factors as demographics, circumstances of the death, and prolonged grief symptoms were taken into account (Holland et al. 2014).

9.4.3 Meaning in Loss Codebook

A complementary approach to meaning assessment is grounded in the qualitative analysis of the narrative responses of a diverse sample of 162 mourners. The study concerned the survivors' attempts to make sense of loss and find some compensatory benefit in the experience. The result was the development of the *Meaning in Loss Codebook*, or MLC (Gillies et al. 2014), a reliable and comprehensive coding system for analyzing meanings made in the wake of the death of a loved one. The MLC encompasses 30 specific categories of meaning made, demonstrating excellent reliability and comprising both negative (e.g., *Lack of Understanding*, *Regret*) and positive (e.g., *Compassion*, *Moving On*) themes that arise. The MLC could thus prove useful in ethnographic or laboratory research on meaning making as expressed in interviews in the wake of political violence or natural disaster, analysis of naturalistic first-person writing about bereavement experiences in grief diaries and blogs, communal accounts of shared losses, and clinical assessment of meanings made in the course of bereavement support or professional intervention. A further advantage of such a narrative coding system is that it does not require literacy (though, like other methods described in this paper, the MLC would require translation and probable adaptation to capture the nuances of meaning-making in different cultural settings).

9.4.4 Assessing Spiritual Struggle

Although we have found general measures of religious coping (Hill and Pargament 2008) useful in studying the spiritual struggle that often follows the death of a loved one, we have ultimately found it valuable to develop a measure specifically validated for use with bereaved populations. The result is the *Inventory of Complicated Spiritual Grief* or ICSG (Burke et al. 2014a). With two diverse samples of bereaved adult Christians (total = 304), we found that the ICSG had strong internal consistency and high test-retest reliability for its constituent subscales in a subsample of participants. Analyses of both samples supported a 2-factor model, with one factor measuring *Insecurity with God* (e.g., "I don't understand why God has made it so hard for me") and the other assessing *Disruption in Religious Practice* (e.g., "I go out of my way to avoid spiritual/religious activities [prayer, worship, Bible reading]"). Analyses further supported the convergent and incremental validity of the 18-item ICSG relative to other theoretically similar instruments and to measures of poor bereavement outcome. This suggests its specific relevance to studying spiritual crisis in bereavement.

Finally, as with our general assessment of meaning systems, we have pursued qualitative research that fleshes out our understanding of the meanings made in the context of spiritual struggle (Burke et al. 2014b). Using 84 participants' written responses to open-ended questions along with systematic exploration of this topic with a focus group, we conducted a directed content analysis. This revealed 17 different themes subsumed in an overarching narrative of resentment and doubt toward God, dissatisfaction with the spiritual support received, and substantial changes in the bereaved person's spiritual beliefs and behaviors. Thus, the study clarified the construct of complicated spiritual grief and laid the groundwork for the development of more specific study and treatment of this condition.

9.5 Conclusion

To an even greater extent than the measures of general meaning making described above, methods bearing on spiritual meaning making are particularly likely to be culture specific. For example, both the ICSG and the qualitative study described here concentrated on the spiritual struggles of Christian samples, both black and white, most of whom presumed a personal relationship with a beneficent deity they construed as watching over them. They were typically quite active, at least prior to the death of their loved one, in their church communities.

The generalization of our findings to other cultural or religious settings can be legitimated only by study of the relevant groups, and should not be assumed in advance. For example, although a sense of anger and betrayal by God following the unjust killing of a loved might characterize survivors from other monotheistic traditions that feature an omnipotent God who hears our prayers—as in Judaism or Islam—spiritual struggle is likely to take different forms in religious traditions such as Buddhism or Hinduism. Similarly, in a world that is increasingly secular, challenges to a world of meaning occasioned by loss are likely to take more psychological, naturalistic, and social forms. Given this, forms of therapeutic intervention relying on a broad range of psychological (Neimeyer 2012) and expressive arts (Thompson and Neimeyer 2014) may prove effective across quite different personal and cultural systems of meaning and to be robust resources in addressing the world of suffering that can follow loss.

In conclusion, my colleagues and I are optimistic about the potential contributions of a meaning systems perspective as an integrative frame for studying the psychology of suffering. We are encouraged by the burgeoning research in this area and hope that our own line of investigation into the quest for meaning and spiritual significance in the wake of loss makes a modest contribution in the understanding and amelioration of suffering.

References

Bonanno, G. A. (2004). Loss, trauma and human resilience. *American Psychologist, 59*, 20–28.

Bonanno, G. A., Wortman, C. B., & Nesse, R. M. (2004). Prospective patterns of resilience and maladjustment during widowhood. *Psychology and Aging, 19*, 260–271.

Burke, L. A., & Neimeyer, R. A. (2014). Complicated spiritual grief I: Relation to complicated grief symptomatology following violent death bereavement. *Death Studies, 38*, 1–9. doi:10.10 80/07481187.2013.829372.

Burke, L. A., Neimeyer, R. A., McDevitt-Murphy, M. E., Ippolito, M. R., & Roberts, J. M. (2011). In the wake of homicide: Spiritual crisis and bereavement distress in an African American sample. *International Journal Psychology of Religion, 21*, 289–307.

Burke, L. A., Neimeyer, R. A., Holland, J. M., Dennard, S., Oliver, L., & Shear, M. K. (2014a). Inventory of complicated spiritual grief: Development and validation of a new measure. *Death Studies, 38*, 1–12. doi:10.1080/07481187.2013.810098.

Burke, L. A., Neimeyer, R. A., Young, A. J., & Piazza-Bonin, E. (2014b). Complicated spiritual grief II: A deductive inquiry following the loss of a loved one. *Death Studies, 38*, 1–14. doi:10.1080/07481187.2013.829373.

Coleman, R. A., & Neimeyer, R. A. (2010). Measuring meaning: Searching for and making sense of spousal loss in later life. *Death Studies, 34*, 804–834.

Currier, J. M., Holland, J. M., & Neimeyer, R. A. (2006). Sense making, grief and the experience of violent loss: Toward a mediational model. *Death Studies, 30*, 403–428.

Currier, J. M., Neimeyer, R. A., & Berman, J. S. (2008). The effectiveness of psychotherapeutic interventions for the bereaved: A comprehensive quantitative review. *Psychological Bulletin, 134*, 648–661.

Currier, J. M., Malott, J., Martinez, T. E., Sandy, C., & Neimeyer, R. A. (2012). Bereavement, religion and posttraumatic growth: A matched control group investigation. *Psychology of Religion and Spirituality, 18*, 65–71.

Gillies, J., Neimeyer, R. A., & Milman, E. (2014). The meaning of loss codebook: Construction of a system for analyzing meanings made in bereavement. *Death Studies, 38*, 1–10. doi:10.1080/ 07481187.2013.829367.

Gundel, H., O'Conner, M., Littrell, L., Fort, C., & Lane, R. (2003). Functional neuroanatomy of grief: An fMRI study. *American Journal of Psychiatry, 160*, 1946–1953.

Hill, P. C., & Pargament, K. I. (2008). Advances in the conceptualization and measurement of religion and spirituality: Implications for physical and mental health research. *Psychology of Religion and Spirituality, 1*, 2–17.

Holland, J. M., Currier, J. M., Coleman, R. A., & Neimeyer, R. A. (2010). The integration of stressful life experiences scale (ISLES): Development and initial validation of a new measure. *International Journal of Stress Management, 17*, 325–352.

Holland, J. M., Currier, J. M., & Neimeyer, R. A. (2014). Validation of the integration of stressful life experiences scale – Short form in a bereaved sample. *Death Studies, 38*, 1–5. doi:10.1080/ 07481187.2013.829369.

Hooghe, A., & Neimeyer, R. A. (2012). Family resilience in the wake of loss: A meaning-oriented contribution. In D. Becvar (Ed.), *Handbook of family resilience*. New York: Springer.

Keesee, N. J., Currier, J. M., & Neimeyer, R. A. (2008). Predictors of grief following the death of one's child: The contribution of finding meaning. *Journal of Clinical Psychology, 64*, 1145–1163.

Kelly, G. A. (1955). *The psychology of personal constructs*. New York: Norton.

Koenig, H. G., Pargament, K. I., & Nielsen, J. (1998). Religious coping and health status in medically ill hospitalized older adults. *Journal of Nervous and Mental Disease, 186*, 513–521.

Lichtenthal, W. G., Currier, J. M., Neimeyer, R. A., & Keesee, N. J. (2010). Sense and significance: A mixed methods examination of meaning-making following the loss of one's child. *Journal of Clinical Psychology, 66*, 791–812.

Lichtenthal, W. G., Neimeyer, R. A., Currier, J. M., Roberts, K., & Jordan, N. (2013). Cause of death and the quest for meaning after the loss of a child. *Death Studies, 37*, 327–342.

McDevitt-Murphy, M. E., Neimeyer, R. A., Burke, L. A., & Williams, J. L. (2012). Assessing the toll of traumatic loss: Psychological symptoms in African Americans bereaved by homicide. *Psychological Trauma, 4*(3), 303–311.

Merleau-Ponty, M. (1962). *Phenomenology of perception*. London: Routledge & Kegan Paul.

Neimeyer, R. A. (2000). Searching for the meaning of meaning: Grief therapy and the process of reconstruction. *Death Studies, 24*, 541–558.

Neimeyer, R. A. (Ed.). (2001). *Meaning reconstruction and the experience of loss*. Washington, DC: American Psychological Association.

Neimeyer, R. A. (2002). *Lessons of loss: A guide to coping*. Memphis: Center for the Study of Loss and Transition.

Neimeyer, R. A. (2004). Fostering posttraumatic growth: A narrative contribution. *Psychological Inquiry, 15*, 53–59.

Neimeyer, R. A. (2006). Widowhood, grief and the quest for meaning: A narrative perspective on resilience. In D. Carr, R. M. Nesse, & C. B. Wortman (Eds.), *Spousal bereavement in late life* (pp. 227–252). New York: Springer.

Neimeyer, R. A. (2009). *Constructivist psychotherapy*. London/New York: Routledge.

Neimeyer, R. A. (2011). Reconstructing the self in the wake of loss: A dialogical contribution. In H. Hermans & T. Gieser (Eds.), *Handbook on the dialogical self*. Cambridge: Cambridge University Press.

Neimeyer, R. A. (Ed.). (2012). *Techniques of grief therapy: Creative practices for counseling the bereaved*. New York: Routledge.

Neimeyer, R. A., & Burke, L. A. (2011). Complicated grief in the aftermath of homicide: Spiritual crisis and distress in an African American sample. *Religions, 2*, 145–164.

Neimeyer, R. A., & Currier, J. M. (2009). Grief therapy: Evidence of efficacy and emerging directions. *Current Directions in Psychological Science, 18*, 252–256.

Neimeyer, R. A., & Sands, D. C. (2011). Meaning reconstruction in bereavement: From principles to practice. In R. A. Neimeyer, H. Winokuer, D. Harris, & G. Thornton (Eds.), *Grief and bereavement in contemporary society: Bridging research and practice*. New York: Routledge.

Neimeyer, R. A., Klass, D., & Dennis, M. R. (2013). Mourning, meaning and memory: Individual, communal and cultural narration of grief. In A. Batthyany & P. Russo-Netzer (Eds.), *Meaning in existential and positive psychology*. New York: Springer.

Paloutzian, R. F., & Park, C. L. (2013). Recent progress and core issues in the science of the psychology of religion and spirituality. In R. F. Paloutzian & C. L. Park (Eds.), *Handbook of the psychology of religion and spirituality* (2nd ed.). New York: Springer.

Park, C. L. (2013). Religion and meaning. In R. F. Paloutzian & C. L. Park (Eds.), *Handbook of the psychology of religion and spirituality* (2nd ed., pp. 357–379). New York: Springer.

Park, C. L., & Paloutzian, R. F. (2013). Directions for the future of the psychology of religion and spirituality. In R. F. Paloutzian & C. L. Park (Eds.), *Handbook of the psychology of religion and spirituality* (2nd ed., pp. 651–665). New York: Springer.

Thompson, B. E., & Neimeyer, R. A. (2014). *Grief and the expressive arts: Practices for creating meaning*. New York: Routledge.

Chapter 10
Coping with the Suffering of Ambiguous Loss

Pauline Boss

10.1 Introduction

Ambiguous loss has no resolution or closure. Unlike with death, there is no official verification of loss, no funeral or rituals of support, and no ending for grief (Boss 1999, 2004, 2006; Boss and Greenberg 1984). There are two types of ambiguous loss. In the first, the missing person is *physically absent* but kept psychologically present in the minds of family and friends, because there is no proof of death and their whereabouts are unknown. Examples are loved ones kidnapped, politically disappeared, vanished in explosions such as New York's 9/11 or from nature's fury—swept away by tsunamis, earthquakes, or landslides. In the second type, a family member is *psychologically absent* while physically present. They are "here, but gone," as in the case of Alzheimer's disease, autism, severe mental illness, or addiction, among others. The first type of ambiguous loss—the *physically missing*—is the subject of this chapter.[1]

Here I address the relentless pain of not knowing the physical whereabouts or fate of a loved one who has been kidnapped or disappeared. With no body to bury or proof that the loss is permanent, families understandably maintain some hope. As a result, grief is frozen, decisions are postponed, and relationships remain in limbo (Boss 1999, 2006). Having to live with such uncertainty embodies a kind of suffering that terrorists now know wounds and tortures families longer than even the horror of a witnessed killing. Unending suffering becomes chronic sorrow (Boss et al. 2011; Roos 2002), often lasting a lifetime or even across generations. Adding to the agony, the family's grief is disenfranchised (Doka 1989), because no one died. In

---

[1] For more information about Type II ambiguous loss, psychologically absent while physically present, see Boss (1999, 2004, 2006); Boss and Dahl (2014).

P. Boss (✉)
Family Social Science Department, University of Minnesota, Minneapolis, MN 55455, USA
e-mail: pboss@umn.edu

© Springer Science+Business Media Dordrecht 2015   125
R.E. Anderson (ed.), *World Suffering and Quality of Life*,
Social Indicators Research Series 56, DOI 10.1007/978-94-017-9670-5_10

the eyes of the law, religious institutions, and the larger community, ambiguous loss is not real. Families cope alone.

The suffering from ambiguous loss is all too often attributed to the pathology of the remaining family members. While individuals often exhibit symptoms of depression and anxiety, and families exhibit more conflict and secrets, the source of pathology lies in the external social context, not in personal deficits, despite how families are treated when suffering ambiguous loss. With no script or rituals for moving forward with ambiguous loss, and with no ending to the loss story, the family's plight is akin to what Frost and Hoggett (2008) call "double suffering": first, a loved one is lost, and second, never found.

Today, this suffering is caused globally by genocide, war, terrorism, crime, and natural disasters (Boss 2006; Faust 2008; Robins 2013; Sluzki 1990, 2003, 2006). Such losses are redoubled by the agonizing doubt that comes with the inability to "know" a loved one's fate. I think of T. S. Eliot who, perhaps because of his wife's institutionalization, wrote, "And what you do not know is the only thing you know."[2] Indeed, this paradox lies at the center of the pain from ambiguous loss.

10.2   Brief Background

The theory of ambiguous loss was introduced to the social sciences in the 1970s (Boss 1977, 1980a, b, 1987; Boss and Greenberg 1984). Since, it has been applied and tested with families of physically missing loved ones, e.g., pilots missing in action (MIA) in Vietnam and Southeast Asia; families of workers who vanished after the 2001 World Trade Center terrorist attacks (Boss 2002; Boss et al. 2003); and most recently, with the villages and families of men and boys kidnapped in Nepal and East Timor (Robins 2010, 2013).

Ideas about ambiguous loss are now linked across disciplines to resilience and trauma (Becvar 2012; Boss 2006) as well as grief and loss (Neimeyer 2015; Neimeyer et al. 2011), chronic sorrow (Boss et al. 2011), and humanitarian work globally (Robins 2010, 2013). Perhaps most important, the theory has been recognized as a model for bridging science and practice (Neimeyer and Harris 2011; Neimeyer et al. 2011).

10.3   Effects of Ambiguous Loss on Families and Individuals

From a systems perspective, ambiguous loss has a negative effect on families *structurally* when parent or spousal roles are ignored, decisions are put on hold, daily tasks are left undone, and family members are fighting or alienated, cut off from one another's support. Customary family rituals and celebrations are cancelled, thus inhibiting essential meaning-making processes. Ambiguous loss has a negative

---

[2] From "Four Quartets." Eliot (1980).

effect on individuals *psychologically* when there are feelings of hopelessness and helplessness that lead to guilt, anxiety, depression, or life-threatening behaviors (Boss 2006).

Overall, the most frequent stressor reported, individually and collectively, is the impossibility of closure. People are held in a state of uncertainty, oscillating between hope and despair. They understandably resist change, because they still hope to find the missing person and continue with life as it was "before." Their lives are frozen in a complexity of loss. Even just a bone providing DNA verification would give some clarity, some measure of peace.

To ease the suffering, a multi-disciplinary stress-based approach is essential. In *sociological* terms, ambiguous loss is a stressor that prevents the maintenance of family boundaries. In *psychoanalytic* terms, it is an uncanny loss that combines the known and the unknown to violate one's trust in reality (Feigelson 1993). In *psychological* terms, it severely complicates the search for meaning, a necessary component in easing the pain of any loss (Boss 2006; Frankl 1963; Neimeyer 2015; Neimeyer and Sands 2011). All of these approaches are valid.

10.4 Cultural Differences

In more Westernized cultures, which tend to be more mastery-oriented, the assumption is that every problem has a solution. This is impossible with ambiguous loss. Instead, we need to increase our tolerance for ambiguity.

After decades of working with families of the missing and training other therapists, I find that the more people are accustomed to mastery, having agency, being in charge, and being able to solve problems, the more they seem to suffer from ambiguous loss. For example, many New Yorkers accustomed to finding answers were stunned and even angry just weeks after 9/11, when families of the missing continued to hope that their loved ones would turn up alive somewhere (a few actually did). Perhaps because the pain was so raw, there was little patience for lingering; New Yorkers wanted closure and the ambiguous grief of others was a constant reminder of something many wanted to move past. A year later, a New York reporter asked me why I thought New Yorkers weren't over 9/11 yet. My answer: "Because you're trying to get over it." Paradoxically, as T. S. Eliot suggests, what we do not know about a missing loved one becomes *all* that we know. Living in this void, those who persist in trying to master ambiguity will suffer more. Another poet, John Keats, recommended in his letters to a young poet that he develop a capability for the void. He called this "negative capability" (Forman 1935).[3]

While Western poets address ambiguity, it is a more integral part of Eastern cultural practices. There, values of mastery, independence, and self-sufficiency are considered barriers to the reduction of suffering. Eastern views encourage us to find a "way beyond the excesses of rationality and individualism" (Mishra 2004: 51).

---

[3] Portions of this paragraph appeared in *The Guardian* Op Ed, "The Pain of Flight MH370 Lies in Its Ambiguity," by Pauline Boss, on March 18, 2014.

This appears to be more useful when individuals' problems are irrational and have no solution. For those who live with ambiguous loss, the goal is not to get rid of suffering, but to allow for its coexistence with some joy in a life well lived.

Recently, Simon Robins with the International Committee of the Red Cross and Red Crescent (ICRC) tested the theory of ambiguous loss in the Eastern cultures of Nepal and East Timor (Robins 2010, 2013). While the theory of ambiguous loss was found more useful than the truth and reconciliation model previously used, he also found that one intervention component, tempering mastery, did not hold in patriarchal cultures where wives of kidnapped men were left without identity or status. Robins concluded that to survive, their mastery did not have to be tempered, but heightened.[4]

What we learn from Robins is that the theory of ambiguous loss, corrected to include his finding, provides a useful framework for guiding interventions with families of the missing in both Eastern as well as Westernized cultures. Where people are more mastery-oriented, their suffering will be eased if interventions lower their expectations for finding clear and absolute solutions. Where people are disenfranchised and have little or no mastery, interventions to ease suffering must empower.

The degree of suffering from ambiguous loss is highly influenced by the cultural belief systems of family members and the community frame (Boss 2006; Goffman 1974; Reiss and Oliveri 1991; Robins 2013). What the powerful demand or what the neighbors think will still influence how families perceive loss and whether they receive social support for living well, despite the ambiguity. Especially with problems that have no solution, human suffering can be lowered if the community as a whole acknowledges that the family's anguish is justifiable. One of the most effective ways is local memorializing (Robins 2013). The names of the missing are displayed in the village square so that families are no longer alone in their suffering and have a sanctioned place to mourn in lieu of a grave. The 9/11 Memorial in Lower Manhattan is a fine example.

10.5   Interventions to Ease the Suffering of Ambiguous Loss

10.5.1   Setting the Stage

10.5.1.1   Family and Community Meetings

For most families experiencing ambiguous loss, the most effective support mechanism is meeting with peers—other families with missing persons (Boss et al. 2003; Robins 2010: 261). For this reason, it is best not to rely solely on medical treatment, and instead, look beyond symptoms of pathology to further assess the social and relational environment. People with missing loved ones often fit the diagnoses of

---

[4] As a result of Robins' findings, I have adjusted Guideline #2, "Tempering Mastery," and re-titled it "Adjusting Mastery," which can mean either raising or lowering one's mastery orientation, depending on the culture.

depression or complicated grief, but they are having a typical reaction to an atypical loss. Diagnostic manuals do list atypical losses, such as suicide or death of a baby, but the atypical loss of ambiguous loss should also be added to this list.[5]

To hold family meetings, find a familiar community setting like a school, church basement, or community hall. In the case of families of New York workers missing after 9/11, it was their labor union hall in Lower Manhattan. Families were self-defined, yet part of the same community (the union) and with the same type of loss. When families travel long distances, offer them food and beverages upon arrival and before leaving for home. The group ideally is comprised of multiple families, often three generations. Early on, it is essential to triage to determine if anyone needs medical treatment. After this, people sit in a large common circle to listen to each other's stories. These narratives, surprisingly, are not just focused on suffering, but also on resilience and survival. The elders in such groups are especially helpful to the younger participants because they know the cultural traditions of the group, and can enlighten, if not guide, the intervention team, and second, having faced hardship and suffering in their earlier years and survived, they know what resilience is and can share what helped them to become stronger despite adversity.

10.5.1.2 The Psychological Family

We are reminded, however, that one's family and community may *not* always be helpful and empowering. Some family members may be judgmental and shaming; others may stay away because they feel helpless in the face of unclear loss. Still others may be part of families and communities where strict social traditions and mores are barriers to coping, especially for women and girls. Without positive support from family members, the person suffering ambiguous loss needs what I have called a *psychological family* (Boss 1999, 2006): a *chosen* family of empathic and supportive peers. With the previously discussed wives of kidnapped men who were now neither wife nor widow, support and empowerment was found only by joining a "psychological family" with other women experiencing the same type of loss (Robins 2013).

10.5.1.3 Dialectical Thinking

With ambiguous loss and its lack of facts, meaning will not emerge from absolute thinking. Rather, it comes from being able to hold two opposing ideas at the same time (Fitzgerald 1945). Dialectical thinking indicates a cognitive shift toward

---

[5]To ease the pain of ambiguous loss, traditional grief therapies are insufficient: the family will resist the fact of death and the idea of closure. They will exhibit symptoms of unresolved grief, but that may reflect a normal sadness, not depression. While the treatment for depression is often medication, the treatment for sadness is human connection. Such connection lies beyond that of therapist and patient; it requires a steady community connection to the people in one's everyday life—relatives, friends, and neighbors (Boss 2006; Landau 2007; Robins 2010; Saul 2013).

multiple meanings—the only way one can make sense of the incongruence of absence and presence. Decades after her boy was kidnapped, a mother says, "He's probably dead… but maybe not." A year after 9/11, the father of a missing electrician told me, "My son has been missing so long now. He's probably dead. But I feel he's here with me and always will be." Such ability to hold conflicting ideas provides the resilience to ease suffering even while ambiguity persists (Boss 2006: 91). Given the absurdity of ambiguous loss, the meaning that promotes emotional growth and well-being comes from holding a complexity of possibilities, not one absolute truth.

10.5.2 Six Guidelines for Living with Ambiguous Loss

The following guidelines are useful both in family meetings and psychotherapy settings. The guidelines are not linear; they can be used in any order. Space allows only a brief description here, but each of the six guidelines is described in depth in Boss (2006).

10.5.2.1 Finding Meaning

When facts are unavailable, perceptions are the only window for change and easing the stress of ambiguity (Boss 1992, 1999, 2006). Families of the missing desperately want an explanation (Robins 2010). Was he killed? Did she suffer? Where is his body? Is she still alive in prison somewhere? Most often, answers are elusive, so meaning has to be socially constructed.

The first step is to name the problem. Keep it simple: "What you are experiencing is an ambiguous loss. It's one of the most stressful kinds of loss because there is no possibility of closure. This is not your fault. The problem is the ambiguity, not you." This is called *externalizing the blame* (White and Epston 1990).

Providing people a name for their pain provides some understanding that it is not their fault and thus allows for movement. As Viktor Frankl said, "Suffering ceases to be suffering as soon as we form a clear and precise picture of it" (1963: 117; in Boss 2006: 90). The picture for these families may not be that clear, but once named, the agonizing doubt can be acknowledged by the larger community. Survivors feel less alone. This is the power of family- and community-based interventions—they provide human connections that, unlike psychotherapy, can continue back in the neighborhood and validate, day-to-day, that one's loss is real.

The beliefs and values of the people we work with usually differ from our own, so always ask: "What does this situation mean to you?" Some believe it is a punishment from God; some believe it is a challenge that they can meet; others believe in fatalism (what will be, will be), destiny, karma, or a spiritual acceptance by trusting and having faith in God or Allah. Still others believe in the harmony of nature and are more sanguine with what they cannot see or prove. Robins (2010) found that for some families in East Timor who believed in a spirit world, the dreams of the healer or a family member erased all doubts about the fate of a missing person: "Many interpreted repeated dreams of the disappeared as evidence that the missing person was still alive and that his spirit was communicating" (Robins 2010: 262).

While such thinking may ease the suffering in the short term, it is likely not useful long term. When religious beliefs are insistent about absolute truth (e.g., alive or dead), the family is more brittle. Missing family members are "closed out" and considered dead and in a "better place" now. Such closure is concocted, however, and can cause even more pain, because secrets and silence are needed to keep the door closed. Sooner or later, a younger family member discovers the story of the family's missing person and feels betrayed for not having been told.

10.5.2.2 Adjusting Mastery

People accustomed to being in charge of their own destinies understandably try to stop pain by seeking closure. They want to stay in charge. They use the best technology, but in the end, their lost person may remain lost. To balance living with the unmanageability of ambiguous loss, we encourage the suffering to find something in their lives that they can control. For empowerment and agency, we must allow people with missing family members "to choose their own forms of both expression and action" (Robins 2013: 172). For example, Robins found that some women from poor and marginalized communities "made the decision to believe that their disappeared husbands were dead and move on with their lives in what appears to be a conscious mastery of ambiguity" (2010: 263). This, too, is a way to empower oneself in the absence of truth.

10.5.2.3 Reconstructing Identity

Ambiguous loss is confusing, and family members no longer know who they are supposed to be. When someone goes missing, they wonder about their roles and status within the family and community. They ask, "Am I still a wife if my husband is missing? Am I still married?" Later on, we ask, "Who are you now? What roles do you play now? What could help you in doing this? Is there any gender, age, or generational discrimination or bias that makes reconstructing your identity more difficult?"

Telling and listening to stories and questions in interaction with others who suffer the same loss sets the stage for one's identity to be relationally changed. Who one "is" becomes gradually reconstructed through the symbolic interaction of language and rituals. Peers serve as "the looking glass" to discover who one is now, understanding that the missing person, in all probability, is not coming back (Boss 2006: 129).

10.5.2.4   Normalizing Ambivalence

Ambivalence, a term originated in 1911 by psychiatrist Eugen Bleuler, refers to conflicted feelings and emotions (Boss 2006: 144). But unlike psychiatric ambivalence, the ambivalence from ambiguous loss is sociological (Merton and Barber 1963). It ruptures relationships and confuses people. As a result, the ambiguity feeds the ambivalence about which action to follow, which decisions to make, what roles to play, and how to feel about the missing person. If feelings are too horrific—such as *wishing* the missing person dead, if only for closure—family members may suffer traumatizing stress.

   Ambivalence is an expected outcome of ambiguous loss. In the social sense, this means recognizing that others feel the same way. Predictably, there is a flood of conflicted emotions such as love for the missing person and also hate toward them, since their absence is causing so much suffering.

10.5.2.5   Revising Attachment

When someone vanishes without a trace, others feel abandoned. Their attachment is severed and now, painfully insecure. Re-connection is not possible, nor is grieving and closure. The family is in a double bind. Anxiety heightens. Revising attachment means using "both-and" thinking to break the immobilization. As we emphasize that closure is not expected, people are relieved to know that they can hang on while also moving forward. We repeat over and over again: There is no *need* for closure. It is, after all, not the attachment that ends, just the relationship as it once was.

10.5.2.6   Finding New Hope

Paradoxically, telling family members that closure is not necessary helps them focus on finding meaning and new hope. This takes time and is best done in the company of others who are experiencing a similar loss. By asking questions and sharing stories, people become more open to new interpretations of their struggle.

   People with missing loved ones often find hope in helping others to prevent such suffering. They discover a greater good and see their plight in a larger frame that can help others, even though they cannot help themselves. The mother of a kidnapped boy begins a national website that revolutionizes the speed at which information about missing children is posted worldwide; the nephew of an MIA WWII soldier renews the search to bring his uncle home, bringing attention to MIA soldiers in today's wars. Finding a greater good in one's life balances the nonsensical with a way to honor the missing person and help others to avoid such pain. The suffering then is not entirely in vain. There is new hope in it.

10.6 Summary

My goal within this chapter is to increase awareness of a unique kind of suffering—ambiguous loss—so that social science researchers and practitioners are more able to recognize this all too common phenomenon, name it, and ease human suffering.

What I see clinically and in the field is that the suffering of ambiguous loss can deepen people's humanity and, thus, their ability to have a good life. They live with the opposing ideas of pain for what they lost and joy for what they still have. While ambiguous loss is cruel, uncanny, irrational, confusing, and unrelenting, we can live well despite unanswered questions. Painful as that may be, especially for those of us accustomed to mastery, this newfound negative capability, as the poet John Keats put it, makes possible the coexistence of human suffering and well-being.

References

Becvar, D. (Ed.). (2012). *Handbook of family resilience*. New York: Springer.

Bleuler, E. (1911). *Dementia praecox oder gruppe der schizophrenien* [Dementia praecox or the group of schizophrenias]. Liepzig/Wien: Franz Deuticke.

Boss, P. (1977). A clarification of the concept of psychological father presence in families experiencing ambiguity of boundary. *Journal of Marriage and the Family, 39*(1), 141–151.

Boss, P. (1980a). Normative family stress: Family boundary changes across the life-span. *Family Relations, 29*(4), 445–450.

Boss, P. (1980b). The relationship of psychological father presence, wife's personal qualities, and wife/family dysfunction in families of missing fathers. *Journal of Marriage and the Family, 42*(3), 541–549.

Boss, P. (1987). Family stress: Perception and context. In M. Sussman & S. Steinmetz (Eds.), *Handbook of marriage and family* (pp. 695–723). New York: Plenum.

Boss, P. (1992). Primacy of perception in family stress theory and measurement. *Journal of Family Psychology, 6*(2), 113–119.

Boss, P. (1999). *Ambiguous loss: Learning to live with unresolved grief*. Cambridge, MA: Harvard University Press.

Boss, P. (2002). Ambiguous loss: Working with the families of the missing. *Family Process, 41*, 14–17.

Boss, P. (2004). Ambiguous loss. In F. Walsh & M. McGoldrick (Eds.), *Living beyond loss: Death in the family* (2nd ed., pp. 237–246). New York: Norton.

Boss, P. (2006). *Loss, trauma, and resilience: Therapeutic work with ambiguous loss*. New York: Norton.

Boss, P. (2014, March 18). The pain of flight MH370 lies in its ambiguity. *The Guardian*. Retrieved from: http://www.theguardian.com/commentisfree/2014/mar/18/flight-mh370-families-grief-ambiguity

Boss, P., & Dahl, C. M. (2014). Family therapy for the unresolved grief of ambiguous loss. In D. W. Kissane & F. Parnes (Eds.), *Bereavement care for families* (pp. 171–182). New York: Routledge.

Boss, P., & Greenberg, J. (1984). Family boundary ambiguity: A new variable in family stress theory. *Family Process, 23*(4), 535–546.

Boss, P., Beaulieu, L., Wieling, E., Turner, W., & LaCruz, S. (2003). Healing loss, ambiguity, and trauma: A community-based intervention with families of union workers missing after the 9/11 attack in New York City. *Journal of Marital and Family Therapy, 29*(4), 455–467.

Boss, P., Roos, S., & Harris, D. L. (2011). Grief in the midst of uncertainty and ambiguity. In R. A. Neimeyer, D. L. Harris, H. R. Winokuer, & G. F. Thornton (Eds.), *Grief and bereavement in contemporary society: Bridging research and practice* (pp. 163–175). New York: Taylor and Francis.

Doka, K. (1989). *Disenfranchised grief: Recognizing hidden sorrow*. New York: Lexington Books.

Eliot, T. S. (1980). *The complete poems and plays: 1909–1950*. New York: Harcourt Brace.

Faust, D. G. (2008). *The republic of suffering*. New York: Vintage Books.

Feigelson, C. (1993). Personality death, object loss, and the uncanny. *International Journal of Psychoanalysis, 74*(2), 331–345.

Fitzgerald, F. S. (1945). *The crack-up*. New York: New Directions.

Forman, M. H. (Ed.). (1935). *The letters of John Keats* (2nd ed.). New York: Oxford University Press.

Frankl, V. (1963). *Man's search for meaning*. New York: Washington Square.

Frost, L., & Hoggett, P. (2008). Human agency and social suffering. *Critical Social Policy, 28*(4), 438–460.

Goffman, E. (1974). *Frame analysis: An essay on the organization of experience*. New York: Harper & Row.

Landau, J. (2007). Enhancing resilience: Families and communities as agents for change. *Family Process, 46*, 351–365.

Merton, R. K., & Barber, E. (1963). Sociological ambivalence. In E. Tiryakian (Ed.), *Sociological theory: Values and sociocultural change* (pp. 91–120). New York: Free Press.

Mishra, P. (2004). *An end to suffering*. New York: Picador, Farrar, Straus, & Giroux.

Neimeyer, R. A. (2015). Meaning in bereavement. In R. E. Anderson (Ed.), *World suffering and quality of life* (pp. 115–124). New York: Springer.

Neimeyer, R. A., & Harris, D. L. (2011). Building bridges in bereavement research and practice: Some concluding reflections. In R. A. Neimeyer, D. L. Harris, H. R. Winokuer, & G. F. Thornton (Eds.), *Grief and bereavement in contemporary society: Bridging research and practice* (pp. 403–418). New York: Taylor and Francis.

Neimeyer, R. A., & Sands, D. C. (2011). Meaning reconstruction in bereavement: From principles to practice. In R. A. Neimeyer, D. L. Harris, H. R. Winokuer, & G. F. Thornton (Eds.), *Grief and bereavement in contemporary society: Bridging research and practice* (pp. 9–22). New York: Taylor and Francis.

Neimeyer, R. A., Harris, D. L., Winokuer, H. R., & Thornton, G. F. (Eds.). (2011). *Grief and bereavement in contemporary society: Bridging research and practice*. New York: Taylor and Francis.

Reiss, D., & Oliveri, M. E. (1991). The family's conception of accountability and competence: A new approach to the conceptualization and assessment of family stress. *Family Process, 30*(2), 193–214.

Robins, S. (2010). Ambiguous loss in a non-Western context: Families of the disappeared in post-conflict Nepal. *Family Relations, 59*, 253–268.

Robins, S. (2013). *Families of the missing: A test for contemporary approaches to transitional justice*. New York/London: Routledge Glasshouse.

Roos, S. (2002). *Chronic sorrow: A living loss*. New York: Brunner-Routledge.

Saul, J. (2013). *Collective trauma, collective healing: Promoting community resilience in the aftermath of disaster*. New York: Routledge.

Sluzki, C. E. (1990). Disappeared: Semantic and somatic effects of political repression in a family seeking therapy. *Family Process, 29*, 131–143. doi:10.1111/j.1545-5300.1990.00131.x.

Sluzki, C. (2003). The process toward reconciliation. In A. Chayes & M. Minow (Eds.), *Imagine coexistence: Restoring humanity after violent ethnic conflict* (pp. 21–31). Cambridge, MA: Jossey-Bass.

Sluzki, C. E. (2006). Foreword. In P. Boss (Ed.), *Loss, trauma, and resilience* (pp. xiii–xv). New York: Norton.

White, M., & Epston, D. (1990). *Narrative means to therapeutic ends*. New York: Norton.

Chapter 11
Social Suffering and an Approach to Professionals' Burnout

Graciela Tonon, Lia Rodriguez-de-la-Vega, and Inés Aristegui

11.1 Helping Professions

In their earliest iterations, professions and occupations of "helping" were associated with religion. Physicians, priests, and lawyers were dedicated to service and believed they had been "chosen." As their practices involved moral rules and values, these professionals often took oaths, such as the Hippocratic Oath, which exhorts physicians to "do no harm." Only in modernity have such professions been emancipated from the religious sphere and become more firmly grounded in autonomous ethics.

There are several characteristics that legitimize a profession: the ability of to provide services—exclusive or not—to certain social demands; the existence of institutions with the capacity to recruit these professionals (Montaño 2000); and additionally, professionals maintain standards of good practice and ethical behavior.

Every profession has a subjective dimension related to the "pride of producer" and includes both rights and duties and the social recognition of those functions (Offe 1982). Of course, money and lifestyle factor into our estimation of professions, as well. Regarding the orientations professionals develop around their working spheres and economic activity, Offe (1982) identifies two mechanisms that regulate the role work plays in personal organization: a pivot of a "proper" life (what should be done) or a necessary condition of survival.

The known "helping professions" differ from other work based on the social, material, and temporal uncertainty of the cases they handle, as well as their

G. Tonon (✉) • L. Rodriguez-de-la-Vega
CICS-Faculty of Social Sciences, Universidad de Palermo, Mario Bravo 1259,
Ciudad Autonoma de Buenos Aires C1175ABW, Argentina
e-mail: gracielatonon@hotmail.com; liadelavega@yahoo.com

I. Aristegui
Psychology Program, Faculty of Social Sciences, Universidad de Palermo,
Mario Bravo 1259, Ciudad Autonoma de Buenos Aires C1175ABW, Argentina

© Springer Science+Business Media Dordrecht 2015
R.E. Anderson (ed.), *World Suffering and Quality of Life*,
Social Indicators Research Series 56, DOI 10.1007/978-94-017-9670-5_11

heterogeneity. Additionally, this work responds to a wholly different set of metrics than most professions. Its utility is not based on technical function or criteria for needs that must be met, largely because the outcomes of such work are often subjective and based on the self-evaluation of quality of life—if a patient or client feels satisfied with the work, the professional "helper" has done their job. Indeed, success in a helping profession may change the client's goals, creating a new marker of success; an improvement in quality of life may allow for new avenues of exploration and growth and change the care relationship.

Another distinguishing feature of the helping professions is that professionals in these areas work with people experiencing personal and social suffering. In this way, care professionals unavoidably experience some level of social suffering, too.

11.2   Method

During the months of July and August of 2013 we conducted an informal, anonymous and voluntary consultation of professionals serving people in situations of suffering. A message was sent by email to 30 medical professionals—psychologists, physicians and social workers- who work at institutions such as hospitals, municipalities, universities and organizations devoted to health care.

The instructions sent to the respondents requested information regarding gender, profession, types of suffering situations addressed and the type of institution where they work. Next, participants were invited to write text answers such questions as these:

- How would you define the concept of suffering considering the personal and social spheres?
- How does the suffering of people you work with affect their quality of life?
- How does the suffering of people you work with affect your quality of life?

After receiving the texts, we analyzed the answers and selected some for in-depth analysis and reporting here to illustrate our findings.

11.3   Defining Suffering

Cassell (1999) states that suffering involves some symptom or process that threatens fear, whether regarding the meaning of the symptom or concerns about the future. Among patients seeking therapy or medical care, suffering can start with anguish over the possibility that if the symptom continues, the person will lose control, and that fear of the future contributes to suffering (Cassell 1999: 531). He further defines suffering as a specific state of distress that occurs when the integrity of the person is threatened or disrupted (Cassell 1999: 531). Though suffering is related to the severity of the affliction, it is measured subjectively, in individuals' own terms. In this sense, suffering is an affliction of the *person*, not the body (Cassell 1999: 532). His implication is that healing professionals must understand the characteristics of the individual to understand their suffering.

While Cassell is the leading voice in defining suffering from the point of view of healing professionals, in the past three decades much research has been done on what has is now called social suffering. Social suffering has come to refer to suffering that is produced primarily by social conditions that damage a collectivity's sense of self-worth, dignity and functioning because they are stigmatized by race, disability, poverty, low social status or other characteristics that should not be relevant (Kleinman et al. 1997). Social institutions typically maintain the status quo that perpetuates the stigma and the socially shared suffering (Bourdieu et al. 2000). Social pain, on the other hand, differs from social suffering in that it is based upon distress inflicted by a primary group, family, friends, or people with whom you might have regular contact. Social pain results from isolation or withdrawal of affection or interaction privileges by others that one cares about (Anderson 2014).

11.4 Helping Professionals Views of Suffering

When we asked professionals about suffering, they said that personal and social suffering are caused by the frustration of losing functions and social positions due to a particular disease and they are surprised how different and subjective this topic is for different people. They frequently observe how suffering is associated with certain individuals' pattern of response, rather than related to a particular disease. Social suffering can be analyzed by personal and social dimensions, some associated with injustice, loneliness, social stigma, vulnerability, or unhappiness.

One professional who assists people who suffer defined suffering "As a situation where the feeling of well-being disappears, giving rise to fears fueled by insecurities and uncertainties; an unpleasant type of sensation related to grief and/or physical or psychological pain." Another said that the causes or levels of intensity are totally subjective, facing the same situation; peoples' responses might be different. It can be assumed that people have a certain threshold and suffering appears beyond that, as they also have levels of tolerance to it. A female psychologist said, "It is like if a bomb had exploded destroying everything that was around and familiar to the person, and used to provide security and containment."

In describing her view of what it is like to suffer, a female physician said in the social sphere, she believes that suffering is what is seen as a common factor by a certain group of people who may be going through the same situation. It can be either the absence of health or the lack of work, as both situations are accompanied by pain, which is reflected in peoples' faces, their listlessness, and lack of interest in what happens around them, which leads some to a total state of lethargy.

A female social worker described suffering as "Appearing when people face certain situations or conflicts but do not have the tools to deal with it or resolve it. Social relationships bring support. Institutions also provide sustenance. In the current crisis situation, with poverty, violence and abandonees people all are vulnerable. Given this situation, those discourses that hold social bond and the symbolic structure that organizes ideals and beliefs are weakening. Thus, there is an impoverishment of the meanings that provide the necessary protection against the incomprehensible and suffering emerges." Another female physician defined suffering as a very subjective state of mind and each individual experiencing it differently, according to his/her personal history, experiences and personality characteristics. Further she wrote,

> Regarding the personal sphere, suffering is experienced in loneliness and sometimes there is no one to accompany that person to cope with it. There are many patients who do not count with someone to share their suffering, especially their emotions, anxiety and fears. Their internal and external stigma, do not allow them to share with their significant others what they are going through, in order to avoid being rejected by them or causing more suffering. In this sense, the professional is the person absorbs patients' anxiety as they do not trust in other people to share what they are experience. This type of patient also requires psychological support in order to better cope with suffering, even to solve it, if that were possible.
>
> Social suffering is more general and broader; one can suffer for the injustice observed every day. Patients tell about how they are treated and discriminated in different fields of their lives, for the children who suffer, for brutal abuse, but this social suffering impacts very differently than personal suffering. Social suffering has such an impact in certain people that generate fight against others' suffering. From a social perspective, there is dissatisfaction or frustration for not being able to relate to others, the loss of opportunities and injustice.

Finally, another female social worker said, "Suffering is the affliction, grief or pain that a person experiences. It can be physical or psychological and it brings unhappiness. Social suffering is mainly related to vulnerable groups in our society to whom public policies fail to address. In the case of people who use drugs, have to do with the inability to have control over their lives, when the addiction is in the foreground, thinking and doing is subordinated to consumption. People stop being the protagonists of their lives becoming an unwitting viewer of something that does not generate satisfaction anymore, but rather causes fear and loneliness. Suffering is a constant feeling in the stories of those who we receive everyday looking for help. Substance abuse affects all spheres of patients' lives, not only individual but also interpersonal relationships within the family, social, and working environments are modified."

The professionals we interviewed referred not only to suffering, but also the places where these stories are told and received. Thus, helping encounters shape not only the scope of what is possible in a narrative of suffering, but also what is impossible—the limits of that story. Suffering is communicable in a framework of social conditions; its meaning varies according to different times and fields; and it involves ethical, political, and epistemic issues for all immersed in this relationship, as well as their social groups.

11.5   Quality of Life and Quality of Working Life

Quality of life refers to the perceptions, aspirations, needs, satisfactions, and social representations members of social group experience in relation to the social dynamics and environments in which they are immersed, including services that are offered and social interventions derived from social policies (Casas 1996: 100). In this way, quality of life considers the citizens' involvement in assessing their needs, and so it gains political significance. Integrating psychological and social measures of subjects' perceptions and evaluations of quality of life contributes to the study of well-being from a physical, psychological, and socio-affective and material needs perspective (Casas 1999). The study of the quality of life also refers to both the physical environment (social welfare) and the psychosocial environment (psychological well-being). The latter is based on the individual's experience and evaluation, including positive and negative measures and an overall perception of his/her life—what is known as *life satisfaction*. It involves both objective and subjective aspects, aggregated in the seven domains operationalized in the quality of life scale (Cummins 1998).

Michalos (2007: 4) states that the quality of life of an individual or a community can be thought of as a function of the current conditions of that life, and it refers to what that subject or community does with those conditions. That function reflects how these conditions are perceived, what the individual or community thinks and feels about those conditions, and which consequences might occur.

Thus, quality of life can conceptually give rise to a new theoretical point of view that involves working from potentialities rather than from deficiencies and emphasizing community by analyzing socio-political context. In this particular perspective, the individual (traditionally considered an "object") becomes the "subject and protagonist" where quality of life is based on the social and political situation, grounded in respect for human rights and prompting integrative work approaches to alleviating suffering (Tonon 2003).

Subjective well-being is based on the conditions in which people's lives develop and refers to an overall balance of life opportunities, social and personal resources, and personal outcomes. Thus, life satisfaction can be defined as the degree to which a person perceives their overall quality of life in a positive way. Quality of *working* life is, to be sure, related to job satisfaction. Individuals have a general expectation of how they think things should be in their jobs and the significant aspects related to that work. When people compare these ideals to actuality, a general evaluation results: an individual assessment of working life satisfaction (Diener et al. 1998). This is one of the classic indicators of people's general attitude toward their careers.

> Besides being a relationship of technical production, is the support to enlist the social structure, establishing a close relationship among the place one occupies in the social division of labor, the social networks and social security systems. (Vélez Restrepo 2004: 88)

Then, if the center of the quality of life is the individual, we can summarize by saying that quality of life recognizes people's perceptions of their living conditions as an entity unto itself, giving it equal or more weight than to the material or objective conditions defined by experts.

11.6   The Social Suffering of Care Professionals

In order to describe how the suffering of the people they work with affects professionals' quality of life, we consulted those caring for people suffering from either a chronic or terminal disease, going through anxious or depressed states, or living in conditions of social emergency, poverty, and unemployment. These professionals mentioned feelings of helplessness and frustration, especially when they see situations that could have been avoided by adequate economic or public policy decisions. A female physician pointed out that she "Feels impotence, when facing the suffering of others and the impossibility of solving the problem over and over every day." A female social worker comments that "Suffering appears by not being able to respond to people's demands and problems because of their lack of material, financial, and human resources."

Feelings of injustice increase when professionals tend to children and youth. Some of them said that they suffer a lot when something happens that could have been avoided, and it "tortures" them to face unfair situations when youth and children suffer at the unnecessary hands of adult family members. What causes the most distress are the situations of injustice and preventable suffering but the helping professional cannot change the course of things. One female physician did point out that she worked to differentiate between her responsibility for providing care and guilt for failing to solve the problem. Others commented on the need for supervision, support and companionship of a team, especially to sustain daily tasks and avoid burnout.

Social support is defined as a source of basic psychological support, a resource for coping, and a stress inhibitor (Maya Jariego 1999: 65). Gil Monte and Peiró (1997) states that social support in work settings increases personal fulfillment, diminishes emotional exhaustion, and decreases negative attitudes and behaviors towards others. This support can be provided by team leaders and co-workers, as well as by the informal social groups generated in everyday working settings (Tonon 2003: 51). In this regard, a female psychologist commented that her "Quality of life is affected by the intensity of the affliction that patients experience." Patients' situations of extreme suffering led her to a state of dejection and hopelessness that she needs to counterbalance by working with other resources that connect her again with a healthy state such as literature, art, meditation, relaxation and healthy bonds. It helps to accept personal limits and reject a sense of omnipotence related to the scope of her interventions. She said, "When working with patients who suffer diseases with high levels of physical and mental pain, we must work on preventing burnout."

"Burnout" can be defined as a response to chronic stressful working situations, particularly among those in the helping professions. While it is not expected that professionals in these areas take *on* the problems of those with whom they work, they *are* required to show an interest in such problems. Transference and exhaustion seem inevitable. Particularly, in countries like Argentina, these professionals are expected to meet the demands of both the individuals they care for and the organizations they work for. Conflict arises when time is limited and the problems are complex (Tonon 2003: 37).

From this perspective, burnout is not only a personal problem, but also a social and political problem. It concerns people from whom these professionals require public-policy decisions that might enable the development of working conditions and preserve the quality of working life of these professionals (Tonon 2003).

The interviewed professionals referred to supervision as necessary; skillful supervision helped them handle the feelings and emotions that working with people in suffering conditions generates: "It is essentially a personal analysis that depends on supervision and networking," says a female psychologist. In this line, Tonon (2004) defines supervision as:

> A theoretical and methodological process which aims to acquiring the necessary new knowledge and skills to the daily professional practice; as well as to provide a space to think about the emotional impact that every situation of care, in which the professional has acted, has on the supervised individual. It is based on a holistic understanding of the situation where theoretical knowledge and practical experience interact (16).

Professionals also expressed the ameliorating effect of focusing on the positive feelings evoked from "success stories" with their clients, as well as focusing on themselves and others as individuals who are capable of producing changes in their lives. They said that is does not always affect them in the same way. Sometimes they can better overcome the feeling of frustration that produce not having enough tools to help that person to resolve what is causing him suffering. Sometimes, they feel distressed when facing suffering and bring those feelings with them to home, in detriment of their quality of life and those around them. The successful cases, although small and individual, give them a positive feedback that helps to overcome failures. They explained that later they try to analyze failures in order to understand what had happened and to learn from their mistakes.

11.7   Yoga to Alleviate Suffering Among Care Workers

Ravettino (2008) has related the practice of some disciplines such as Yoga with a "light" lifestyle and highlights how major business organizations are increasingly incorporating physical activity into working settings through a wide range of fitness and relaxation sessions. Several Argentinean companies are offering these to employees during working hours, with the intention of reducing absenteeism and boosting performance.

As Halpern (2011) and others (Kellner et al. 2002; Coulter and Willis 2004) argued, "alternative techniques" for wellness are now common practice in Western cultures. Yoga is one of the most well-known and frequently practiced techniques for alleviating stress and promoting resilience. It includes physical practices (postures or *asanas*, breathing exercises, relaxation, and meditation) as well as philosophical formulations regarding reality and consistent lifestyles.

The word "yoga" comes from the root *yuj* (to join or to yoke) and is used to refer to "any technique for asceticism and any method of meditation" (Eliade 1988: 18). However, there is a classic Yoga, a system of philosophy (*darshana*) expressed by Patanjali in his *Yoga-Sutra* (the best known formulation in the West), as well as countless other popular forms.

Besides its practical, physical benefits as a movement or exercise regimen, a useful feature of Yoga is its initiation structure. The practice is learned under the guidance of a teacher (or guru), akin to other Indian philosophical systems. Thus, Yoga has an initiatory and oral. As yogis begin to the profane world (family, society) and become dedicated to exceeding the behaviors and values of mundane human behavior as guided by a teacher, it is said that this practice involves both death (of an "old" way of being) and rebirth (or release) (Eliade 1988). Of course, much of the rejection aspects of a yogic approach must been seen as symbolic; a person who practices Yoga need not reject family or society, but may learn to adapt their interactions with family and society in a new, more open and peaceful way. They may learn to release stress and unnecessary attachment, each of which produces suffering.

As it is expressed in the *Yoga Sutra*, mere existence is associated with suffering: "everything is sorrow for the wise" (*Yoga-Sutra* ll: 15). However, this universal suffering (of all living beings) has a positive, intrinsic value: it can spur practitioners toward liberation.

In the *Yoga Sutra*, the author enumerates the eightfold path of yoga (or *Ashtanga Yoga* in Sanskrit):

1. *Yama* (control of the body and mind)
2. *Niyama* (ethical principles to promote well-being through self-discipline)
3. *Asana* (control of body postures and functions)
4. *Pranayama* (the regulation of breathing, energy, and mental processes)
5. *Pratyahara* (withdrawal of the senses)
6. *Dharana* (concentration)
7. *Dhyana* (meditation and contemplation)
8. *Samadhi* (total merging with the object of meditation)
(Iyengar 2002; Lorenzen and Preciado Solis 2003)

There are many approaches with regard to yogic practices, although they differ in their quality, populations, and methods. While some of these approaches consider effects on the overall quality of life, others address the effects on the quality of the *working* life from different perspectives, particularly the therapeutic one (Asuero et al. 2013; Araiza Díaz 2009; Duro Martín 2002; Fajardo Pulido 2009; Janakiramaiah et al. 2000; Raub 2002; Shannahoff-Khalsa 2006; Taylor Gura 2002).

Valente and Marotta (2005) have explored the impact of regular Yoga practice on the personal and professional life of psychotherapists, categorizing their perceptions into four areas of therapists' professional growth and self-care behavior: self-awareness, balance, self-acceptance and acceptance of others, and yoga as a way of life.

Consistently, Hartfield et al. (2011) shows the effectiveness of yogic practice in improving resilience and well-being in the workplace. Their sample of university employees who practiced 6 weeks of yoga reported feeling more confidence in stressful situations, higher levels of energy, and an increase in their life satisfaction and sense of purpose. These findings have been replicated in several studies conducted with different populations (Granath et al. 2006; McDonald et al. 2006).

Furthermore, Nikolic-Ristanovic (2011) considers the application of Yoga practice to work with crime victims, including victims of war. Here, yoga is used not only to provide support to the victims, but also to prevent the burnout of the professionals who work with them. From her personal experience, the author highlights the following positive effects: increased capacity to cope with the experiences of victims; greater ability to facilitate the perception of a traumatic experience within a broader life experience and better aptitude in separating from victims' experiences. Nikolic-Ristanovic also argues that these professionals become better at establishing good communication and empathic expression among themselves, making them better able to recognize the signs of burnout (2011). Although Nikolic-Ristanovic (2011) posits the need for more detailed studies on the topic, she believes yogic practice holds value for care workers: "Yoga, then, apparently, has a positive effect on the quality of the overall relationship with the victim and the provided support, while simultaneously reducing the negative effects on researchers, and providers of assistance" (159).

11.8 Conclusions

Quality of working life is related to job satisfaction, and individuals have a general expectation of how things should be in their jobs, as well as significant aspects of their work. Those in the helping professions work with people experiencing personal and social suffering, and their own discourses reveal personal and social suffering, too. They suffer alongside those they help, dealing with senses of injustice, loneliness, social stigma, vulnerability, and unhappiness. Care workers speak of helplessness and frustration, especially in those suffering situations that might have been avoided by suitable economic or public policy decisions. To continue working with people in suffering conditions, professionals report the need for professional support and companionship in a team. These supports help workers in their daily tasks and to avoid burnout.

In this regard, the practice of Yoga appears as an opportunity and alternative to improve quality of life and general resilient capabilities. In research in working settings, in particular, Yoga serves to decrease stressful situations, strengthen personal abilities, and the opportunities for a joint construction. Further, similar, alternative practices among workers not only hold promise for those qualities that make for a "better" worker: yoga and other contemplative physical and emotional practices also provide moments for the deep consideration of ethical, political, and epistemic issues that relate to the construction of social relationships and social suffering.

References

Anderson, R. E. (2014). *Human suffering and quality of life – Conceptualizing stories and statistics*. New York: Springer.

Araiza Díaz, A. (2009). *Conocer y Ser a través de la práctica del Yoga: una propuesta feminista de investigación performativa*. Doctoral thesis, Universitat Autònoma de Barcelona. Retrieved from http://www.tdx.cat/bitstream/handle/10803/5474/aa1de1.pdf;jsessionid=D2682BFBC06 C9F499F36CC7A4FA0099F.tdx2?sequence=1

Asuero, A. M., Rodriguez Blanco, T., Pujol-Ribera, E., Berenguera, A., & Moix Queraltó, J. (2013). Evaluación de la efectividad de un programa de mindfulness en profesionales de atención primaria. *Gac Sanit*. http://dx.doi.org/10.1016/j.gaceta.2013.04.007

Bourdieu, P., et al. (2000). Understanding. In P. Bourdieu et al. (Eds.), *The weight of the world: Social suffering in contemporary society*. Stanford: Stanford University Press.

Casas, F. (1996). *Bienestar Social. Una introducción psicosociológica*. Barcelona: Editorial PPU.

Casas, F. (1999). Calidad de vida y calidad humana. *Revista Papeles del Psicólogo, 74*. Madrid. Retrieved from http://www.papelesdelpsicologo.es/vernumero.asp?id=812

Cassell, E. (1999). Diagnosis suffering: A perspective. *Annals of Internal Medicine, 131*, 531–534.

Coulter, I. D., & Willis, E. M. (2004). The rise and rise of complementary and alternative medicine: A sociological perspective. *Medical Journal of Australia, 180*(11), 587–589. https://www.mja.com.au/journal/2004/180/11/rise-and-rise-complementary-and-alternative-medicine-sociological-perspective

Cummins, R. (1998). *Comprehensive quality of life scale*. Melbourne: A.C.Q.O.L.

Diener, E., Suh, E., & Oishi, S. (1998). Recent findings on subjective well-being. *Indian Journal of Clinical Psychology, 24*, 25–41.

Duro Martín, A. (2002). Calidad de vida laboral y Psicología Social de la Salud en el Trabajo: Hacia un modelo de componentes comunes para explicar el bienestar laboral psicológico y la salud mental laboral de origen psicosocial. Resultados preliminares. *Revista del Ministerio de Trabajo y Asuntos Sociales, 56*, 57–98. Retrieved from www.empleo.gob.es/es/publica/pub_electronicas/.../56/Inf02.pdf

Eliade, M. (1988). *Yoga, inmortalidad y libertad*. Buenos Aires: La Pléyade.

Fajardo Pulido, J. A. (2009). Yoga, cuerpo e imagen: espiritualidad y bienestar, de la terapia a la publicidad. *Universitas Humanística, 68*, 33–47.

Gil Monte, P., & Peiró, J. (1997). *Desgaste psíquico en el trabajo: El síndrome de quemarse*. Madrid: Editorial Síntesis.

Granath, J., Ingvarsson, S., Von Thiele, U., & Lundberg, U. (2006). Stress management: A randomized study of cognitive behavioural therapy and yoga. *Cognitive Behavioral Therapy, 35*(1), 3–10.

Halpern, J. S. (2011). *Yoga for improving sleep quality and quality of life in older adults in a Western cultural setting*. Bachelor thesis. Escuela de Ciencias de la Salud, Colegio de Ciencia, Ingeniería y Salud, Universidad R. M. I. T, Victoria, Australia.

Hartfiel, N., Havenhand, J., Khalsa, S. B., Clarke, G., & Krayer, A. (2011). The effectiveness of yoga for the improvement of well-being and resilience to stress in the workplace. *Scandinavian Journal of Work, Environment & Health, 37*(1), 70–76.

Iyengar, B. K. S. (2002). *Light on the Sutras of Patanjali*. London: Thornsons/Harper Collins.

Janakiramaiah, N., Gangadhar, B. N., Naga, V., Murthy, P. J., Harish, M. G., Subbakrishna, D. K., et al. (2000). Antidepressant efficacy of Sudarshan Kriya Yoga (SKY) in melancholia: A randomized comparison with electroconvulsive therapy (ECT) and imipramine. *Journal of Affective Disorders, 57*(1–3), 255–259.

Kellner, M. J., Boon, H., Wellman, B., & Welsh, S. (2002). Complementary and alternative groups contemplate the need for effectiveness, safety and cost-effectiveness research. *Complementary Therapies in Medicine, 10*, 235–239.

Kleinman, A., Das, V., & Lock, M. (Eds.). (1997). *Social suffering*. Berkeley: University of California Press.

Lorenzen, D. N., y Preciado Solís, B. (2003). *Atadura y Liberación. Las religiones de la India.* México: El Colegio de México.

Maya Jariego, I. (1999). *Análisis de los recursos de apoyo social de los inmigrantes africanos y latinoamericanos en Andalucía.* Tesis de doctorado en Psicología Social. Universidad de Sevilla. España.

McDonald, A., Burjan, E., & Martin, S. (2006). Yoga for patients and carers in a palliative day care setting. *International Journal of Palliative Nursing, 12*(11), 519–523.

Michalos, A. (2007). *Education, happiness and well-being.* International conference on 'Is happiness measurable and what do those measures mean for public policy?' at Rome, 2–3 April 2007, University of Rome 'Tor Vergata', organized by the Joint Research Centre of the European Commission, OECD, Centre for Economic and International Studies and the Bank of Italy.

Montaño, C. (2000). *La naturaleza del Servicio Social* (Biblioteca Latinoamericana de Servicio Social). Sao Paulo, Brasil: Cortez Editora.

Nikolic-Ristanovic, V. (2011). Possible application of yoga in victimology. En: P. Nikic (Ed.), *Proceedings "Yoga – The Light of Microuniverse" of the International Interdisciplinary Scientific Conference "Yoga in Science – Future and Perspectives", September 23–24, 2010, Belgrade, Serbia* (pp. 156–161). Belgrade: Yoga Federation of Serbia. Retrieved from http://yoga-science.rs/eng/sciarticles/17-vesna-nikolic-ristanovic.pdf

Offe, C. (1982). *¿Es el trabajo una categoría sociológica clave?* Conferencia Inaugural. XI Congreso de Sociología. Bamberg.

Raub, J. A. (2002). Psychophysiologic effects of Hatha Yoga on musculoskeletal and cardiopulmonary function: A literature review. *The Journal of Alternative and Complementary Medicine, 8*(6), 797–812.

Ravettino, A. J. (2008). El estilo de vida *light.* Hábitos y patrones de consumo. *Revista Científica de UCES, XII*(1), 103–117.

Shannahoff-Khalsa, D. (2006). *Kundalini yoga meditation: Techniques specific form psychiatric disorders, couples therapy, and personal growth.* New York/London: W. W. Norton & Company.

Taylor Gura, S. (2002). Yoga for stress reduction and injury prevention at work. *Work: A Journal of Prevention, Assessment and Rehabilitation, 19*(1), 3–7.

Tonon, G. (2003). *Calidad de vida y desgaste profesional: una mirada del síndrome de burnout.* Bs. As: Espacio Editorial.

Tonon, G. (2004). *La supervisión como cuestión profesional y académica.* Bs. As: Espacio Editorial.

Valente, V., & Marotta, A. (2005). The impact of yoga on the professional and personal life of the psychotherapist. *Contemporary Family Therapy, 27*(1), 65–80.

Vélez Restrepo, O. (2004). *Reconfigurando el Trabajo Social. Perspectivas y tendencias contemporáneas.* Bs. As: Espacio Editorial.

Chapter 12
The Invisible Suffering of HIV and AIDS Caregivers in Botswana

Gloria Jacques

12.1 Introduction

Barnett and Whiteside (2002: 14–15) claim that the worst impact of HIV and AIDS is felt in households where "social reproduction occurs at its deepest level." They also note that "government(s) and (the) international community have most difficulty responding" to the home care dimensions of the pandemic.

HIV and AIDS have decimated many societies (especially in southern Africa) since the early 1980s. With the pandemic has come isolation, discrimination, and a severe threat to the quality of life of individuals and families largely due to the sexual and intimacy-related implications of the disease and the rapidity of its spread. Family care and responsibility, cornerstones of African culture, seemed a logical resource in addressing the demands of the situation. However, a significant ingredient of a holistic approach to the issue has to be an understanding that care for HIV and AIDS patients should also include care and support for their families, especially the caregivers, throughout the process, including – significantly – the bereavement stage (Stegling 2000). This ideal practice should encapsulate: counseling of patients and family members in the home environment; material support; home visits by health workers; and co-ordination of the work of hospitals, clinics, social welfare organizations, community groups, and families. Furthermore, it is essential that caregivers be specifically trained in the intricacies of HIV and AIDS support in order that the patient receives quality care and caregivers know how to protect themselves (Botswana Ministry of Health 2005). This, in Africa, has not always been the case. This chapter considers the case of the southern African nation of Botswana as representative of the tragic HIV and AIDS pandemic in southern Africa. To some extent, it applies globally as well.

G. Jacques (✉)
Department of Social Work, University of Botswana, Private Bag 0022, Gaborone, Botswana
e-mail: jacques@mopipi.ub.bw

© Springer Science+Business Media Dordrecht 2015   147
R.E. Anderson (ed.), *World Suffering and Quality of Life*,
Social Indicators Research Series 56, DOI 10.1007/978-94-017-9670-5_12

12.2 Research on HIV and AIDS and Home Care in Southern Africa

In African communities, home-based care has been acclaimed as advantageous in dealing with the HIV and AIDS crisis through its apparent enhancement of the process of dying and death for both patients and family caregivers. Uys (2003), in a study of seven South African communities, found that many affected families preferred that their relatives die with dignity at home rather than in hospitals, despite the burden that HIV and AIDS impose on households (Barnett and Whiteside 2002).

Family caregiving is especially important in poor rural settings where health care services are virtually nonexistent (Kipp et al. 2006). However, with few other support systems in place, this can be stressful for the caregivers. Brouwer et al. (2000) stressed the problems for Buganda women in Uganda associated with caring for their HIV positive relatives, especially children. They also identified lack of training for family caregivers in Kenya. Research in the Democratic Republic of Congo by Kipp et al. (2006) found that caregiving responsibilities included feeding, bathing, and medicating patients while only 25 % of caregivers interviewed reported receiving support from significant others, linking this directly to the issue of stigma. Ostracism and reduction in social contact exacerbated the situation culminating in a pervasive feeling of unhappiness and little interest in life. As dire as these findings appear, the caregivers (mostly women) were, in fact, being given some support through community home-based care programs. Many more in Africa do not receive any assistance; thus caregiver support needs to be a funded component of all HIV and AIDS programming.

HIV-related caregiving very often has a deleterious effect on the physical and mental health of caregivers. A study in Tanzania by Nnuko et al. (2000) indicated that family caregivers spent 3–7 h a day in care-related activities and that this constituted a considerable socio-economic burden for them. In a cultural context, women are disproportionately affected through societal expectations of having to fulfill caring roles especially in HIV- and AIDS-affected households (Steinberg et al. 2002; Lindsay et al. 2003). The research by Nnuko et al. (2000) established that most men were unwilling to care for the sick. Gender approaches relate to society's expectations, social roles, behaviors, and attitudes of men and women. These are defined by cultural norms and social mores intersected with variables such as economic status, religion, race, ethnicity, and age, culminating in a tsunami of attitudes and opinion. In the care economy women predominate, and this cross cuts generations (Elson 2002) with particular reference to HIV- and AIDS-affected households (Budlender 2004).

Home care in an African context involves the transfer of medical supervision from a formal institution to the patient's family in a community setting. Ideally this includes other professional and non-professional actors (Jacques and Stegling 2004; Ngwenya and Butale 2005). In theory the envisaged goals of community home-based care programs are to provide appropriate care to patients and their families in a home setting and to help families to maintain their independence and achieve the best possible quality of life (WHO 2002). Social support networks are, therefore, crucial for emotional and spiritual wellbeing of caregivers and their patients for, without this essential element, the effect is one of social isolation (at best) and (at worst) ostracism.

In a South African study on gendered home-based care (Akintola 2006) the burdens of care expected of women included the physical (disability and illness); the cultural (declining the use of protective clothing such as gloves, seen as a barrier to love); the emotional (feelings of guilt, distress, and fear of death); and socioeconomic hardships. Highly emotional experiences included watching their loved ones die (usually without the support of significant male others), particularly during the grieving process both before and after death. Furthermore, the risk of contracting HIV is heightened among primary caregivers who have had little or no training in providing hands-on care (Ndaba-Mbata and Seloilwe 2000; Akintola 2006).

A study of the psychosocial impact on caregivers of people living with HIV and AIDS in South Africa (Orner 2006) found that poverty, prejudice, and gender bias constituted extreme challenges. These considerations should, it was recommended, inform home-based care policies, programs, and interventions. Furthermore, caregivers did not always have money for transport and thus had to walk long distances to collect medication from clinics leading to high levels of emotional distress. Many suffered disruption of work and social patterns culminating in loneliness, despair, and diminished quality of life. Orner (2006) recommended care training to enable optimal contribution to the needs of the patient, as well as positive support for the caregiver.

African countries supporting home-based care have incorporated variations of the methodology depending upon perceived need and interpretation of its underlying philosophy. In Rwanda, services are provided through volunteer networks in the community with assistance from nongovernmental organizations' staff. Both patients *and* caregivers benefit from psychosocial support, stigma reduction, income-generating activities, and assistance with school fees for the children of those living with HIV and AIDS (Chandler et al. 2004). In Uganda caregivers derive significant benefit from monthly support group meetings organized by program counselors and social workers where issues relating to health education, HIV prevention, and nutrition are discussed (Mmopelwa et al. 2013).

In Malawi, a study by Pindani et al. (2013) found that the program was perceived to be beneficial by people living with HIV and AIDS although affected by challenges such as lack of transport to health facilities and limited resources and knowledge on the part of caregivers. They found that, despite its benefits, the "noble task" of caring for people living with HIV and AIDS had been left to family members who were frequently overburdened with, and overwhelmed by, the responsibility. Another issue of concern was that caregiver support structures, such as group work for education and sharing of concerns related to caring, were located principally in urban centers denying access to those in more remote areas. Furthermore, in Malawi, young girls missed school to assist in the caregiving process producing a vicious cycle of poverty and poor physical and mental health, which increased the risk of HIV infection of caregivers themselves and negatively affected their quality of life (Chikalipo 2007).

12.3 Botswana and Its HIV and AIDS Epidemic

As stated in the previous section, the practice of home based care for people living with HIV and AIDS is commonly accepted in the countries of sub-Saharan Africa where the pandemic has reached crisis stages. Botswana is one of those countries and, with a prevalence rate for 15- through 49-year-olds of 24.8 %, is second only to Swaziland. Botswana is an upper middle income country (nominal GDP per capita $7,096 in 2009) with a stable government, which has implemented effective development policies since independence in 1966 (CIA World Factbook 2013; NACA and US Government 2010–2014). Prior to independence the country was a British Protectorate. As a result of wealth, largely related to diamonds, combined with the government's commitment to democracy and the rule of law, there has been significant growth and major reduction in poverty levels over the past 40 years. Key areas of health progress include: 97 % antenatal care coverage; 94 % deliveries attended by a skilled health worker; 97 % of 1-year-old children fully immunized for DPT3; and 100 % facilities providing antenatal care also provide HIV testing and counseling (NACA and US Government 2010–2014).

Notwithstanding these statistics, HIV and AIDS threatens the future of the country. Furthermore, despite the foundation of a relatively strong health system, human resources and infrastructure are severely stressed necessitating focus on cost-effectiveness of service delivery, human resources, and financial management of the epidemic.

The Botswana government confronted the issue by developing a National Strategic Framework and introducing, in 2001, the Masa (New Dawn) program providing free reliable antiretroviral drugs and counseling to citizens. Similarly the Prevention of Mother-to-Child Transmission initiative has reduced the rate of transmission of the virus to less than 3 % of those enrolled in the program. Nongovernmental, community based, and civil society organizations are active partners in the fight against HIV and AIDS related suffering at national and local levels (Jacques and Mmatli 2013).

As early as 1992 the National AIDS Control Program (NACP) developed operational guidelines on community home-based care for people with AIDS in Botswana; these were revised in 1996 by the Ministry of Health's AIDS/STD Unit (NACP 30) and form the basis for the ongoing program of home-based care in the country. The rationale for the program was that the extended family is traditionally considered to be the greatest resource for people in need of care and support due to long term illness. Members are capable of sharing responsibility for care with social welfare workers and health personnel but the main responsibility lies with the family (NACP 30, 1996, 2001, 2005).

The overall goal of the Community Home Based Care (CHBC) Program is to prevent HIV transmission in society and reduce the impact of HIV and AIDS on those infected and affected. Specific objectives include: ensuring an optimum level of care; offering nursing care in a homely and familiar setting; extending ongoing counseling services to patients and their families; and establishing functional referral systems between hospitals, district health teams, and clinics, (NACP 30, 2005). Specific and comprehensive CHBC activities include: health related needs assessments of patients and their families; the development of a plan of action for identified needs; provision of continuing support and care to patients and their families; identification of community support groups; education and training of social welfare officers, patients, and community caregivers on home care management; and establishment of a comprehensive referral system to ensure continuity of care (ibid).

Notwithstanding the country's commitment to controlling the epidemic and reporting no new cases by 2016, the 2008 Botswana AIDS Impact Survey (BAIS III) found that the national HIV and AIDS prevalence rate was 17.6 % (20.4 % for females and 14.2 % for males) (Botswana Ministry of Health 2009). The Survey further established that only 23 % of men and 10.4 % of women reported having multiple sexual partners. Furthermore, only 45.8 % of men and 34.6 % of women used condoms in nonregular relationships. In 2010 studies by CoBaSyS & UB TARSC (2011) found that the percentage of people voluntarily testing in public facilities had decreased. A consequential study in Old Naledi (a high-density, low-income suburb of the capital city, Gaborone) established that community response in HIV and AIDS treatment, care, and support was compromised in many ways. The research found that health services required improved resource allocation including vehicles for ambulatory services. One astounding observation was that, at times, caregivers had to transport patients to health centers in wheelbarrows, which is painful and demeaning for both. Mobile clinics for dispensing antiretroviral drugs were also needed. Furthermore, the community felt that health workers required more relevant and in-depth training to enhance the quality of life of people living with HIV and AIDS and their caregivers.

12.4   Home Care in Botswana

The HBC program encompasses, ideally, the provision of health care to ailing persons in their homes by family or non-family members supported by skilled nonmedical professionals such as social welfare officers and community volunteers (Mmopelwa et al. 2013). In the context of Botswana, a home-based care "patient" is a person who has been medically diagnosed as terminally or chronically ill (including HIV- and AIDS-related illnesses) and who, after evaluation of their socioeconomic status, is found to be in need of material assistance on medical grounds (Botswana Ministry of Health 2005).

In resource-rich environments where antiretroviral drugs (ARVs) are available, HIV and AIDS are conceptualized as a chronic condition. In sub-Saharan Africa, where most are poor, it is a terminal condition. However, Botswana has been a pioneer in the provision of medication free of charge to the population. Furthermore, the adoption of the philosophy of routine testing as part of general medical care has served to demystify the disease to some extent (Jacques 2004).

The concept of life expectancy at birth is a measure of overall quality of life in a country and may be conceptualized as indicating the potential return on a state's investment in human capital (Browning 2008). Life expectancy in Botswana has, as a result of HIV and AIDS, fallen from 65 in 1995 to 40 in 2005 but rose to 55 in 2013 (CIA World Factbook 2013).

Caregivers require personal support in this physically and emotionally challenging situation. When a holistic approach is adopted, including (essentially) care for the caregiver, the program can yield significant health and social benefits (Jacques and Stegling 2004). This was reinforced by a 2004 study by Akintola of home care for people living with HIV and AIDS in South Africa that found female caregivers tended to suffer from exhaustion, malnourishment, and psychological distress. Jacques and Stegling (2004: 191) conclude that: "Home-based care, while politically correct, expedient, and culturally relevant, embodies the germ of exacerbated human suffering for patients and caregivers alike, unless vigorously controlled and supported through appropriate allocation of material and psychosocial resources."

This form of care in Botswana is conceptualized and implemented in a variety of ways throughout the country as programs and communities have access to different resources. Although the range of services differs, it generally includes (ideally) counseling and psychosocial support; social services (financial, legal, and material); and medical/nursing care (Ogden et al. 2004). However, in a country sampling of urban and rural CHBC programs, Browning (2008) identified poverty and financial restraints, stigma and discrimination (linked to sexually transmitted diseases and same sex practices), overburdening of family members, and inadequate support structures for caregivers to be threatening the efficacy of the initiative. Many households lacked basic facilities such as toilets and regular collection of solid waste. This led to improper handling of soiled laundry and inadequate ventilation, increasing caregivers' risk of infection. Botswana's fragile, drought-affected environment also challenges regular bathing of patients, threatening the health status of both patients and caregivers (Ngwenya and Kgathi 2006).

Protective clothing is not always included in care packages for informal caregivers and arrangements for disposal of clinical waste are, at times, erratic. Furthermore, exposure to infection carries no compensation for family caregivers as it does for professionals such as nurses, for example (Kang'ethe 2010). Community volunteers, when present, spend less time with patients and more on attempting to earn a living as the government stipend is insufficient for their needs. This further threatens the wellbeing and quality of life of family caregivers (Browning 2008).

12.5   Gender and Care in Botswana

There is a robust association between gender equality and development as measured by the UNDP's Human Development Index (HDI) (Anderson 2014). Unless female caregivers are appreciated and supported, the care system is likely to fail.

Kang'ethe (2010), in one program in Kanye in the South East District of Botswana, found that 98 % of the caregivers were women who felt that they were community scapegoats. They complained that the process of caregiving subjected them to physical and emotional pain with inadequate government or societal recognition, support services, supervision, counseling or care packages. Lack of necessary equipment created stress compromising their psychological and emotional health and wellbeing or quality of life.

Other studies found female caregivers in Botswana unable to discharge their roles due to old age or disability (Jacques and Stegling 2004). Specific challenges for women associated with caring for HIV and AIDS patients include feelings of helplessness, insomnia, unresolved grief, despondency, and hopelessness (Uys and Cameron 2003; Kang'ethe 2010). Furthermore, the Kanye study identified that the majority were over 50 and crippled by poverty. Seventy-four percent (74 %) had never attended school and 88 % had no source of income, largely due to their caregiving responsibilities. Stipends and other support services are thus urgently needed for caregivers (Kang'ethe 2010).

Anecdotal evidence supports the fact that elderly caregivers may themselves become HIV positive through transmission of the virus during the caring process. A study in Botswana by Ndaba-Mbata and Seloilwe (2000) of caregivers' perceptions of their situation pointed to a sense of isolation, feeling drained economically and emotionally, dealing with distressing symptoms including pain, and not being aware of the nature of the patient's illness. The latter is related to the controversial issue of human rights in the context of health care and the needs of the sick. Competing rights and responsibilities are becoming more openly discussed and evaluated, especially in Botswana, where the 2013 Public Health Act has generated a strong debate over issues of confidentiality and "the need to know." The Act makes provision for health professionals to inform significant others of HIV-positive patients of the health status of those for whom they are responsible and through whom they could be at risk (Botswana Ministry of Health 2013).

It is estimated that up to 49 % of all households in the country are likely to have at least one member infected with the virus (Botswana Ministry of Health 2009). Although support mechanisms are in place for family caregivers, they do not adequately ease their burden of care (Mmopelwa et al. 2013). A study conducted in the North West District of Botswana found that female parents were most commonly caregivers to their ailing children of all ages. A majority of these primary caregivers was also from households with no cash income. This constituted a heavy burden for those caring for critically ill patients, involving (apart from care-related tasks) collecting firewood, drawing water, cleaning the physical environment, and washing the patients' children (Ngwenya and Kgathi 2006).

One of the measurements of cost used in the study by Mmopelwa et al. (2013) was the wellbeing valuation method, which calculates the cost of loss of wellbeing (quality of life) of the caregiver (Phaladze et al. 2005). This includes the level of happiness experienced in the pursuit of caregiving and the balance between cost and benefit. The research found that care was burdensome because it involved terminal illness, fulltime care, and, possibly, more than one patient. Hidden costs subsisted in reduced quality of life, and the researchers recommended that this could be addressed, in part, through increasing the budget for community "volunteers" and organizing regular support group meetings based on a successful Ugandan initiative which contributed significantly to allaying suffering and improving quality of life.

In Botswana, the understanding is that primary caregivers are family members (almost all female) while community caregivers (so-called "volunteers") assist them and move from home to home within a specific geographical area (Kang'ethe 2013). Although modification of cultural beliefs and practices is a lengthy process it is essential in the face of life threatening forces. Uys and Cameron (2003) recommend that ongoing training and refresher courses, stress management sessions, and development seminars be provided to hone and upgrade family and community caregivers' skills and knowledge. Kang'ethe (2013) also suggests that the government of Botswana follow the lead of the state in Mozambique, whose policy is to pay community caregivers 60 % of the country's minimum wage rate to encourage greater participation in supporting family caregivers. Furthermore, as in many child foster care programs in developed societies, a system of respite care by community members may provide opportunities for recharging of caregivers' emotional and physical batteries, thereby enhancing the quality of life and of care for both patients and care providers.

Another significant issue for some female caregivers in Botswana is their paid employment outside the home. In a study on the spill-over effects on work and family wellbeing for employed HIV caregivers in Botswana, Rajaraman et al. (2008) found that they were more likely than other caregivers to take leave from work, for longer periods, and at an unpaid level. This led to job loss in some cases with negative consequences for household economic security and quality of life for all concerned (Heymann 2006). The 2008 study also found that HIV and AIDS caregivers who were in employment faced a greater burden of care as a result of needs of the sick being exacerbated by the absence of the caregiver. They also had less time to spend with their own children leading to the latters' poorer academic and behavioral outcomes. Where the caregivers themselves were HIV positive, the physical, emotional, and financial burdens were immense.

12.6   HIV and AIDS and Stigma in Botswana

The ongoing stigma associated with HIV and AIDS results in caregivers and families becoming isolated and alienated from their communities. Browning's 2008 study found that they experienced loneliness and isolation as people did not want to associate with them. This in turn led to many complaining of exhaustion, depression, and distress. Young female caregivers reported dropping out of school, partly because of prejudicial attitudes of others, and participating in illegal activities such as commercial sex work to provide economic support to the family (Lindsey et al. 2003; Browning 2008). Browning's research established that, in general, caregivers expressed feelings of helplessness, guilt, anger, and alienation. Since caregiving is location-oriented social mobility of a caregiver is reliant on external social support and palliative care from friends and neighbors (Ngwenya and Kgathi 2006). If this is not available due to stigma and exclusion, the role of the caregiver is further compromised. Research into HIV- and AIDS-related stigma in Africa generally (and Botswana in particular), focusing specifically on home-based care, recommends the development of income-generating projects and food security initiatives to increase stability and improve the quality of life for caregivers. Also needed are greater allocations of state funding for support services; educational programming demystifying HIV and AIDS at the community level; closer collaboration between professionals and household members; and planned emotional and psychosocial support for those involved in caregiving (Lindsey et al. 2003; Browning 2008).

Considering the dynamics of the HIV and AIDS situation in sub-Saharan Africa, Campbell (2003) suggests that the social capital perspective constitutes a relevant framework for the construction of a health enabling community context. This perspective emphasizes specific processes among people and organizations, especially collaboration and trust, in pursuing mutually beneficial goals. These networks have to operate effectively within households, communities, and with outside institutions. Thus, quality of life is achieved if both the cared *for* and the care*givers* are cared *about* by others.

12.7 Conclusion

Some consider quality of life as perceived by the individual and not by what their life means to others in the society. Alleyne (2001) believes that a life of quality should also be measured by the extent to which those touched by that life are enhanced in some manner. A holistic approach embraces both perspectives as caregivers are also sufferers and sufferers, caregivers.

Adequate support for home caregivers is critical for the survival, as well as the quality of life, of southern Africa because it is afflicted by one of the most catastrophic health challenges of the modern era. As considerable strides have already been made in countries such as Botswana, there is reason to hope that long-term progress will be assured. The alternative is unacceptable.

References

Akintola, O. (2006). Gendered home-based care in South Africa: More trouble for the troubled. *African Journal of AIDS Research, 5*(3), 237–247.

Alleyne, G. (2001). *Health and the quality of life*. http://www.paho.org/english/dbi/es/Alleyne.pdf. Accessed 11 Jan 2014.

Anderson, R. (2014). *Human suffering and quality of life: Conceptualising stories and statistics*. New York: Springer.

Barnett, T., & Whiteside, A. (2002). *AIDS in the twenty-first century: Disease and globalization*. New York: Palgrave Macmillan.

Botswana Ministry of Health. (2005). *Community home-based care for people with AIDS in Botswana: Operational guidelines.* The AIDS/STD Unit, National AIDS Control Programme. Republic of Botswana.

Botswana Ministry of Health. (2009). *Botswana AIDS impact survey* (BAIS 111). Republic of Botswana, Central Statistics Office, Gaborone.

Botswana Ministry of Health. (2013, September). Public Health Act No.11 of 2013. *Government Gazette,* Vol. *L11* No. *48.*

Brouwer, C. N., Lok, C. L., Wolffers, I., & Sebagalla, S. (2000). Psychosocial and economic aspects of HIV/AIDS and counselling of caretakers of HIV – Infected children in Uganda. *AIDS Care, 12*, 535–540.

Browning, E. (2008). Bringing HIV/AIDS care home: Investigating the value and impact of community home-based care in Botswana. *Independent study on society and culture in Africa in association with Associated Colleges of the Midwest, U.S.A.*

Budlender, D. (2004). Why should we care about unpaid work? *A guidebook prepared for the UNIFEM Southern Africa Region Office.* UNIFEM: Harare.

Campbell, C. (2003). *Letting them die: Why HIV prevention programmes fail.* Cape Town: Juta. Oxford: James Currey/Bloomington: Indiana University Press.

Chandler, R., Decker, C., & Nziyige, B. (2004). *Estimating the cost of preventing home based care for HIV/AIDS in Rwanda.* Bethesda: The Partners for Health Reformplus Project, Abt Associates.

Chikalipo, M. (2007). *Analysis of community home based care in Malawi.* MSc thesis, Queen Margaret University, Edinburgh.

CIA World Factbook. (2013). *Botswana.* https://www.cia.gov/library/publications/the-world-factbook/. Accessed 12 Jan 2014.

CoBaSys (Community Based Systems in HIV Treatment) Programme & UB TARSC (University of Botswana Training and Research Support Centre). (2011). *Strengthening community health systems for HIV treatment, support and care – Old Naledi, Gaborone, Botswana.* Report. (Support from the European Commission).

Elson, D. (2002). Macroeconomics and macroeconomic policy from a gender perspective. *Public Hearing Commission on Globalisation of the World Economy – Challenges and Responses.* Deutscher Bundestag.

Heymann, J. (2006). *Forgotten families: Ending the growing crisis confronting children and working parents in the global economy.* New York: Oxford University Press.

Jacques, G. (2004). Routine testing for HIV in Botswana: Public health panacea or human rights fiasco? A social work perspective. In G. Jacques, G. Lesetedi, & K. Osei-Hwedie (Eds.), *Human rights and social development in southern Africa* (pp. 283–303). Gaborone: Bay Publishing.

Jacques, G., & Mmatli, T. O. (2013). Addressing ethical non-sequiturs in Botswana's HIV and AIDS policies: Harmonising the halo effect. *Journal of Ethics and Social Welfare.* doi:10.1080/17496535.2013.768071.

Jacques, G., & Stegling, C. (2004). HIV/AIDS and home based care in Botswana: Panacea or perfidy? In A. Metteri, T. Kroger, A. Pohjola, & P.-L. Rauhala (Eds.), *Social work approaches in health and mental health from around the globe* (pp. 175–193). Binghamton/New York: The Haworth Social Work Practice Press.

Kang'ethe, S. (2010). Human rights perspectives on caregiving of people with HIV: The case for the Kanye home-based care programme, Botswana. *African Journal of AIDS Research, 9*(2), 193–203. doi:10.2989/16085906.2010.517489.

Kang'ethe, S. M. (2013). Feminization of poverty in palliative care giving of people living with HIV and AIDS and other debilitating diseases in Botswana: A literature review. *Journal of Virology and Microbiology,* Article ID772210. doi:10.5171/2013.772210.

Kipp, W., Nkosi, T. M., Laing, L., & Jhangri, G. S. (2006). Care burden and self-reported health status of informal women care-givers of HIV/AIDS patients in Kinshasa, Democratic Republic of Congo. *AIDS Care, 18*(7), 694–697.

Lindsey, E., Hirshfeld, M., Tlou, S., & Ncube, E. (2003). Home-based care in Botswana: Experiences of older women and young girls. *Health Care for Women International, 24*(6), 486–501.

Mmopelwa, G., Ngwenya, B. N., Sinha, N., & Sanders, J. B. P. (2013). Caregiver characteristics and economic cost of home-based care: A case study of Maun and Gumare Villages in North West District, Botswana. *Chronic Illness, 9*(1), 3–15.

NACA (National AIDS Co-ordinating Agency) and Government of the United States of America. (2010). *Partnership framework for HIV/AIDS 2010–2014.* Government of Botswana and Government of the United States of America.

National AIDS Control Programme (NACP) 30. (1996/2001/2005). Government of Botswana.

Ndaba-Mbata, R. D., & Seloilwe, E. S. (2000). Home-based care of the terminally ill in Botswana: Knowledge and perceptions. *International Council of Nurses, International Nursing Review, 47*(4), 218–223.

Ngwenya, B. N., & Butale, B. M. (2005). HIV/AIDS, intrafamily resources capacity and home care in Maun. *Botswana Notes and Records, 37,* 138–160.

Ngwenya, B. N., & Kgathi, D. L. (2006). HIV/AIDS and access to water: A case study of home-based care in Ngamiland, Botswana. *Physics and Chemistry of the Earth, 31,* 669–680.

Nnuko, S., Chiduo, B., Wilson, F., Msuya, W., & Mwaluko, G. (2000). Tanzania: AIDS care – Learning from experience. *Review of African Political Economy, 27*(86), 547–557.

Ogden, J., Esim, S., & Grown, C. (2004). Expanding the care continuum for HIV/AIDS: Bringing caregivers into focus. *Horizons Report.* Washington, DC: Population Council and International Centre for Research on Women.

Orner, P. (2006). Psychosocial impacts on caregivers of people living with AIDS. *AIDS Care: Psychological and Socio-medical Aspects of AIDS/HIV, 18*(3), 236–240.

Phaladze, N. A., Human, S., Dlamini, S. B., Hulela, E. B., Hadebe, I. M., Sukati, N. A., Makoae, L. N., Sebone, N. M., Moleko, M., & Holzemer, W. L. (2005). Quality of life and the concept of "living well" with HIV/AIDS in sub-Saharan Africa. *Journal of Nursing Scholarship, 37*(2), 120–126.

Pindani, M., Maluwa, A., Nkondo, M., Nyasulu, B. M., & Chilemba, W. (2013). Perception of people living with HIV and AIDS regarding home based care in Malawi. *Journal of AIDS and Clinical Research.* ISSN*: 2155–6113 JAR an open access journal, 4*(3), 1000201.

Rajaraman, D., Earle, A., & Heymann, S. J. (2008). Working HIV caregivers in Botswana: Spill-over effects on work and family wellbeing. *Community, Work & Family, 11*(1), 1–17.

Stegling, C. (2000). *Current challenges of HIV/AIDS in Botswana* (Working paper No. 1). Gaborone: Department of Sociology, University of Botswana.

Steinberg, M., Johnson, S., Schierhout, G., & Ndegwa, D. (2002). *Hitting home. How households cope with the impact of the HIV/AIDS epidemic: A survey of households affected by HIV/AIDS in South Africa.* Menlo Park: Henry J. Kauser Family Foundation, Publication no. 6059.

Uys, L. R. (2003). Aspects of the care of people with HIV/AIDS in South Africa. *Public Health Nursing, 20*(4), 271–280.

Uys, L. R., & Cameron, E. (2003). *Home-based HIV/AIDS care.* Cape Town: Oxford University Press.

WHO (World Health Organization). (2002). *Community home-based care in resource-limited settings: A framework for action.* Geneva: World Health Organization.

Chapter 13
Loneliness as Social Suffering: Social Participation, Quality of Life, and Chronic Stroke

Narelle Warren and Darshini Ayton

13.1 Introduction

Stroke is a catastrophic health event that, similar to many other long-term conditions, blurs the distinction between disability and chronicity (Manderson and Smith-Morris 2010; Warren and Manderson 2013), leading to long-term cognitive, physical, and social impairments. This occurs in multiple ways. Stroke is disabling by nature: it leads to changes in the physical capacity of the body. This can be seen immediately after stroke when the person affected may experience a wide range of mental and bodily symptoms including (but not limited to) weakness, balance problems, difficulty controlling movement or speech, issues with swallowing, or loss of proprioception. At the same time, stroke causes ongoing disability and may lead to limitations in mobility (e.g., requiring a wheeled walker or wheelchair), communication, or functional ability to undertake the activities of daily living, including self-care. As with other disabilities, the physical (or biological) and social dimensions of stroke, individually and in composite, are central to the production of individuals' suffering (Manderson and Smith-Morris 2010).

In this chapter, we posit that recovery from stroke is a profoundly social experience, though it has been largely emphasised as an acute biomedical process. Most improvements, centred on ideas of regaining "functioning" and resuming activities of daily living, occur in the first 3 months post-stroke (Teasell et al. 2012). After this

N. Warren (✉)
School of Social Sciences, Monash University, Clayton,
VIC 3800, Australia
e-mail: Narelle.Warren@monash.edu

D. Ayton
School of Public Health and Preventive Medicine, Monash University,
Clayton, VIC 3004, Australia
e-mail: Darshini.Ayton@monash.edu

© Springer Science+Business Media Dordrecht 2015
R.E. Anderson (ed.), *World Suffering and Quality of Life*,
Social Indicators Research Series 56, DOI 10.1007/978-94-017-9670-5_13

point, fewer functional gains are made, and stroke enters the realm of chronicity. Most people are discharged to home or a long-term care facility (such as a nursing home). Recovery extends over months and years (Aziz et al. 2008; Legg and Penn 2013; Teasell et al. 2012). Psychological, social, and psychosocial recovery is primarily achieved during this chronic phase, when the longer-term effects of stroke are felt, realized, and lived (Gallagher 2011; Wottrich et al. 2012).

This transition in the site of stroke recovery, from the hospital or clinic to the home or care setting, is foregrounded against a series of losses that accompany or follow stroke. While biomedical and rehabilitative efforts have concentrated on the functional (e.g., in terms of speech or movement) and cognitive (e.g., changes in memory, concentration, or affect) capacity changes that occur around the stroke event, longer term, more subtle losses in personal identity and social participation coexist. These losses contribute essentially to a keen type of social suffering, marked by distress and sadness (Rock 2003). The various stroke-related losses may be intertwined, with one type of loss pre-empting another. For instance, since changes in communicative abilities are common after stroke, especially within the context of aphasia, there may then be profound challenges for the maintenance of friendships (Davidson et al. 2008; Hilari et al. 2010). Similarly, impaired cognitive functioning may act to inhibit social engagement if the stroke sufferer is unable to maintain conversation or contribute meaningfully to interactions (Davidson et al. 2008); limited physical mobility may mean that opportunities for social participation are reduced (McKevitt et al. 2011). Alone or in concert, all these factors may act together to produce a profound sense of social isolation and loneliness.

In Charmaz's (1983) still-relevant report, suffering occurs through changes in self-image and the loss of self following the onset of a chronic condition. Here, suffering has its basis in four interconnected sources. First, *living a restricted life* occurs when one is housebound due to an illness. Illness becomes the focus of everyday life, restricting opportunities to reconstruct the self as an autonomous individual. Dependency is a focus of this restriction. Second, *social isolation* occurs as people's opportunities to share social worlds with others wanes. The reciprocity of social relations (predicated on equal effort expended by all parties in the interaction) is disrupted. This serves to weaken social ties, heightening isolation from former networks. Charmaz's third source, *discrediting definitions of the self*, relates to the loss of past positive self-image. Illness prevents people from fulfilling obligations or meeting the expectations of others; illness-determined limitations are then interpreted by others as some sort of personal frailty. Social isolation is, in this condition, "chosen" as a strategy to preserve a sense of self. Finally, *becoming a burden* reflects progressive reliance on others through dependence on others, including in terms of mobility.

These four dimensions speak to the known parameters of social life following stroke. For the most part, stroke renders the affected person necessarily reliant on others to move around the home or the community (Mayo et al. 2002), increases the need for someone to provide care, and reduces the size and range of a person's social networks (Northcott and Hilari 2011). Suffering in this context is relational: it is derived from, interpreted through, and tested and (sometimes) contested by social interactions.

13.2 Suffering, Quality of Life, and Capabilities

People aspire to live a life they perceive as meaningful and as having "quality" (Warren and Manderson 2013), even where their bodily or health context does not appear to support this. Following stroke, people employ multiple strategies to enhance their quality of life. This often involves a reordering or reinterpretation of their priorities as well as a greater reliance on their resources, especially their social support networks (Clarke and Black 2005). Precisely how they make these changes extends beyond the individual social and bodily contexts, and is influenced by sociocultural, economic, political, environmental, and psychological factors.

Expanding on this idea, the central question examined in this chapter is: How do people reconstruct their lives in the face of such social suffering to attain a sense of quality in their lives? To answer this question, we draw on the capabilities approach (Nussbaum 2005; Sen 1987) which conceptualizes quality of life as a person-centred concept. The *capability* of a particular person, or their ability to live a life that they perceive as having "quality," reflects their access to certain types of *functionings*, shaped by the *resources* available to them (Warren and Manderson 2013).

Resources can be both instrumental (related to material things that people can use, such as nutritional food, a wheelchair, walking stick, commode chair, and so forth) and affective (related to psychosocial aspects of existence, such as the presence of a supportive social network). While Sen (1987) argues that the notion of resources extends beyond the level of income, financial resources are undoubtedly important. They shape individuals' access to affective resources by providing a buffer against the socially isolating effects of poverty, as Mills and Zavaleta poignantly demonstrate in this volume.

Functionings are perceived as the range of "beings and doings" that the individual can choose from and understand as valuable; yet, as Robeyns (2006) argues, these remain underspecified and difficult to understand in an applied sense. Individuals can *be* or *do* in a range of ways. Being healthy, active, lonely, safe, educated, a burden, mobile, or a good friend are varying types of being important to this chapter. Within the context of the present research, "doings" could include communication, mobility, social participation, subjective well-being, or even symptom control. In more conventional approaches to quality of life, "functionings" might be understood as outcomes.

Quality of life (or well-being) can be derived from both capabilities—a person's abilities, opportunities, or "possibilities" (as termed by Sen 1987)—and functionings (what people can achieve through these capabilities). Extending this approach to social suffering in the context of chronic stroke, we posit that suffering operates by impeding a person's access to or mobilization of their social resources (i.e., it shapes their capabilities). The shrinking social networks experienced by people after stroke (i.e. limited resources) also *contribute* to suffering by reducing individuals' ability to achieve a specific set of functionings around social participation.

Through a series of short case studies, this chapter describes how people with stroke and their caregivers have actively sought to deploy their available social resources (usually social relations) to achieve specific sets of doings. For some, this was constrained by a lack of material resources. Our data, therefore, provide the ground to evaluate the utility of the capabilities approach for examining how the concepts of suffering and quality of life intersect for people recovering from chronic stroke.

13.3   The Ethnographic Study of Chronic Illnesses

The research on which this chapter is based was conducted as part of a larger ethnographic study on the social influences shaping the management of stroke and Parkinson's disease over time in the state of Victoria (Australia). We draw on a subset of data exploring the experiences of people who had experienced a stroke in the previous 5 years and the experiences of their family caregivers. Between 2011 and 2014, participants living in urban and regional parts of the state took part in three in-depth interviews: at recruitment, 6 months later, and then 9 months after that. Interview data were supplemented with photo elicitation (Allotey et al. 2003) and observational methods in an attempt to identify factors of which we were otherwise unaware. Recruitment was purposive, supplemented by a network sampling technique ("snowball sampling"), and occurred through advertisements placed in community newspapers, online noticeboards, and support organization newsletters; several participants also contacted the research team after attending a presentation about the study.

Overall, 20 people who had experienced a stroke and 19 informal caregivers participated in this study. With some exceptions, participants were over 70 years old and living in their own home, receiving care from a family member. All were of European descent (Anglo-Australian) and many were receiving some sort of governmental assistance (either through subsidised health care or age-related welfare). Most interviews were undertaken as "dyad" interviews, whereby both the person who had experienced stroke and their primary caregiver took part together. This enabled the involvement of people with greater levels of disablement, particularly those with ongoing memory and communication issues, and followed recommendations on interviewing people with cognitive impairment (Paterson and Scott-Findlay 2002). In some instances, the caregiver took part in an additional, separate interview. Consent was negotiated immediately prior to each interview to ensure that participation was voluntary.

During interviews, we sought to gain participants' narratives of stroke and attempted to capture their experiences of stroke, how they understood their (or their family member's) stroke, what it was like for them during the acute phases, how it impacted their lives in the longer term, as well as their care arrangements, engagement with health professionals, self-management strategies, psychosocial issues, access to formal and informal social support, and concerns for the future. Data collection was iterative within and between each interview, allowing the researchers to follow up on any unexpected or novel topics raised by participants. All interviews were audio-recorded and later transcribed verbatim.

Data were analyzed via a grounded theory approach, using the constant comparison method outlined by Markovic (2006). Working together through the initial phases of analysis, we identified and named the thematic concerns (codes) that were expressed during participants' accounts. Coding occurred at two levels: while some codes were identified based on what the participants had actually said (*semantic themes*, Braun and Clarke 2006), other codes represented our awareness of a deeper meaning or mechanism at play. Such *latent themes* (Braun and Clarke 2006) form the theoretical foundation of this chapter. The excerpts from interviews selected here demonstrate the different ways in which we see social relations impacting people's experience of social suffering following stroke. Each excerpt provides insights into the relationship between suffering and quality of life. All participants are referred to by pseudonyms. Ethical approval for the conduct of the study was obtained from the Monash University Human Research Ethics Committee.

13.4 Our Findings

13.4.1 Suffering as a Consequence of Reduced Resources

For all participants in our study, stroke had profound and lasting effects on social participation. This caused considerable distress and led to a sense of loneliness; we conceptualized this as a form of social suffering. Many described how they had fewer friends in the years following their stroke; the long-term physical effects of stroke had social implications. For example, a number of participants became progressively more isolated as a result of ongoing fatigue. They tired easily, and over time they had less energy or interest in going out and socialising. Indeed, participants typically reported that their primary reason for leaving the home was to attend medical appointments or to undertake chores such as grocery shopping. In this way, their lives gradually become more focused on the home environment (speaking to Charmaz's 1983 definition of the *restricted life* in chronic illness) and eventually participants had access to fewer social resources. This, in turn, reduced the person's opportunities for socialization (leading to *social isolation*) and often prompted a restriction in the *functionings* available to participants. In addition, that most participants relied on others for help with their day-to-day life echoed Charmaz's *being a burden* aspect of suffering, impacting on the functionings available to caregivers.

The cognitive impairments associated with stroke left many participants feeling overwhelmed in social situations, as they often felt unable to "keep up" with conversations or express themselves properly. Eileen said, "I have trouble when I want to say something, [my brain] doesn't process it." Gus found that he was unable to express himself properly in social settings: "I used to be able talk alright but now I get tongue-tied and forgetful." Participants found it difficult to sustain concentration and required social assistance from their family caregiver, as this excerpt from an interview with Arthur (person with stroke) and Joan (his wife) illustrates:

Interviewer:	What's it like for you having Joan to help you with eating and bathing?
Arthur:	I can't keep up with anybody else.
Joan:	[She] said, do you mind I've got to help you?
Arthur:	No, I don't mind.
Joan:	Do you like it? Do you like me helping you?
Arthur:	No, I don't mind.
Joan:	You wished you could do it yourself.
Arthur:	Yeah.
Joan:	Sometimes he tries to do things and he has several falls doing that. He thinks he'll help me, and of course he can't manage and then we've got to scoop you up, haven't we?
Arthur:	What?
Joan:	[I've] got to pick you up.
Arthur:	Yeah. That's hard to do. You wouldn't do it.

In "losing track" of conversations like Arthur, participants often felt self-conscious and reluctant to take part in social activities, ultimately choosing to stay home in order to avoid the awkwardness of many interactions.

Where participants experienced difficulties in communication, their sense of social restriction was heightened. Following his stroke, Jamie was left aphasic and communicated through the use of a digital speech device. Even with the device, it was often difficult to understand what he was trying to communicate, as his sister Sharon explained: "Jamie's communication is quite good now, even single words." This reflected Charmaz's (1983) concern with *discrediting definitions of the self*, whereby participants (both those who experienced stroke and their carers) struggled with their inability to behave in socially normative ways. Nicholas had continence issues and required assistance in toileting after his stroke:

> He was incontinent… This is a condition that you have after a stroke. Nobody talks about it… I could have been sitting next to him and by the time he could verbalise [his need to use a toilet], it was too late… But the brain obviously couldn't verbalise it in time and often when I looked at him after a disaster happened… he had this foggy look on his face as if to say he couldn't really see what was the problem. (Evka, Nicholas's partner and carer)

Bodily changes, as well as changes in motor skills or emotional responses, shaped how participants chose to engage with others socially. Many participants in our study described how their ongoing challenges with swallowing or feeding themselves led them to deliberately avoid particular social settings. Experiences of unexpected or random crying also shaped social participation. Eileen, for example, described how her increased emotionality after stroke led others to avoid her as a way of managing their own inability to respond appropriately:

> I'm still very emotional, like when you've had a stroke, you can cry and you don't know why… One of the things that really, really upset me [was that] a lot of people who haven't had strokes can't cope. [My friends have] all gone, never come back. I can count my friends on [one hand] now and that, you know… at times I cry about it… I know they don't understand it. Maybe they find it hard looking [at me] when I get [emotional – *Eileen is weeping*]. When I think of them, it just gets to me.

Gus, too, became very emotional after his stroke. He related this both to the associated cognitive changes and to his struggle with his lost independence:

Gus: I cry, and I can't control it. Doesn't matter if I go somewhere. [I was out] the other night and a guy asked me about the stroke and I burst out crying. It's something that just happens.
Interviewer: Is it something that relates to you just feeling sad about the stroke?
Gus: Yeah, it's [also] about my life sort of thing.

Not long after his first of five strokes, Gus's wife left him and he was forced to retire. Since then, one of his children had stopped talking with him. He described how these factors, combined with his lingering hurt over his child and inability to understand what had caused the rift, left him feeling very lonely and unable to find a sense of well-being:

> I was lonely too, being here on my own… You like to be able turn around and say good day [to someone], it makes you lonely… After stroke… you [have to] learn to start life all over again. And its like you are going backwards. [So] to stop work dead and you got no hope, what do you do? That's where loneliness sets in as well. You've got to stay in touch with people.

In addition, Gus found that the loss of his driver's licence further impacted on his quality of life as he became more reliant on others to drive distances:

> I have to get someone else to drive. Which means you've got to rely on someone else. That's a problem, relying on someone else… I like being independent.

Gus, however, was able to combat his loneliness through several means. First, he enjoyed being social, but not dependent on others, and sought out opportunities for socialization: "There's not many people that I can't ring up and go and have a coffee with or sit down and chat to." In addition, he became involved in several stroke and brain injury support groups, which provided further opportunities for interactions. He also turned to the Internet to develop new connections. In this way, Gus used his sociability as a resource (a type of functioning), and that heightened his quality of life.

13.4.2   Alleviating Suffering Through Redeploying or Finding New Resources

Despite feeling socially isolated and unable to participate in social life in the same way that they had before stroke, participants described how they used social resources to achieve a sense of quality of life. This occurred in two ways: through the development of new resources, such as support groups, and the redeployment of pre-existing social relations, which involved the transformation of existing relationships into a new form.

Like Gus, some participants in our study looked for new types of resources that they could employ to achieve their desired goals around social participation (i.e. new functionings). For many, this involved participation in a support group or other types of organized socialising. For Jamie, aphasia both contributed to his social isolation and presented a challenge for his family in trying to alleviate his suffering and distress:

Sharon: Our biggest hiccup this year has probably been when you had your low patch at the end of winter, wasn't it Jamie? But you're feeling better again now, aren't you?
Jamie: Yes yes
Sharon: Jamie managed to communicate to a carer that he'd been feeling suicidal and that he was… just been bored a lot and I think a long winter in this [aged care institution]… It was just driving you crazy, wasn't it Jamie?
Jamie: Yes yes

Sharon and her siblings worked to increase Jamie's opportunities for social participation in order to help him feel better about life. As a result, he became actively involved in a stroke support group and developed new friendships; he started going out for dinner regularly and attended sporting events. Involvement in these social activities allowed Jamie to feel more independent and as though he was important in the lives of others; in response, his suicidal ideation ceased.

Stroke support groups were, as may be evident already, especially important, as they formed a new type of resource for social interactions that was accepting of the limitations of the post-stroke body. The groups alleviated the potential for being discredited that concerned some participants. Joan and Arthur, among others, perceived support groups as an ideal way to balance their desire for social interactions against managing potentially embarrassing situations:

Joan: We made new friends going to the stroke support group, because they are understanding and it's very relevant to be among other stroke victims. Some [are] worse than Arthur, some [are] better than Arthur, some you wouldn't know had a stroke. We've certainly made new friends…
Arthur: It's quite a friendly one. We go every month.
Joan: Every month. It doesn't matter if you need to eat your food with a spoon or be fed or need your meals cut up, everyone's the same, everyone understands… Generally, I have to help [Arthur] sometimes. But I always make sure it's [what he wants].

The sense of safety and lack of judgement truly supported participants, both those who experienced stroke and their caregivers, in attaining a sense of well-being and social participation. In this way, support groups acted as a resource to alleviate participants' isolation and formed a new type of functioning. They alleviated some of the social suffering around stroke.

Support groups also provided participants with an opportunity to reclaim their independence through being a "safe space". They encouraged participants, regardless of marital status, to get out of the house and move forward in their recovery. As Samantha, who has had a stroke, explained:

> [After stroke,] you do sit around in a bit of self-pity. Which quite rightfully, you are allowed to I suppose, but I am not one of them people. So I found that very hard to cope with. But you think, well you are very lucky, get on with life. Found [stroke group] quite good actually… I just go along by myself. It's good because… I had really lost all my confidence as well… Just going out and doing things by yourself [helps].

Although she had become increasingly reliant on her husband, Samantha believed that doing things on her own was a significant step in her recovery.

Close family members and friends became a more important resource than ever for giving participants, especially the caregivers, a sense of social engagement. Still, the role these connections took in the lives of our participants (regardless of whether they had stroke or were a carer) was fundamentally transformed by stroke. After stroke, social ties as resources were used in a different way: they transformed from a reciprocal to a more unidirectional style of relation. Limited mobility following stroke meant that friends and family members often had to visit participants in their home. This did prompt a shedding of some social relations, as Walter (person with stroke) explained:

Interviewer: What about your friends, have they given you much support?
Walter: Not really. It's amazing how they disappear. Probably only one or
              two kept up the [contact]… Really and truly, [most people] don't
              want to know. They expect you to be a dribbling idiot. I really
              haven't had [much contact with my old friends]. The friends I have
              now are probably stroke people… Probably only one or two [old
              friends keep in touch], whereas before we had heaps of people.

While Joan and Arthur experienced a similar process, Joan explained how the important people in their lives had stayed in touch: "We don't see some of our friends as much now of course. But on the whole, our real friends, will still be our real friends." Their interview was heavily focused on the social impacts of stroke and, during it, Joan clearly described how they had redeployed their existing relations:

> We can't get to church anymore. We just can't. Arthur can't cope anymore. So we have a visitor coming every few weeks [who] tells us what's happening. Things like that. [There are] not many days, consecutive days, when someone hasn't called in. The family ring every day. So, we have lots going on still.

Pre-illness membership of groups, such as church groups, appeared to play an important role in participants' ability to transform their social relationships into new and lasting types of resources.

13.4.3 Suffering and Reduced Social Connectedness Due to Limited Finances

For a number of study participants, changes in employment status led to a reduction in opportunities for socializing with friends and family. After a series of mild strokes in her early 40s, Allie left work. Due to ongoing fatigue and concentration issues, she was unable to return to work, even though she had made a "good" recovery. She had to live on a disability pension. As her interview illustrates, Allie lost contact with many friends and instead became reliant on a good friend, her children, and the stroke support group:

> [The benefits from the support group relate to] just getting out and meeting people, just getting out of the house. 'Cos I can't work, so I've lost all that contact with people that I used to see every day or whatever. I still see like one girl that I used to work with… Um, I saw her a couple of months ago out at the market place. And that's the first time I'd seen her in about three years. So you just lose contact with everyone.

The cost and effort required to go to restaurants, to the movies, or on a holiday was often out of reach for those on a carer's allowance or disability pension. All of our participants were living on some form of welfare following their stroke; only one person with stroke (Samantha) and two carers had contemplated returning to work. Their accounts describing reduced opportunities for social participation occurred in the context of limited financial resources; although we did not explore it here, finances may also underscore the importance of stroke support groups: participation was often free or minimal. Similarly, participants' lower incomes may have prompted their retreat from engaging with friends and family, which has implications for their well-being. As the effects of stroke persist, people often do not recover fully; similarly, the losses of social connections were neither transient nor short term.

13.5 Conclusion

Ultimately, this chapter tells stories of hope. Our participants related accounts about how they used a range of strategies to attempt to overcome their sense of social isolation and the associated suffering. Many were successful in alleviating their suffering to some extent, although the lingering social isolation caused by their persistent disabilities continued to resonate for many. The older age of our participants is likely to be influential here. Through increased likelihood of disability and the shrinking of social networks due to mortality, longevity itself may contribute to suffering (Anderson, Chaps. 1 and 32, this volume).

By applying a capabilities approach lens, this chapter highlights the ways in which social (presence of friends and family members, availability of support groups, and access to technologies) and economic resources mediate experiences of social suffering. Social resources supported our respondents in achieving a range of social functionings, evidenced by their engagement in supportive social environments and close relationships with others. These provided a sense of quality in patient and caregivers' lives. In contrast, and although it is not explored in detail here, the low incomes of participants may have prevented them from achieving their full functionings and capabilities.

The contribution of an ethnographic approach to this volume lies in its detail of the intimate ties between suffering and social relations. In particular, the relations of care evidenced in and through participants' accounts highlights the ways in which people actively resist or attempt to reframe suffering. Carers especially sought, through their actions and their ethos of care, to alleviate the suffering of their loved one, often making compromises in their own lives to ensure that the person with a stroke was able to achieve quality of life through an *engagement* in life (see Manderson and Warren 2013).

The concept of compromise is central here; people make decisions based on the best options available to them. These facets of experience are complex and nuanced. While they may be partly captured through the capabilities approach, we believe that it overlooks the affective dimensions of care relations in responding to suffering and enhancing quality of life. In this way, our findings reflect Dean's (2009) critique of the method: he argues that the capabilities approach is unable to reflect the realities of the interdependency in human interactions precisely because of its emphasises on the independence of individuals. Instead, Dean highlights the pervasive vulnerability that characterizes human relationships and, thus, the drive for connection. As he points out and as we have illustrated here, people negotiate, struggle, and deal with competing priorities in order to achieve a "good life".

Regardless of our participants' outcomes, meaning and quality in their lives was achieved through a sense of connection with others. Samantha's account highlights how the alleviation of suffering relies on a premise of simultaneous interdependence and autonomy (Dean 2009). Central to all of these accounts is the difficulty of defining the concept of love, overlooked by the capabilities approach and oft-maligned elsewhere. With an understanding that they are loved and cared about by someone, usually their spouse, our participants' suffering was conquerable, even in the face of considerable physical, cognitive, and communication difficulties.

References

Allotey, P. A., Reidpath, D. D., Kouame, A., & Cummins, R. (2003). The DALY, context and the determinants of the severity of disease: An exploratory comparison of paraplegia in Australia and Cameroon. *Social Science and Medicine, 57*(5), 949–958.

Aziz, N. A., Leonardi-Bee, J., Phillips, M., Gladman, J. R., Legg, L., & Walker, M. F. (2008, April 16). Therapy-based rehabilitation services for patients living at home more than one year after stroke. *Cochrane Database Systematic Reviews* (2), CD005952.

Braun, V., & Clarke, V. (2006). Using thematic analysis in psychology. *Qualitative Research in Psychology, 3*(2), 77–101. doi:10.1191/1478088706qp063oa.

Charmaz, K. (1983). Loss of self: A fundamental form of suffering in the chronically ill. *Sociology of Health & Illness, 5*(2), 168–195. doi:10.1111/1467-9566.ep10491512.

Clarke, P., & Black, S. E. (2005). Quality of life following stroke: Negotiating disability, identity, andresources.*JournalofAppliedGerontology,24*(4),319–336.doi:10.1177/0733464805277976.

Davidson, B., Howe, T., Worrall, L., Hickson, L., & Togher, L. (2008). Social participation for older people with aphasia: The impact of communication disability on friendships. *Topics in Stroke Rehabilitation, 15*(4), 325–340. doi:10.1310/tsr1504-325.

Dean, H. (2009). Critiquing capabilities: The distractions of a beguiling concept. *Critical Social Policy, 29*(2), 261–273.

Gallagher, P. (2011). Becoming normal: A grounded theory study on the emotional process of stroke recovery. *Canadian Journal of Neuroscience Nursing, 33*(3), 24–32.

Hilari, K., Northcott, S., Roy, P., Marshall, J., Wiggins, R. D., Chataway, J., & Ames, D. (2010). Psychological distress after stroke and aphasia: The first six months. *Clinical Rehabilitation, 24*(2), 181–190. doi:10.1177/0269215509346090.

Legg, C., & Penn, C. (2013). Uncertainty, vulnerability, and isolation: Factors framing quality of life with aphasia in a South African township. In N. Warren & L. Manderson (Eds.), *Reframing disability and quality of life: A global perspective* (pp. 17–38). Dordrecht: Springer.

Manderson, L., & Smith-Morris, C. (2010). Introduction. On chronicity: Unsettling biomedical binaries and attending to context. In L. Manderson & C. Smith-Morris (Eds.), *Chronic conditions, fluid states: Chronicity and the anthropology of illness* (pp. 1–18). New Brunswick: Rutgers University Press.

Manderson, L., & Warren, N. (2013). "Caring for" and "caring about": Embedded interdependence and quality of life. In N. Warren & L. Manderson (Eds.), *Reframing disability and quality of life: A global perspective* (pp. 179–194). Dordrecht: Springer.

Markovic, M. (2006). Analyzing qualitative data: Health care experiences of women with gynecological cancer. *Field Methods, 18*(4), 413–429. doi:10.1177/1525822x06293126.

Mayo, N. E., Wood-Dauphinee, S., Durcan, L., & Carlton, J. (2002). Activity, participation, and quality of life 6 months poststroke. *Archives of Physical Medicine and Rehabilitation, 83*(8), 1035–1042.

McKevitt, C., Fudge, N., Redfern, J., Sheldenkar, A., Crichton, S., Rudd, A. R., et al. (2011). Self-reported long-term needs after stroke. *Stroke, 42*(5), 1398–1403.

Northcott, S., & Hilari, K. (2011). Why do people lose their friends after a stroke? *International Journal of Language and Communication Disorders, 46*(5), 524–534. doi:10.1111/j.1460-6984.2011.00079.x.

Nussbaum, M. C. (2005). Wellbeing, contracts and capabilities. In L. Manderson (Ed.), *Rethinking wellbeing* (pp. 27–44). Perth: API Network.

Paterson, B., & Scott-Findlay, S. (2002). Critical issues in interviewing people with traumatic brain injury. *Qualitative Health Research, 12*(3), 399–409.

Robeyns, I. (2006). The capability approach in practice. *Journal of Political Philosophy, 14*(3), 351–376.

Rock, M. (2003). Sweet blood and social suffering: Rethinking cause-effect relationships in diabetes, distress, and duress. *Medical Anthropology, 22*(2), 131–174. doi:10.1080/01459740306764.

Sen, A. K. (1987). *The standard of living: The Tanner lectures*. Cambridge: Cambridge University Press.

Teasell, R., Mehta, S., Pereira, S., McIntyre, A., Janzen, S., Allen, L., et al. (2012). Time to rethink long-term rehabilitation management of stroke patients. *Topics in Stroke Rehabilitation, 19*(6), 457–462. doi:10.1310/tsr1906-457.

Warren, N., & Manderson, L. (2013). Reframing disability and quality of life: Contextual nuances. In N. Warren & L. Manderson (Eds.), *Reframing disability and quality of life* (pp. 1–16). Dordrecht/New York: Springer.

Wottrich, A. W., Astrom, K., & Lofgren, M. (2012). On parallel tracks: Newly home from hospital–people with stroke describe their expectations. *Disability and Rehabilitation, 34*(14), 1218–1224. doi:10.3109/09638288.2011.640381.

Part III
Quality of Life: Global, Community, and Personal

Chapter 14
Child Well-Being and Child Suffering

Kenneth C. Land, Vicki L. Lamb, and Qiang Fu

14.1   Introduction

Child well-being research stems from the social indicators movement of the 1960s and 1970s (Lamb and Land 2015), and it has received increasing attention since UNICEF's annual reports on *The Progress of Nations* began in 1993. The reports were designed to monitor the well-being of children across the globe in order to chart the changes and advances made since the 1990 World Summit for Children (UNICEF 1997). The very existence of the reports documents that the available indicators were not adequate for monitoring children even in the developed world. The reports also recognized that suffering is a barrier to the realization of child well-being and happiness, whether in the form of physical suffering, mental suffering, or social suffering (Anderson 2014: 10).

This chapter describes the well-being research literature and the extent to which it can be used to infer about child suffering. It commences with a review of the objective and subjective approaches to measuring well-being and moves into a look at the United Nations Convention on the Rights of the Child and how it has been referenced in cross-national studies of child well-being. This leads to a descriptive

K.C. Land (✉)
Department of Sociology, Faculty of Sociology, Duke University,
268 Soc-Psych, Durham, Box 90088, NC 27708-0989, USA
e-mail: kland@soc.duke.edu

V.L. Lamb
Department of Human Sciences, Faculty of Human Sciences, North Carolina Central
University, 203 Dent Human Sciences Bldg., Durham, NC 27707, USA
e-mail: vlamb@nccu.edu

Q. Fu
Department of Sociology, Duke University, 346, Soc-Psych Bldg,
90088, Durham, NC 27708-0989, USA
e-mail: fu.qiangsoc@gmail.com

© Springer Science+Business Media Dordrecht 2015   173
R.E. Anderson (ed.), *World Suffering and Quality of Life*,
Social Indicators Research Series 56, DOI 10.1007/978-94-017-9670-5_14

analysis of country-specific indicators of child suffering in relation to corresponding values of the Human Development Index and consideration of what this tells us about child suffering in relation to human development. We conclude with future directions for advancing the global monitoring of child suffering.

14.2   Approaches to Well-Being Measurement

Researchers approach measurements of child well-being both objectively and subjectively.[1] Objective measures focus on the state or status of the child, whereas subjective views focus on the expression of opinions, behaviors, beliefs, feelings, or experiences.

Objective measures of child well-being are based on available statistical data and can include indicators associated with health (e.g., infant mortality or low birth weight), education (e.g., completion or graduation rates), economy (e.g., child poverty), or behaviors (e.g., teen pregnancy rates). Such measures generate reports on the "State of the Child" and have been produced for children of varied age-groups and from different population settings including local, state or sub-regional, national, and multinational regions. Literature reviews have revealed that such reports date back to the 1950s, although the majority of early reports are singular reports rather than a series of reports (Ben-Arieh and Goerge 2001; Ben-Arieh 2006, 2012). However, there are notable series reporting objective measures of children. These include UNICEF's *State of the World's Children* reports since 1979 and *The Progress of Nations* reports published since 1993. In the United States, the Annie E. Casey Foundation has published the *KIDS COUNT Databook* since 1990, ranking and comparing the 50 U.S. states on ten negative, objective indicators of child well-being and the U.S. Federal Interagency Forum on Child and Youth Statistics has issued reports entitled *America's Children: Key National Indicators of Well-Being* since 1997.

Subjective measures or indicators of child well-being are usually obtained through sample surveys designed to measure opinions, attitudes, or responses from children or adults speaking on behalf of children. These metrics are important for more fully understanding expressed or experienced notions of well-being. Efforts to harmonize comparisons across nations have yielded survey instruments used in various countries. In Europe, child well-being indicators from sample surveys of children include the Program for International Student Assessment (PISA), the Health Behavior in School-aged Children (HBSC), European School Survey Project on Alcohol and other Drugs (ESPAD), and indicators regularly collected via surveys by international organizations such as UNICEF, the World Bank, and the World Health Organization. As the titles indicate, such surveys are usually collected for

---

[1] This review of approaches to well-being measurement is based on Lamb and Land (2015), which can be consulted for more details.

specific reasons, yet also yield important indicators for comparative research of child well-being.

The term *social indicators* was coined in the early 1960s to refer to efforts to detect social change and to evaluate the impact of specific programs, such as the U.S. space program. The basic social indicator question is "How are we doing?" (Land 2000). Work on social indicators during the 1960s and 1970s followed two basic traditions. One was the *development of objective measures* through the review of available data to provide descriptive evaluations of the status of society and to recommend unmet data needs for such evaluations. The other direction was the *development of subjective indicators of well-being and quality of life*. Both traditions have impacted the monitoring and measurement of child well-being (Land et al. 2007).

In the tradition of subjective indicators, Cummins (1996) conducted a review of empirical studies of adult quality of life (QOL). He found that a vast majority of the total reported data could be grouped into seven domains of life, subjectively reported in focus groups, case studies, clinical studies, and sample surveys: (1) economic or material well-being; (2) health; (3) safety; (4) productive activity (e.g., employment, job, work, schooling); (5) place in community or community engagement (e.g., education and job status, community involvement, self-esteem, and empowerment); (6) intimacy (e.g., relationships with family and friends); and (7) emotional well-being (e.g., mental health, morale, spiritual well-being). According to Cummins, the empirical studies indicate that all seven domains are relevant to the overall concept of subjective well-being or QOL. As recommended in a comprehensive review of numerous QOL indices (Hagerty et al. 2001), these domains identified can and should be used to guide the selection and classification of indices of QOL based on *objective* data.

14.3   The United Nations Convention on the Rights of the Child

In 1989, the United Nations (UN) adopted the Convention on the Rights of the Child (CRC) (United Nations 1989),[2] which has been ratified by all UN countries except the United States and Somalia. Prior to 1989, a number of other international resolutions and declarations regarding children included the Geneva Declaration of the Rights of the Child of 1924, the Declaration of the Rights of the Child adopted by the UN General Assembly in 1959, plus International Covenants on Civil and Political Rights and on Economic, Social, and Cultural Rights adopted in 1976. The CRC was formulated to recognize that children are citizens of society in their own right, rather than merely future adults; thus, the overriding purpose was to grant children the full range of human rights including: the right to survival; to develop to

---

[2] See Lamb and Land (2015) for additional materials on the CRC and cross-national studies using concepts and measures based on the CRC.

the fullest; to protection from harmful influences, abuse and exploitation; and to participate fully in family, cultural, and social life (UNICEF n.d.).

There are four core principles in the CRC that encompass the human rights to be held by all children:

1. non-discrimination (*Article 2*),
2. devotion to the best interests of the child (*Article 3*),
3. the right to life, survival, and development (*Article 6*), and
4. respect for the views of the child (*Article 12*) (United Nations 1989).

Under the CRC, children are to be recognized as active members of a society with entitled rights (though also family dependents) and the international community is to establish criteria regarding the improvement of child well-being and child QOL (Casas 1997).

According to Article 1 of the Convention, a child is defined as "every human being below the age of 18 years unless, under the law applicable to the child, majority is attained earlier" (United Nations 1989: 2). The CRC indicates that childhood should be recognized as a *separate phase* in life, and children are *active members* of the society. Part I of the Convention on the Rights of Children lists 41 articles that define the numerous rights of children. In addition to the four core principles listed above, the CRC includes other specific rights:

- citizenship, and an identity that is separate from adults (*Articles 7, 8*),
- the implementation and legal protection of children's rights including when arrested, imprisoned, or accused of infringing penal law (*Articles 4, 16, 37, 40*),
- freedom of thought, religion, and other basic freedoms (*Articles 13, 14, 15*),
- access to "the highest attainable standard" of health care and health facilities, which include accommodation for children with disabilities or in institutions due to physical and/or mental health needs (*Articles 23, 24, 25*),
- the right to a standard of living that promotes proper "physical, mental, spiritual, moral and social" development as well as equal access to education at all levels (*Articles 27, 28*),
- protection from child trafficking, economic exploitation, sexual exploitation and abuse, and other exploitation that adversely affects the child's welfare (*Articles 11, 32, 34, 35, 36*), as well as
- respect for parents and family and the duties they fulfill in nurturing and protection of children (*Articles 5, 9, 10, 18*).

The fourth CRC core principle impacted the development of indicators and methodologies in the study of child well-being. It is important that children's voices are heard and understood, as their perspectives may differ from those of adults. This emphasis on respecting children as persons can contribute to informing policymakers and child advocacy concerns, and children can become better informed about legal and political issues that directly affect their lives (Ben-Arieh 2005). In fulfilling these obligations, an increasing number of countries, particularly European countries, are collecting data or reviewing available data to establish the baseline rights and concerns of children as outlined in the CRC.

14.4 Cross-National Studies of Child Well-Being Using the CRC Approach

Several recent, cross-national studies of child well-being have emerged from the CRC. Starting with the credo *"to improve something, first measure it,"* and incorporating the CRC in the conceptualization and interpretation of child well-being, UNICEF (2007) conducted a study of child well-being across Organisation for Economic Cooperation and Development (OECD) countries. The results were published in an *Innocenti Report Card* on *Child Well-Being in Rich Countries* (UNICEF 2007) in which multiple domains of child well-being were calculated—a vast improvement over UNICEF's earlier use of income and poverty as a proxy. The ranking of countries varied across the domains, demonstrating that no one indicator could serve as such a unilateral proxy.

Jonathan Bradshaw and colleagues Petra Hoelscher and Dominic Richardson were members of the group of external advisors for the UNICEF Report Card 7. This team has conducted a number of cross-sectional, cross-national studies of the well-being of children, one of which was a report in conjunction with the 2007 UNICEF report. In comparing child well-being in OECD countries, Bradshaw et al. (2007a) provided additional information regarding the selection of indicators and a more detailed explanation regarding the methodology used to develop the rankings. In the same year, Bradshaw and colleagues (2007b) published a multi-dimensional child well-being index for the 25 European Union countries (EU25). This study was more detailed due to the availability of indicators for the EU25 countries as compared with the OECD nations. Bradshaw and Richardson (2009) went on to conduct another study of child well-being in 27 EU countries plus Iceland and Norway. The results were similar to those in their EU25 study: In general, the Nordic countries (the Netherlands, Sweden, Finland, and Denmark) ranked in the top third, and the former Eastern bloc countries, except Slovenia, were in the bottom third. Iceland and Norway, when included in the second model, ranked third and fourth in child well-being (respectively), between Sweden, ranked second, and Finland, ranked fifth (Bradshaw and Richardson 2009).

Richardson et al. (2008) expanded their global multidimensional study of child well-being by focusing on 21 countries from Central and Eastern Europe (CEE) and the Commonwealth of Independent States (CIS), covering the first decade of the twenty-first century. As the authors explained, "the CEE/CIS region is very heterogeneous in terms of geography and natural resources, demographic structure, economic and political developments" (2008: 212). All the countries were experiencing social changes, particularly in demographic reforms and economic structures, so they emphasized the importance of studying child well-being amid such transitions. Richardson et al. (2008) identified trends in the ranking of dimensions: Belarus, Bulgaria, and Russia ranked high in dimensions associated with standard public services, such as economic and material situation, child health, and education, but ranked poorly on personal and social relationships and indicators of risk and safety behaviors. The opposite was evident for countries that in turmoil, such as Bosnia

Herzegovina, Uzbekistan, and Azerbaijan. For example, ethnic conflict and divisions in Bosnia Herzegovina stalled the establishment of public services to support the diverse population, and thus, poverty rates were high along and the country had many displaced persons. The new EU members Romania and Bulgaria ranked in the middle and lower third, respectively, indicating that children in these countries have yet to benefit from their countries' EU membership. The authors' research also aimed to determine how influential a country's wealth, or GDP per capita, was when associated with overall rankings of the CEE/CIS countries; wealth only explained about a third of the variation in ranking of child well-being in the countries studied (Richardson et al. 2008).

For their part, Lau and Bradshaw (2010) evaluated children's well-being in 13 countries at various levels of successful economic growth and development in the Pacific Rim. A number of countries – Australia, Japan, New Zealand and the Asian newly developing economies of Singapore, Hong Kong, and South Korea – ranked highly on the global HDI,[3] whereas Malaysia, Thailand, China, the Philippines, Indonesia, and Vietnam had high to medium HDI rankings (Lau and Bradshaw 2010). By comparison, Japan, Singapore, Taiwan, Hong Kong, and New Zealand were the five top-ranking countries in overall child well-being. As with other multinational studies of child well-being, no Pacific Rim country was consistent in its ranking among the seven domains. Indonesia and the Philippines, at the bottom of the overall rankings, each scored high for subjective well-being. Thailand ranked high for living environment. Wealthier countries were associated with higher scores ($R^2 = 0.54$), although there were some notable exceptions: Australia and South Korea (Lau and Bradshaw 2010).

Existing cross-national comparisons of child well-being notably omits the systematic study of child well-being in Africa, Central and South America, and South and West Asia. There are international publications of objective indicators of the state of the child, such as the aforementioned UNICEF reports and indicators published by the World Bank, but, to date, there has been no systematic study of the available data for child well-being in these parts of the world.

14.5   Child Suffering and Human Development

The main emphasis of recent cross-national studies of the condition of children has been on measures of well-being, the positive end of a suffering-to-well-being scale. The question to which we now turn is the extent to which existing sources of cross-national data can be used to assess the suffering end of this spectrum for children.

Insofar as we seek comprehensive comparisons across large numbers of countries that range from developed to less developed, the available indicators of child suffering are very limited, concentrated among indicators of health and education. Thus, we focus our analysis on the extent to which cross-national indicators of child

---

[3] The Human Development Index is to be discussed more fully in the next section of this chapter.

suffering correlate with human development indicators (specifically, the HDI). The HDI is a composite social indicator and well-being index based on life expectancy, education, and income statistics at the country or national level. Its objective is to rank as many countries as possible on a scale of human development. The following is a brief summary of its conceptual and methodological foundations.[4]

The HDI has been produced and updated yearly since 1990 by the United Nations Human Development Programme (UNDP). See http://www.undp.org/content/undp/en/home.html. In 2013, the UNDP operated in 177 countries, working to help each draw on the UN's resources to find its own solutions to development challenges. As an executive board within the UN General Assembly, the UNDP's Administrator is the third highest-ranking official in the UN. The UNDP works in four main areas: poverty reduction and achieving the Millennium Development Goals (MDGs; United Nations 2000); democratic governance; crisis prevention and recovery; and environment and sustainable development. The Millennium Development goals are to, by the year 2015:

1. eradicate extreme poverty and hunger;
2. achieve universal primary education;
3. promote gender equality and empower women;
4. reduce child mortality;
5. improve maternal health;
6. combat HIV/AIDS, malaria, and other diseases;
7. ensure environmental sustainability; and
8. develop a global partnership for development.

With the institutional sponsorship and consistent support of the UNDP and the efforts of the HDI project team to update and improve the index, the HDI has become one of the most well known composite social indicators.

Conceptually, the HDI is based on the work of Sen and Nussbaum (Nussbaum and Sen 1992; Sen 1987), who developed the *capabilities approach to human well-being*, which focuses what human beings can do and be, instead of on what they have. Sen and Nussbaum defined *capabilities* as individuals' abilities and the power to do certain things, obtain what they desire, achieve desired states of being, utilize the resources they have in the way they desire, and be who they want to be (Stanton 2007: 9). Capabilities facilitate using goods in ways that are meaningful to individuals. Sen used the term *functionings* for the capabilities that individuals actually used or participated in, while the more comprehensive capabilities term refers to the full set of functionings that are feasible or can be used by a given individual or group of individuals. Capabilities also can have intrinsic value by adding worthwhile options or positive freedoms to individual's lives (Sen 1999; Crocker 1992, 1995).

Based on the Sen-Nussbaum capabilities conceptualizations, Mahbub ul Haq directed the "human development project" of the UNDP in the late 1980s. This project sought to develop a new conceptualization of human well-being that went beyond national income and measures such as GDP to make well-being measures

---

[4]For a more detailed exposition and assessment of the HDI, see Land (2015).

based on the new definition available. The project produced its first *Human Development Report (HDR 1990*, UNDP) in 1990 (and a new volume has followed every year). *HDR 1990* stated that the human development process is one of enlarging people's choices.

With the 2010 HDI Report, the HDI was revised. It combined the following statistical measures of the three dimensions:

- A long and healthy life as measured by life expectancy at birth (LE)
- Education index as measured by mean years of schooling (MYS) and expected years of schooling (EYS)
- A decent standard of living as measured by Gross National Income per capita (GNI_{pc}) in purchasing power parity with the United States dollar (PPP US$)

For a calendar year for which the HDI is calculated, country-level measures are scaled as proportions of the maximum observed value for that year in that category. Prior to the *HDR 2010*, the scaled values of each of the education statistics were arithmetically averaged to calculate a country-level arithmetic mean Education Index, and then the scaled values for each of the three component dimensions were arithmetically averaged to yield country-level HDI values. Beginning with the *HDR 2010*, the arithmetic means were replaced with geometric means, less affected by extreme values on any one of the three component indices of the HDI (see, e.g., Hines 1983). Thus, the Revised HDI geometric mean formula places more emphasis on consistency across a country's three HDI component statistics and makes an extremely large or small value on any one of the three components less influential.

The *HDR 2010* contains HDI numerical values and rankings for a total of 186 countries. These are grouped into quartiles: Very High Human Development, High Human Development, Medium Human Development, and Low Human Development.

Now we can ask, what is the cross-national relationship of the HDI to indicators of child suffering? At this inclusive, global level of cross-national comparisons, in contrast to the region-specific studies of child well-being reviewed above, the available indicators of child suffering are very limited and concentrated among indicators of health and education.

Figure 14.1 shows cross-national scatterplots of six child suffering indicators (on the vertical axes) for 2010 or 2011 with HDI values (on the horizontal axes) for 2010. The HDI values are bounded by 0.34 and 0.955. The first three panels show scatterplots of bivariate relationships between health statistics that are indicative of early childhood suffering. Panel A plots the infant mortality rate (deaths between birth and age 1 per 1,000 live births) for 2010 and the HDI. The infant mortality rates range from a low of 3 to a high of 114; overall, countries scoring in the Very High and High quartiles have relatively low infant mortality rates. The overall relationship is a reverse J-curve as the HDI ranges from lower to higher levels. The scatterplot also shows evidence of heteroscedasticity, with countries in the lower quartiles having a larger range of infant mortality rates than countries in the higher quartiles. These properties of the Panel A scatterplot are evident in the next two graphs as well. Panel B shows the scatterplot of the child mortality rate for children ages zero to 5 per 1,000 live births in 2010 and the HDI values. Again, the relationship is heteroscedastic with larger variance among the rates at lower levels of human development. The relationship is strongly negative in that higher HDI levels are associated with lower child mortality rates. Panel C displays the scatterplot of the percentage of children under age 5 who are moderately or severely underweight for their age in 2010 and the HDIs. Data for this statistic is missing for 77 countries. Nonetheless, the scatterplot shows a reverse J-curve, heteroscedastic relationship between levels of human development and this health indicator of child suffering.

Panels D and E in Fig. 14.1 show relationships between the HDI and measures of public health immunizations against childhood diseases. Panel D contains plots of the percent of children with DTP (Diphtheria, Tetanus, and Pertussis/ Whooping Cough) immunization in 2010 and the HDIs. Panel E gives similar data for measles vaccinations. These scatterplots show quite different cross-national relationships. In Panel D, it is evident that DTP immunization coverage is 90 % or above for countries at Very High and High levels of the HDI. At Medium and Low HDI levels, all countries have DTP immunization percentages of 60 % or greater and many are at the 80 % or greater level. The measles immunization percentages plotted in Panel E are more dispersed – at all levels of the HDI, there are countries with percentages of coverage below 80 %. The numbers of such countries are larger at Low to Medium HDI levels.

In addition to the health indicators of child suffering in Panels A through E of Fig. 14.1, another indicator for which there are data on is the combined (both sexes) gross enrollment in primary educational institutions percentage plotted in Panel F.[5] Higher education levels can be associated with lower levels of child suffering, in the sense that more education opportunities are indicative of lower levels of social suffering in Anderson's (2014: 10) conceptualization. The scatterplot of school enrollment and HDI statistics in Panel F show a positive linear relationship, with higher levels of human development associated with higher percentages enrolled. This positive relationship is to be expected, since Education is one of the three dimensions of the HDI. At the same time, the plot also evidences some heteroscedasticity at the Very High and High levels of the HDI, with some countries having percentages enrolled in the 60–80 % range even though most countries at this level of development have enrollment percentages of 80 % or more. There also is some heteroscedasticity at the Low end of the HDI scale, with some countries having percentages enrolled in the 20–40 % range even though most countries at this human development level are in the 40–70 % range. In sum, Panel F shows that higher levels of human development as measured by the HDI are associated with greater educational experiences of children and, by inference, lower levels of social suffering.

---

[5] While this statistic is defined as the number of students enrolled in primary, secondary and tertiary levels of education, regardless of age, as a percentage of the population of school age for the three levels for each country, values range up to 105 % due to inconsistencies in the enrollment and/or population data (UNESCO 2009).

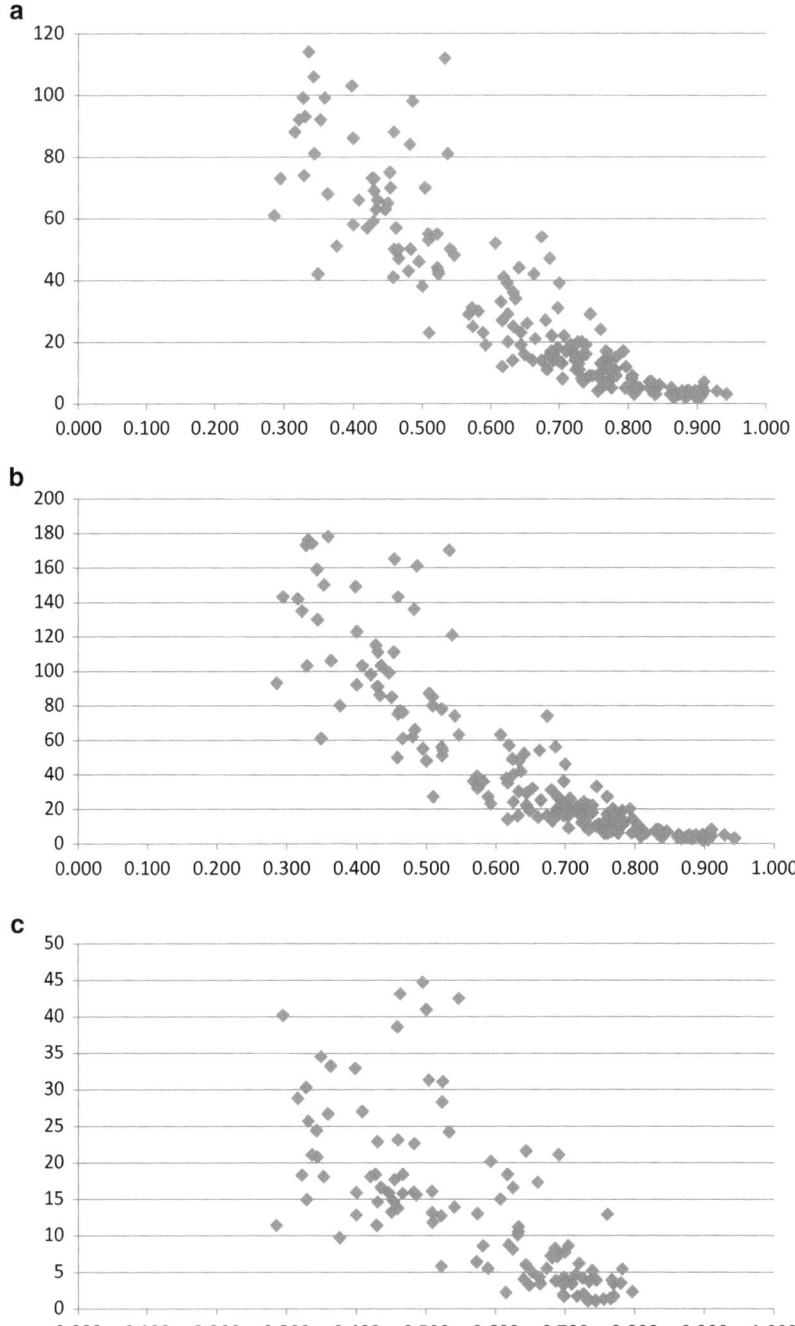

Fig. 14.1 Cross-national scatterplots of relationships between 2010 Human Development Index Values (Horizontal Axes) and Measures of Child Suffering (Vertical Axes) (**a**) Infant Mortality Rate (Deaths Between Birth and Age 1 per 1,000 Live Births), 2010, (**b**) Under Age 5 Mortality (per 1,000 Live Births), 2010, (**c**) Children Under Age 5 Who Are Underweight For Their Age

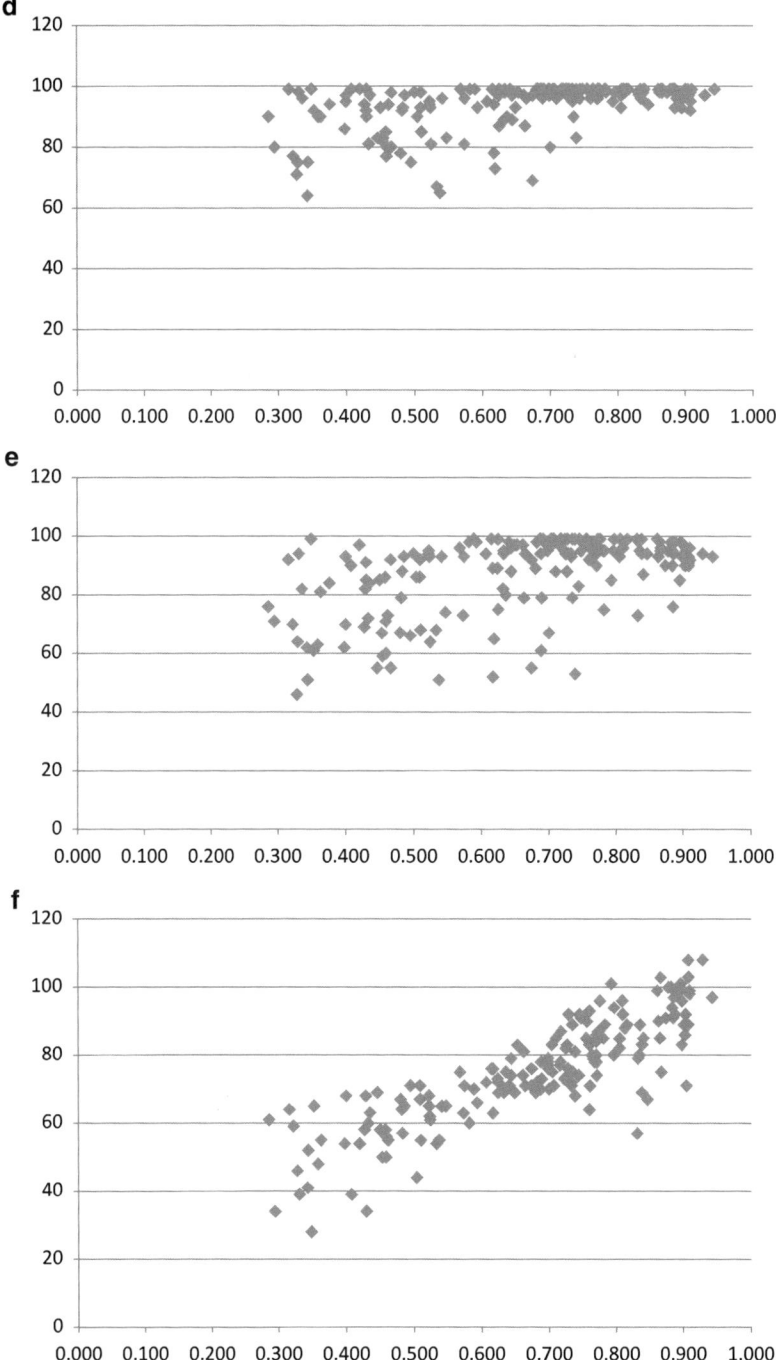

Fig. 14.1 (continued) (Moderate or Severe, Percent), 2010, (**d**) DTP (Diphtheria, Tetanus, and Pertussis (Whooping Cough)) Immunization Coverage (Percent), 2010, (**e**) Measles Immunization Coverage (Percent), 2010, (**f**) Combined (Both Sexes) Gross Enrollment in Education (Percent of a Theoretical School Age Population), 2011

14.6   Conclusion: What Needs to Be Done

We began this chapter by noting Anderson's (2014: 10) conceptualization of suffering as including physical, mental, and social stress. We also noted that suffering is the negative end of a suffering-to-well-being spectrum or dimension along which individuals, countries, and other units of analysis can be arrayed. With a focus on children, our review and summary shows that much research has pursued a well-being, rather than a suffering, perspective, at least among the more developed countries of the world. It also is clear, however, that the absence of child suffering, and indicators thereof, are very much consistent with the principles and rights identified in the CRC.

We have described international comparisons of several country-specific indicators of child suffering in relation to corresponding values of the HDI. On the basis of these analyses, two tentative generalizations can be made. First, national level (and likely, subnational level) indicators of the incidence or prevalence of child physical, mental, or social suffering generally decline as human development, conceptualized in the human capabilities terms of Sen and Nussbaum and as measured by the HDI, increase. For some indicators, the nature of the functional relationship to the HDI will take the form of a reverse J-curve, with large decreases in child suffering as human development increases from the Low to the Medium and High levels of the HDI. Others will exhibit a linear functional relationship. Second, for those countries for which sufficient statistical data are available to construct a broad array of child well-being indicators, there generally will be a negative relationship between increases in the child well-being indices and indicators of child suffering.

Does this mean that we need not work to develop a more complete array of indicators of child suffering at the national level? Not at all. To begin with, a systematic application of Anderson's physical, mental, or social suffering constructs to develop a more complete array of country-level indicators is a clear starting point. The few examples of child suffering indicators we have presented in this chapter are only illustrative. A systematic identification of a full range of such indicators, especially in conjunction with the CRC, would be most desirable. In addition, while the general negative functional relationships of national level child suffering indicators with the HDI and with indices of child well-being stated in the previous paragraph might hold on the whole, there are likely a number of indicators of specific forms of child suffering that deviate from the general cross-national functional forms, providing additional information and courses of action to prevent child suffering. In this way, the child suffering perspective can advance the global monitoring of child suffering and add value to existing HDI and well-being data and analyses.

References

Anderson, R. E. (2014). *Human suffering and quality of life conceptualizing stories and statistics.* Dordrecht: Springer.

Ben-Arieh, A. (2005). Where are the children? Children's role in measuring and monitoring their well-being. *Social Indicators Research, 74*, 573–596.

Ben-Arieh, A. (2006). Is the study of the "State of our children" changing? Revisiting after 5 years. *Children and Youth Services Review, 28*, 799–811.

Ben-Arieh, A. (2012). How do we measure and monitor the "state of our children"? Revisiting the topic in honor of Sheila B. Kamerman. *Children and Youth Services Review, 34*, 569–575.

Ben-Arieh, A., & Goerge, R. (2001). Beyond the numbers: How do we monitor the state of our children? *Children and Youth Services Review, 23*(8), 603–631.

Bradshaw, J., & Richardson, D. (2009). An index of child well-being in Europe. *Child Indicators Research, 2*, 319–351.

Bradshaw, J., Hoelscher, P., & Richardson, D. (2007a). *Comparing child well-being in OECD countries: Concepts and methods.* Florence: UNICEF Innocenti Research Centre.

Bradshaw, J., Hoelscher, P., & Richardson, D. (2007b). An index of child well-being in the European Union. *Social Indicators Research, 80*, 133–177.

Casas, F. (1997). Children's rights and children's quality of life: Conceptual and practical issues. *Social Indicators Research, 42*, 283–298.

Crocker, D. (1992). Functioning and capability: The foundation of Sen's and Nussbaum's development ethic. *Political Theory, 20*, 584–612.

Crocker, D. (1995). Functioning and capability: The foundation of Sen's and Nussbaum's development ethic. In M. Nussbaum & J. Glover (Eds.), *Women, culture, and development: A study of human capabilities* (pp. 153–198). Oxford: Oxford University Press.

Cummins, R. A. (1996). The domains of life satisfaction: An attempt to order chaos. *Social Indicators Research, 38*, 303–328.

Federal Interagency Forum on Child and Family Statistics. (1997). *America's children: Key national indicators of well-being.* Washington, DC: Federal Interagency Forum on Child and Family Statistics.

Hagerty, M. R., Cummins, R. A., Ferris, A. L., Land, K. C., Michalos, A., Peterson, M., Sharpe, A., Sirgy, J., & Vogel, J. (2001). Quality of life indexes for national policy: Review and agenda for research. *Social Indicators Research, 55*, 1–96.

Hines, W. G. S. (1983). Geometric mean. In S. Kotz & N. L. Johnson (Eds.), *Encyclopedia of statistical sciences* (pp. 397–400). New York: Wiley-Interscience.

Lamb, V. L., & Land, K. C. (2015). Worldwide view of child well-being. In W. Glatzer (Ed.), *Global handbook of quality of life and well-being.* New York: Springer.

Land, K. C. (2000). Social indicators. In F. B. Edgar & R. V. Montgomery (Eds.), *Encyclopedia of sociology* (pp. 2682–2690). New York: Macmillan.

Land, K. C. (2015). The human development index. In W. Glatzer (Ed.), *Global handbook of quality of life and well-being.* New York: Springer.

Land, K. C., Lamb, V. L., Meadows, S. O., & Taylor, A. (2007). Measuring trends in child well-being: An evidence-based approach. *Social Indicators Research, 80*(1), 105–132.

Lau, M., & Bradshaw, J. (2010). Child well-being in the Pacific Rim. *Child Indicators Research, 3*, 367–383.

Nussbaum, M., & Sen, A. (Eds.). (1992). *The quality of life.* Oxford: Clarendon.

Richardson, D., Hoelscher, P., & Bradshaw, J. (2008). Child well-being in Central and Eastern European countries and the Commonwealth of Independent States. *Child Indicators Research, 1*, 211–250.

Sen, A. (1987). *The standard of living.* Cambridge: Cambridge University Press.

Sen, A. (1999). *Commodities and capabilities.* New York: Oxford University Press.

Stanton, E. A. (2007). *The human development index: A history* (Working paper series, number 127). Amherst: Political Economy Research Institute, University of Massachusetts. www.peri. umass.edu

UNDP (United Nations Development Programme). (1990 through 2011, and 2013). *Human development report*. New York: UNDP.

UNESCO (United Nations Educational, Scientific, and Cultural Organization). (2009). *Education indicators technical guidelines*. Paris: UNESCO Institute for Statistics.

UNICEF (United Nations Children's Fund). (1997). *The progress of nations 1997*. http://www. unicef.org/pon97. Retrieved July 19, 2013.

UNICEF (United Nations Children's Fund). (2007). *Child poverty in perspective: An overview of child well-being in rich countries*. Florence: UNICEF Innocenti Research Centre.

UNICEF (United Nations Children's Fund). (n.d.). *Convention on the rights of the child*. http:// www.unicef.org/crc. Retrieved July 10, 2012.

United Nations. (1989). *Convention on the rights of the child*. Geneva: United Nations.

United Nations. (2000). *United Nations millennium declaration*. New York: United Nations.

Chapter 15
Felt-Suffering and Its Social Variations in China

Yanjie Bian and Jing Shen

15.1 Introduction

In this chapter we measure "felt-suffering" and examine its social variations in China. Quality of life (QOL) is directly impacted by individuals' physical and mental suffering in a variety of ways (Anderson 2014). By using the 2005 and 2010 Chinese General Social Surveys (CGSS), we conceptualize felt-suffering as feeling limited in daily life, due to physical and mental conditions. We measure felt-suffering on three indicators: poor health, physical suffering, and mental suffering. We are particularly interested in the uneven distribution of felt-suffering among different social groups in contemporary China. We ask: How does the level of risks of felt-suffering vary among different social groups? Which groups are the most vulnerable to felt-suffering? And are there any changes in the level of felt-suffering for each of the social groups in the second half of the 2000s?

The authors are grateful to Ron Anderson and Susan McDaniel for their helpful comments on an earlier draft.

Y. Bian (✉)
Department of Sociology, Faculty of Sociology, University of Minnesota,
Minneapolis, MN 55455, USA

Faculty of Sociology, Xi'an Jiaotong University, Xi'an, China
e-mail: bianx001@umn.edu

J. Shen
The Prentice Institute for Global Population and Economy, University of Lethbridge,
4401 University Drive West, Lethbridge, AB T1K 3M4, Canada
e-mail: jing.shen@uleth.ca

© Springer Science+Business Media Dordrecht 2015
R.E. Anderson (ed.), *World Suffering and Quality of Life*,
Social Indicators Research Series 56, DOI 10.1007/978-94-017-9670-5_15

15.2 Existing Studies on Suffering

While all human societies pursue happiness and well-being as the ultimate goal, suffering is the perpetual barrier that makes this goal not always, and sometimes rarely, achievable. The study of suffering and solutions to it has thus increasingly become a pressing issue. An analysis of the 2000–2003 National Health and Nutrition Examination Survey shows a chronic pain level of 10 % among adults in the USA (Hardt et al. 2008). A more recent Institute of Medicine report estimated that 45 % of adults in the USA, or 100 million, are at risk of chronic pain. Beyond the United States, Harstall and Ospina (2003) evaluated 13 major studies of chronic pain in Europe, Canada, Australia, and Israel. Across these 13 large studies, the prevalence of chronic pain ranged from 10 to 50 % in adult populations, with a weighted average of 31 % across developed countries. In *Human Suffering and Quality of Life*, Anderson (2014: 10) defined suffering as "perceived threat or damage to a sense of self," and "distress resulting from threat or damage to one's body or self-identity." This includes distress resulting from threat or damage to one's physical being (i.e., physical suffering), distress originating in one's cognitive or affective self-identity (mental suffering), and distress cumulating from threat or damage to one's social identity (social suffering).

Although physical and mental suffering usually refer to inner discomforts of a human body while social suffering is often caused by external forces, these two sides are inherently correlated. Social suffering impacts an individual by either or both physical and mental means, so that social suffering is ultimately shown as either physical or mental suffering—or both. Physical and mental suffering do not just concern individuals, but constitute a social issue that needs to be dealt with at the societal level. As Wilkinson (2005) argued, suffering is a social result of individuals' loss of the sense of worth and humanity. Kleinman (2009) also emphasized social institutions, global systems, and culture as causes of human suffering. From a sociological viewpoint, Anderson (2014) has related suffering to the interpretation of the meaning of modern history and an inhuman state produced by institutions and policies. This points to the importance of the roles of societal factors in causing—as well as relieving—human suffering.

Following these scholars, we do not distinguish social suffering from physical and mental suffering in our measures of felt-suffering. In fact, we *focus* on social factors in our analysis of the variation of felt-suffering.

In addition to individuals' demographic differences (such as gender, age, race, and ethnicity), social factors of suffering have been explored in the existing literature. In Lelkes' (2013) policy analysis, religion, marital status, education, employment, and income were taken into account as effective aspects to minimize suffering. These variables were also included in studies of happiness, subjective well-being, and QOL. Following the existing studies, we will use social factors relevant to China to study social variations in the Chinese's felt-suffering. Despite the pervasive existence of suffering in human societies, studies directly focusing on suffering are still scarce, particularly in developing countries. Suffering is not evenly distributed across the globe. Individuals in the Global South are more likely to suffer from poor and worsening living conditions resulting from the lack of abilities to cope with natural and human disasters, poor economies, and the deteriorating environment (Anderson 2014). Studying the case of China is thus of great empirical and theoretical importance, for it helps identify the sources of human suffering within the context of a rapid economic growth.

15.3 Suffering in a Transitional Context: Research Hypotheses

Since market-oriented reforms were launched at the end of the 1970s, China has made impressive progress in socioeconomic development. During the past three decades, an estimated 400 million people have been lifted out of poverty. The average years of schooling among adult Chinese aged 15–64 rose from 5 to 9 years, and life expectancy extended from 67 years in 1980 to 75 years in 2013 (WHO[1] and World Bank[2] websites as of January 2014). Still, as China has officially become the world's second largest economy, the improvement of Chinese health has taken a much slower pace, according to the report titled *China: Health, Poverty, and Economic Development* by World Health Organization and China State Council Development Research Center (2005). Despite Chinese people's positive feelings towards the rapid economic growth (Liu et al. 2012; Bian et al. 2014), negative consequences of the socioeconomic changes and an aging population have generated new sources of social suffering. We focus on the impacts of the demographic change, the increase in social inequality, and the changing social relations on the level of felt-suffering among Chinese citizens.

15.3.1 Elders and Women as the Most Vulnerable Demographic Groups

In 2009, China's population aged 65 years and above reached 113.1 million, or 8.5 % of its total population. This indicates China's formal international classification as an "aging society" (Sun et al. 2011). Within this aging population, the subgroup of elders aged 80 and above—known as the "oldest old"—is the fastest growing group. Based on data released by the National Bureau of Statistics of China (2002), by 2000, the size of the oldest-old population had already reached approximately

---

[1] Retrieved on January 20, 2014: http://www.who.int/countries/chn/en/

[2] Retrieved on January 20, 2014: http://search.worldbank.org/data?qterm=life+expectancy+in+China+2013&language=EN&op=

11.5 million and accounted for nearly 9 % of all elders aged 60 years and older. One demographic study predicts China's population aged 60 years and older will represent approximately 25 % of the total population by the year of 2050 (Zeng et al. 2010). The two CGSS datasets used in this study reflect this fast aging trend of the Chinese population. Changes in proportions of all other age groups have been mild between 2005 and 2010, but the proportion of respondents aged 60 and above increased from 17.9 % in 2005 to 23.2 % in 2010. This represents a nearly 6 % increase in the population of elders within 5 years.

The supply of long-term care for elders lags far behind the growth of the elder population. Traditionally, care for elders in China is almost solely provided by offspring, other family members, relatives, or informal (unpaid) caregivers (Wu et al. 2008). As the size of the usual Chinese family decreases (not only due to the implementation of the one-child policy, but also, increasingly, because of the high costs of living and education), it has become more difficult for the elderly to rely on the care and support of adult children/grandchildren (Bartlett and Phillips 1997). Unfortunately, institutional care for elders is still underdeveloped, despite its quick growth in recent decades. At the end of 2004, institutional beds were available only for 0.9 % of elders aged 60 and above, and elders who suffered from physical and/ or mental disabilities were most likely to be denied admittance to such an institution (Wu et al. 2008). Taken together, these facts indicate that Chinese people have an increasing risk of felt-suffering with age.

The other salient demographic change lies in the shrinkage of the female population in the labor market from 2005 to 2010. The proportion of working women consistently constituted above 40 % of the labor force in the first half of the 2000s. For example, the proportion of working women represented 42.4 % and 44.7 % of the total population in the labor market, in 2002 and 2004, respectively; and around 46 % of new employees were women each year in the same period. However, the proportion of employed women reduced to about 37 % in 2010.[3] The lingering impacts of the global economic recession and the reform in the higher education system in the early 2000s, among other factors, created the tightest ever labor market since the start of the socioeconomic reform. Consequently, women have increasingly been marginalized in the Chinese labor market. Those women who are able to actively participate in the labor market face rising discrimination, unjustifiably demanding working conditions, and increasing difficulties to balance work and family obligations (He and Wong 2011; Zuo and Bian 2005). We expect the following:

Hypothesis 1: Women and older people are more likely to feel suffering than men and younger people, respectively.

---

[3] Computations were based on information from China Labor Statistical Yearbooks in 2003, 2005, and 2011.

15.3.2 Suffering Deepened by Increasing Social Inequality

Existing studies on the sense of happiness have documented the positive impacts of economic development on Chinese citizens' subjective well-being. According to data issued by the government-run social media, the percentage of "happy" Chinese people increased from 44.8 % in 2010 to 47.9 % in 2012.[4] Using CGSS data from 2003 to 2010, Liu et al. (2012) confirmed the positive association between economic development and the sense of happiness among the Chinese. A similar trend was also found in Bian et al.'s 2014 study, based on data collected from 12 provinces in West China. However, the measure of the sense of happiness used in those studies seems to focus heavily on respondents' perceptions of changes in living standards as measured by a variety of subjective material criteria. To the best of our knowledge, no study has focused directly on physical and mental suffering that Chinese people have encountered in the context of a rapid economic growth (though negative impacts of economic development on individuals' well-being have gradually drawn scholarly attention).

The most obvious consequence of a rapid economic growth may lie in environmental costs. As Kan (2009) pointed out, China's environmental problems (including outdoor and indoor air pollution, water shortages and pollution, desertification, and soil pollution) have become more pronounced and damaging to the health of Chinese residents in recent years. According to estimations made by the WHO, each year, approximately 300,000 premature deaths are caused by outdoor air pollution and 420,000 premature deaths are caused by the use of solid fuels in China (Smith et al. 2004). The World Bank estimated that the health cost of cancers and diarrhea associated with water pollution reached approximately $8 billion (all dollar amounts in US dollars) in rural areas of China in 2003 (Kan 2009). In 2008, the government spent $66 billion (1.49 % of the national GDP) to cope with pollution (National Bureau of Statistics of China 2009). Risks of suffering resulting from environmental problems are visible and have drawn public attention.

Increasing social inequality, another consequence of fast-paced economic development, is less visible. Social disparities are as great as, if not more severe than, the impacts of environmental issues on individuals' levels of felt-suffering. Thus, in this study, we pay particular attention to how the changing trend in the level of felt-suffering can be explained by the increase in social inequality.

Although under-studied, the association between economic development and social members' physical and mental health can be seen in a few studies regarding Asian countries. Friedman and Thomas (2009) used data from the Indonesia Family Life Survey to examine the impact of the 1997 Asian financial crisis on individuals' psychological well-being. Their findings show that the economic crisis was detrimental to psychological well-being (measured by depression, anxiety, and lowered aspirations) across all age groups. Liang et al. (2000) found a socioeconomic

---

[4] Retrieved from the Financial Channel, CCTV, March 7, 2012: http://finance.jrj.com.cn/2012/03/07132012427439.shtml

gradient in old age mortality in China and Taiwan. Using multiple health outcome measures for data collected in Thailand, Zimmer and Amorbsirisomboon (2001) found strong socioeconomic associations with self-assessed health and functional limitation. They did not, however, find a significant association between one's socioeconomic status (SES) and self-reported chronic health conditions, such as cardiovascular diseases.

Following the conventional wisdom, we consider education and self-reported social class position as the measures of one's SES. In today's China, as in many societies, education is directly associated with income. This is rather accurately reflected by one's self-assessed social class position (particularly when an accurate report about income is not available). Those who experience improvement in their SES tend to have higher subjective well-being scores (Xing 2012; Steele and Lynch 2013; Bian et al. 2014). Lowered SES causes suffering from the scarcity of resources and opportunities. Thus, using education and self-reported social class position as indicators, we hypothesize that:

Hypothesis 2: Individuals who have lower socioeconomic statuses tend to suffer to a greater extent, compared to their counterparts who have higher socioeconomic statuses.

We distinguish two measures of one's SES:

Hypothesis 2(a): Poorly educated individuals are more likely than highly educated ones to suffer.
Hypothesis 2(b): Individuals who perceive themselves at lower social classes are more likely than those perceiving themselves at higher social classes to suffer.

In addition to the SES dimension, social inequality in China's context is also often observed in a spatial dimension. China has long struggled with the urban-rural division and regional disparities. While two-thirds of the total population reside in rural areas, resources are concentrated in the cities. Urbanites enjoy significantly higher earnings and standards of living, as well as easier access to the government's medical insurance plans and better healthcare facilities. By contrast, rural healthcare has been described as often administered by "barefoot doctors," practitioners briefly trained to provide frontline service and often on a part-time basis (Sidel 1993). In other words, the rapid economic growth due to China's transition has significanlty benefited the healthcare system in urban areas, but not in rural areas. Particularly, the community aspects of healthcare in rural China have been slowly dismantled in the process of privatization of healthcare, which has further exacerbated the unequal opportunities for healthcare between rural and urban citizens.

Increasing social inequality has also been driven by the imbalanced economic development across Chinese regions. In the beginning of the reform, east coastal areas along the Pacific were given priority in practicing market mechanisms by attracting foreign investments directly (Naughton 2007). Almost two decades later, the market economy was established in the western regions, where poor peasants and ethnic minority groups constituted the majority of the population (Bian et al. 2014). While the government successfully led the nation through the transitional process by opening up regional markets step by step, this differential developmental strategy deepened regional gaps in economic development and income distribution. We hypothesize that social inequality, shown as the urban-rural division and regional disparities, would have a significant impact on the Chinese citizens' well-being. In brief,

Hypothesis 3: Urbanites are less likely than rural residents to suffer, and individuals living in highly developed regions are less likely to suffer than those living in less developed regions.

15.3.3 Social Disconnection: A Source of Suffering in Modern Society

Suffering due to social disconnection has often been seen as a by-product of industrialization in developed countries. Using data drawn from the 1985 General Social Survey in the United States, Marsden (1987) found a decreasing trend in the network size of an average American. Physical and mental suffering occurred in people who had fewer contacts to discuss important matters. This argument was echoed by Putnam's influential book *Bowling Alone* (2000), which expressed concern for Americans' well-being in a time of social isolation, identified by their shrinking social connections with the government, the church, the community, and even the family.

Recent studies using Chinese data revealed similar findings about the importance of social connection for happiness (Bian et al. 2014), particularly among elders (Sun et al. 2011). Based on data from the 2008 National Household Health Survey (NHHS), Sun et al. found that elders who lived alone were significantly more likely to report problems with mobility, pain/discomfort, and anxiety/depression. However, if those elders retained close relationships with their relatives and/or friends, their likelihood of reporting health-related problems decreased significantly. Similarly, in another study about rural elders in China, Zhen and Silverstein (2008) found those who retained positive relationships with their daughters-in-law were more likely to report high scores in both physical and mental health. Socially isolated individuals are more likely to feel unhappy, which may in turn increase their chances of developing physical problems. Our hypothesis is thus as follows:

Hypothesis 4: Individuals who are integrated to the society through marital and/or social relations are less likely to feel suffering than those who lack these types of social connections.

15.4 Research Design

Data In this study, we used data from the Chinese General Social Surveys (CGSS) in 2005 and 2010. The CGSSs are large, cross-sectional household surveys using the countrywide representative sampling frame. Excepting Tibet, all provinces and regions of China are covered. Only civilian residences are sampled. A mapping method is used to randomly sample households, ensuring that "migrant population" residents in the cities and towns are sampled with equal probability as permanent residents with urban household registration. Data collection is based on the use of structured questionnaires through face-to-face interviews. A detailed methodlogical report of the CGSSs can be found elsewhere (Bian and Li 2012).

Because of the rapidly increasing social inequality in the second half of the 2000s, we chose to focus on the survey data collected in 2005 and 2010. Another advantage of using data from these two years is that similar questions about physical and mental limitations in one's daily life were asked in both surveys. A similar sampling frame was also used in both years, resulting in similar sample sizes between these two surveys. In 2005, 10,372 Chinese adults, aged between 18 and 94, were sampled, including 4,919 men and 5,453 women. In 2010, the total sample size was 11,783, among which 5,677 were men and 6,106 were women, with an age range of 17–96. The comparable samples between the two years offer fairly robust evidence to test our hypotheses.

Felt-Suffering We measured the concept of felt-suffering by three dichotomous variables. Based on a 5-point measure of self-reported general health conditions, we generated the first measure—"poor health" (with "yes" coded as 1 and "no" coded as 0) to measure if there were identifiable causes of one's suffering. Respondents who reported that their general health status was "excellent," "good," or "OK" were included in the group of "0", while those who reported that their general health status was either "poor" or "very poor" were included in the group of "1". People with poor general health are expected to be more likely to feel suffering in their daily lives.

The second measure is physical suffering. Similar to the Integrated Health Interview Series database used in Anderson's (2014) study, the CGSSs measured physical suffering by the extent to which the respondent felt limited in his or her daily routine activities. In our study, we coded physical suffering as "yes" (=1), if the respondent reported that their physical conditions bothered their daily routine activities, either "sometimes," or "often," or "always." We coded physical suffering as "no" (=0), if the respondent reported that their physical conditions did not at all bother, or seldom bothered their daily routine activities.

The third measure, mental suffering, was coded in a similar way. The group of "yes" (=1) includes respondents who reported that their daily routine activities were interrupted by their emotional problems (i.e., anxiety and depression), either "sometimes," or "often," or "always". The group of "no" (=0) includes respondents who reported that their daily routine activities were not at all interrupted, or seldom interrupted by their emotional problems.

Social Factors We used two demographic variables: gender (male = 1; female = 0) and age (coded in year). Our socioeconomic status (SES) variables include education (coded in year) and self-assessed SES (lower = 1; lower-middle = 2; middle = 3; upper-middle = 4; and upper = 5). In the regression analysis that follows shortly, squared age and education were also used to control over possible quadratic effects of age and education, respectively. To take into account social inequality in the spatial dimension, we used two locality variables. "Urban" is a dichotomous variable referring to the location of a respondent's residence, with urban areas coded 1 and rural areas coded 0. We generated the variable of "region", based on GDP per capita[5] across province-level units: 3 units (Beijing, Tianjin, Shanghai), in which GDP per capita was above 20,000 *yuan*, were coded as the highly developed region; 7 units along the coastal line, where GDP per capita was between 10,000 and 20,000 *yuan*, were coded as the fairly developed region; and all the remaining units, where GDP per capita was below 10,000 *yuan*, was coded as the least developed region. For the convenience of coding, we named the three categories high, medium, and low developmental regions. Finally, we used two variables to measure one's social connections. Marital status is a dichotomous variable, with living with a partner coded 1 and otherwise coded 0. We also considered the strength of ties one had with family members, relatives, and friends. All respondents were categorized into two groups: "pro-social" (coded as 1) and "anti-social" (coded as 0). Respondents who reported that they were not at all close to, or not very close to, anyone else were considered anti-social; all other respondents were categorized into the pro-social group.

Analytic Strategy Following descriptive statistics, Binary Logit Regression models were used to estimate the three dichotomous dependent variables. We pooled the 2005 and 2010 CGSS datasets together by using the survey year as a binary variable (with the year of 2010 coded 1, and the year of 2005 coded 0). We also controlled over the interaction effects between all independent variables and the binary variable of the survey year, so that we were able to distinguish the average effect of an independent variable from its changing effect between 2005 and 2010.

15.5 Results

Level of Suffering Figure 15.1 presents the three measures of suffering in 2005 and 2010. In 2005, about 16 % of respondents reported poor health. The percentages of reported physical suffering and mental suffering are higher, around 23 % and 30 %, respectively. In 2010, the percentages of reported suffering went up in all three measures. More than 18 % of respondents reported poor health, 29 % physical suffering, and 34 % mental suffering. While existing studies show a slight increase in Chinese people's sense of happiness or subjective well-being in the 2000s (Xing 2012; Steele and Lynch 2013), there seems to be an increasing level of health-related suffering among the Chinese from 2005 to 2010.

In Fig. 15.2, we presented a series of binary cross-tabulation results. Descriptive statistics show that the proportions of women who felt suffering were greater than

---

[5] Information was collected from Table 3–9 in China Statistical Yearbook 2003, complied by National Bureau of Statistics of China.

Fig. 15.1 Distribution of three measures of felt-suffering, CGSS 2005–2010

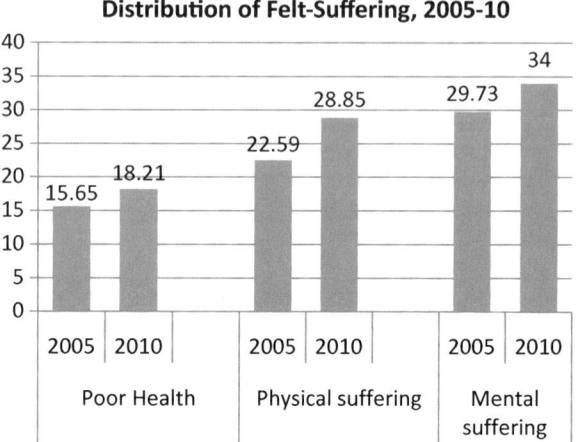

those of men in all the three measures and in both years. Moreover, from 2005 to 2010, more respondents reported the feeling of suffering in all the three measures and in both genders. Similar trends are generally observed in the dimensions of age, urban-rural division, relationship status, education, and self-reported SES. In general, higher proportions of individuals who reported suffering were observed in the groups of elders, rural residents, individuals living without partners, the poorly-educated, and those who ranked themselves at lower social classes, in all the three measures and in both years. The proportions also increased in general overall during the 5 years. Interestingly, however, the distribution of suffering by the self-reported SES seems to display a "U-shape" relationship. The lowest level of suffering was not found in the upper class, but rather, in the upper-middle class, across three measures. Also, while more individuals seemed to suffer in 2010, fewer individuals aged under 40 reported poor health in 2010, compared to the numbers of individuals with poor health in the corresponding age groups in 2005. In 2010, individuals with some post-secondary education also reported poor health less often than their counterparts in 2005.

Demographic Attributes We further examined the impacts of social factors on the likelihoods for one to feel suffering in three measures. Table 15.1 confirms a clear gender gap in all three measures of suffering, with women having a significantly higher probability of having poor health, and feeling suffering physically as well as mentally than men. The non-significant interaction effects show that this gender gap is persistent and unchanged between 2005 and 2010. In both years, men were 33 % (coef. = −0.401) less likely than women to report poor health, 31 % (coef. = −0.365) less likely to report physical suffering, and 18 % (coef. = −0.201) less likely to report mental suffering. In terms of age, one's risk of having poor health increases by 9 % (coef. = 0.088) for every year increase in age. The statistically positive yet extremely small coefficient of the quadratic term indicates that although aging could have a

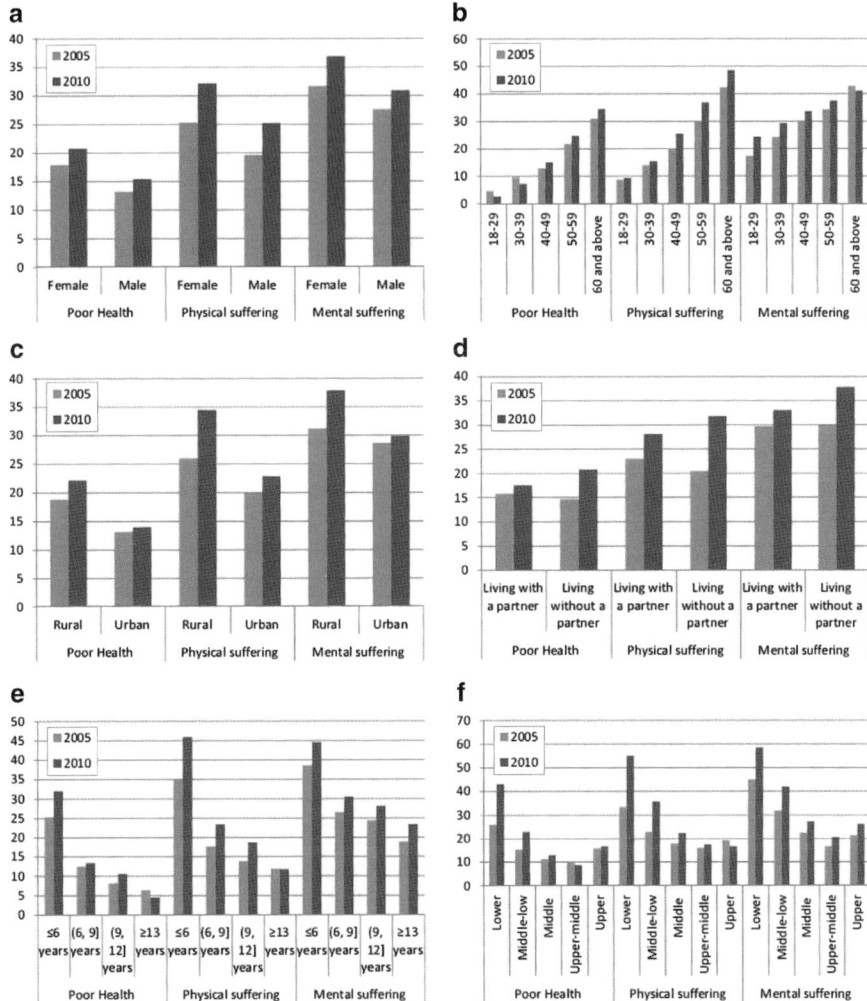

Fig. 15.2 Distribution of three measures of felt-suffering by individual traits, CGSSs 2005–2010. (**a**) By gender (**b**) By age (**c**) By urban-rural division (**d**) By relationship status (**e**) By education (**f**) By self-reported SES

positive impact on one's well-being, the positive effect of aging would not occur in a reasonable lifespan of human beings. Turning to the interaction effects, we observed that the risk of poor health became much higher in 2010 than in 2005. The patterns of risks for physical and mental suffering were similar. Other covariates being equal, older people have higher risks of feeling physical and mental suffering in both 2005 and 2010; for every year of increase in age, physical suffering went up by 7 % (coef.=0.066), and mental suffering went up by 5 % (coef.=0.047). The gender and age effects confirm that Chinese women and older people are indeed

Table 15.1 Binary logit regression of general, physical, and mental suffering

Independent variables	Poor health		Physical suffering		Mental suffering	
	Main effect	Interaction with year	Main effect	Interaction with year	Main effect	Interaction with year
Year (2010=1)	−1.417***		0.075		0.787**	
	(0.541)		(0.426)		(0.350)	
Demographic attributes						
Male	−0.401***	0.056	−0.365***	0.030	−0.201***	−0.013
	(0.061)	(0.082)	(0.053)	(0.071)	(0.047)	(0.063)
Age	0.088***	0.065***	0.066***	0.025	0.047***	−0.006
	(0.014)	(0.019)	(0.011)	(0.015)	(0.010)	(0.013)
Age square	−0.0004***	−0.001***	−0.0002**	−0.0002	−0.0002**	−0.000
	(0.0001)	(0.000)	(0.0001)	(0.0002)	(0.000)	(0.000)
Socioeconomic status						
Education	−0.014	−0.019	−0.066***	0.014	−0.045***	−0.029
	(0.020)	(0.027)	(0.018)	(0.024)	(0.016)	(0.022)
Education square	−0.003*	−0.001	0.001	−0.001	0.0001	0.002
	(0.001)	(0.002)	(0.001)	(0.002)	(0.001)	(0.001)
Lower-middle SES	−0.507***	−0.194*	−0.380***	−0.193*	−0.442***	−0.097
	(0.073)	(0.113)	(0.066)	(0.106)	(0.059)	(0.098)
Middle SES	−0.830***	−0.455***	−0.674***	−0.474***	−0.896***	−0.233**
	(0.073)	(0.114)	(0.065)	(0.105)	(0.059)	(0.098)
Middle-upper SES	−0.910***	−0.650***	−0.799***	−0.574***	−1.275***	−0.181
	(0.140)	(0.200)	(0.120)	(0.170)	(0.113)	(0.159)
Upper SES	−0.472	−0.499	−0.620**	−0.918*	−0.987***	−0.132
	(0.311)	(0.560)	(0.288)	(0.541)	(0.269)	(0.463)
Locality						
Urban	−0.287***	0.202**	−0.215***	−0.076	0.001	−0.022
	(0.069)	(0.095)	(0.061)	(0.083)	(0.054)	(0.075)
Fairly-developed	0.242**	−0.284*	0.220**	−0.134	0.241***	−0.111
	(0.119)	(0.161)	(0.099)	(0.134)	(0.086)	(0.118)
Least-developed	0.473***	0.018	0.406***	0.067	0.513***	0.022
	(0.114)	(0.154)	(0.094)	(0.128)	(0.082)	(0.114)
Social connections						
Living with a partner	−0.128	−0.012	−0.087	−0.130	−0.233***	−0.027
	(0.090)	(0.118)	(0.081)	(0.106)	(0.071)	(0.094)
Pro-social	−0.427***	0.114	−0.188*	−0.085	−0.396***	0.229**
	(0.112)	(0.125)	(0.106)	(0.116)	(0.096)	(0.106)
Constant	−3.522***		−2.729***		−1.332***	
	(0.376)		(0.317)		(0.263)	
N	21,418		21,387		21,394	

Note: Presented in the table are regression coefficients followed by standard errors in parentheses.
Two detailed level of significance: ***p<0.001, **p<0.01, *p<0.05, +p<0.1

more likely to be in poor health conditions, and feel suffering physically and mentally. These findings are in support of Hypothesis 1.

Socioeconomic Status Both education and self-perceived SES generate consistent results for a negative association with the risks of suffering. That is, the risks of suffering were lower for a highly educated or higher-status person. While education presented a curvilinear, negative effect on the risk of poor health, its effects on physical and mental suffering were linear and negative. The effects of education did not change from 2005 to 2010, as education-year interactions were not significant. SES exerted more consistent effects and the cross-year changes were also rather significant: The higher the social status at which one ranked him- or herself, the lower the risk was for one to report poor health, and feelings of physical and mental suffering. One exception is the non-significant effect of being at the upper class on the risk of poor health. However, the risks of suffering steadily decreased as one's social status increased. The significant interaction effects show that gaps in the risks of suffering widened between the lower class and other social classes, indicating the sharp increase in the feeling of suffering among the most socioeconomically disadvantaged individuals. Overall, the results of educational and SES effects on suffering are in strong support of Hypothesis 2. Namely, socioeconomic status makes great differences in individuals' risks of suffering in all the three health-related measures.

Locality Effects Urbanites were 25 % (coef.=−0.287) less likely than rural residents to report poor health in 2005, and this difference was further enlarged by 19 % in 2010 (the urban-year interaction coef.=−0.202). Urbanites were also 20 % (coef.=−0.215) less likely than their rural counterparts to feel physical suffering, and this effect did not change from 2005 to 2010. There was no urban-rural difference in mental suffering. Furthermore, levels of poor health, physical, and mental suffering were highly associated with economic development of the region where the respondent resided. Compared to those in the region with the highest level of economic development, individuals in fairly-developed provinces were about 25–27 % more likely to report poor health, physical, and mental suffering; and individuals in least-developed provinces were about 50–67 % more likely to report suffering in the three measures. Interaction terms show that these estimated differential margins remained the same between 2005 and 2010, other than one exception. Altogether, the general tendency is that urbanization and economic development reduce the risks of suffering, in support of Hypothesis 3.

Social Connections Living with a partner did not make a difference in one's risk of having poor health and feeling physical suffering in 2005 or 2010, but it made a great difference in mental suffering in both years at a similar level. A person who lived with a partner was 21 % (coef.=−0.233) less likely to suffer mentally than a person who shared similarities in other characteristics but did not live with a partner. On the other hand, pro-social individuals had significantly lower risks of suffering in all three dimensions. Compared to those who did not have close relationships with anyone else, individuals who reported close relationships with family members, relatives, or friends were 35 % (coef.=−0.427) less likely to report poor health,

18 % (coef. = −.188) less likely to feel physical suffering, and 23 % (coef. = −.396) less likely to feel mental suffering. While the positive effect was reduced on mental suffering in 2010, effects on the risks of poor health and physical suffering were the same between the two years. These findings thus support Hypothesis 4 mainly when mental suffering is considered.

Between-Year Change We now revisit trends in the increase in the levels of suffering in all three measures from 2005 to 2010, as shown in Figs. 15.1 and 15.2. It is evident that the between-year increase in poor health resulted mostly from the fact that from 2005 to 2010, health worsened for older people, lower-status ones, and those who lived in less-developed regions, implying worsening living conditions for these groups due to the increase in social inequality over the 5-year span. The increases in physical and mental suffering, on the other hand, were due mostly to the greater effects of one's socioeconomic status in 2010 than in 2005.

15.6   Conclusion

Our analysis shows that the relative levels of poor health, physical suffering, and mental suffering increased in China from 2005 to 2010. A number of social factors might have contributed to this increase.

Gender, education, level of economic development of the region, partner status, and social connections were found to exert generally consistent effects on felt-suffering among the three measures in both 2005 and 2010. Namely, being male, being more educated, living in the highly developed region, living with a partner, and having close social connections significantly reduce risks of felt-suffering. These results have three implications for how suffering can be reduced in the future. First, the increase in higher education and economic growth in less developed regions will significantly reduce the risks of suffering. Second, social justice and social equality between men and women will reduce the risks of suffering, especially for women. Finally, China must increase quality of marital and social life in order to maintain a low level of suffering among citizens.

Age, rural-vs.-urban residence, and self-perceived socioeconomic status also affected one's felt-suffering in all three measures, and the effects of these factors varied from 2005 to 2010. First, the risk of poor health increased with age and the age effect nearly doubled in 2010. This implies that living conditions and social support system for Chinese elders must be improved in order to prevent them from suffering from poor health. Second, compared to rural residents, urbanites were significantly less likely to report poor health in 2005, but this urban-rural difference nearly disappeared in 2010. Whether this was due to the improved rural living conditions or the worsening living conditions in the cities should be a research task for future studies. Third, socioeconomic status has a significantly positive effect on all three measures of suffering, and the effect was much stronger in 2010 than in 2005. This indicates that as a fast-growing economy, China must actively improve living standards for the poor and constrain the rich from benefitting in an already very unequal distribution of income and wealth.

The increase in all three of our suffering measures should be further studied with a much greater effort than we could give in this chapter. If suffering were to continue to rise at the rate we found, that would indicate serious problems for China, a second largest economy of the world. Does the rise imply a rise in expectations of freedom from suffering due to higher income and wealth in more recent years? Could the rise be that increasing environmental problems caused certain physical and/or mental issues, which were formerly not labeled as suffering, to become identified as suffering? Might the rise be caused by some other unknown factors? Also, can the rise be replicated in newer studies? These questions need be taken seriously in future studies.

References

Anderson, R. E. (2014). *Human suffering and quality of life conceptualizing stories and statistics*. Springer. www.springer.com

Bartlett, H., & Phillips, D. R. (1997). Ageing and aged care in the People's Republic of China: National and local issues and perspectives. *Health & Place, 3*(3), 149–159.

Bian, Y. J., & Li, L. L. (2012). The Chinese General Social Survey (2003–2008): Sample designs and data evaluation. *Chinese Sociological Review, 45*(1), 70–97.

Bian, Y. J., Zhang, L., Yang, Z. K., Guo, X. X., & Lei, M. (2014). Subject well-being in China: A multifaceted view. *Social Indicators Research*. doi:10.1007/s11205-014-0626-6.

Friedman, J., & Thomas, D. (2009). Psychological health before, during, and after an economic crisis: Results from Indonesia, 1993–2000. *The World Bank Economic Review, 23*(1), 57–76.

Hardt, J., Jacobsen, C., Goldberg, J., Nickel, R., & Buchwald, D. (2008). Prevalence of chronic pain in a representative sample in the United States. *Pain Medicine, 9*(7), 803–812.

Harstall, C., & Ospina, M. (2003). How prevalent is chronic pain? *Pain Clinical Updates, 11*(2), 1–4. Seattle: International Association for the Study of Pain.

He, X., & Wong, D. (2011). A comparison of female migrant workers' mental health in four cities in China. *International Journal of Social Psychiatry, 59*(2), 114–122.

Kan, H. (2009). Environment and health in China: Challenges and opportunities. *Environmental Health Perspectives, 117*(12), A530.

Kleinman, A. (2009). *Unpacking global health: A critical sociology of knowledge III. Slide presentation*. http://www.scribd.com/doc/90989880/Lecture-2-Unpacking-Global-Health-II. Accessed 20 Jan 2013.

Lelkes, O. (2013). Minimising misery: A new strategy for public policies instead of maximising happiness? *Social Indicators Research, 114*, 121–137.

Liang, J., McCarthy, J. F., Jain, A., Krause, N., Bennett, J. M., & Gu, S. (2000). Socioeconomic gradient in old age mortality in Wuhan, China. *Journal of Gerontology: Social Sciences, 55B*, S222–S233.

Liu, J. X., Xiong, M. L., & Su, Y. (2012). National happiness at a time of economic growth: A tracking study based on CGSS data. *Social Sciences in China, 12*, 102–125.

Marsden, P. (1987). Core discussion networks of Americans. *American Sociological Review, 52*(1), 122–131.

National Bureau of Statistics of China. (2002). *China statistical yearbook 2002*. Beijing: China Statistics Press.

National Bureau of Statistics of China. (2009). *China statistical yearbook 2009*. Beijing: China Statistics Press.

Naughton, B. (2007). *The Chinese economy: Transitions and growth*. Cambridge, MA: MIT Press.

Putnam, R. (2000). *Bowling alone*. New York: Simon and Schuster.

Sidel, V. W. (1993). New lessons from China: Equity and economics in rural health care. *American Journal of Public Health, 83*, 1665–1666.

Smith, K., Mehta, S., & Feuz, M. (2004). Indoor smoke from household solid fuels. In M. Ezzati, A. D. Rodgers, A. D. Lopez, & C. Murray (Eds.), *Comparative quantification of health risks: Global and regional burden of disease due to selected major risk factors* (Vol. 2). Geneva: World Health Organization.

Steele, L. G., & Lynch, S. M. (2013). The pursuit of happiness in China: Individualism, collectivism, and subjective well-being during China's economic and social transformation. *Social Indicators Research, 114*, 441–451.

Sun, X., Lucas, H., & Meng, Q. (2011). Associations between living arrangements and health-related quality of life of urban elderly people: A study from China. *Quality of Life Research, 20*, 359–369.

Wilkinson, I. (2005). *Suffering: A sociological introduction*. Indianapolis: Polity.

World Health Organization and China State Council Development Research Center. (2005). *China: Health, poverty, and economic development*. Report is available via: http://www.who.int/macrohealth/action/CMH_China.pdf?ua=1

Wu, B., Mao, Z., & Xu, Q. (2008). Institutional care for elders in rural China. *Journal of Aging and Social Policy, 20*(2), 218–239.

Xing, Z. (2012). A study of the relationship between income and subjective well-being in China. *Sociological Research, 1*, 196–219.

Zeng, Y. C., Ching, S. S., & Loke, A. Y. (2010). Quality of life measurement in women with cervical cancer: Implications for Chinese cervical cancer survivors. *Health and Quality of Life Outcomes, 8*(1), 30.

Zhen, C., & Silverstein, M. (2008). Intergenerational support and depression among elders in rural China: Do daughters-in-law matter? *Journal of Marriage and Family, 70*, 599–612.

Zimmer, Z., & Amorbsirisomboon, P. (2001). Socioeconomic status and health among older adults in Thailand: An examination using multiple indicators. *Social Science and Medicine, 52*(8), 1297–1311.

Zuo, J., & Bian, Y. (2005). Beyond resources and patriarchy: Family decision-making power in a Chinese city. *Journal of Comparative Family Studies, 36*(4), 601–627.

Chapter 16
Suffering Ailments and Addiction Problems in the Family

Mariano Rojas

16.1 Introduction

The family is an ancient and essential human institution; family members often constitute a close and intimate network of ties that systematically constitute major socializing effects on all members. Even though well-being is a personal experience, it is important to recognize that well-being does not exist in a bubble—that is, it is not independent of what happens to those we care about. Family could be understood as the first-level human ecosystem in the generation and sustainability of people's well-being (Bronfenbrenner 1979).

Unfortunately, many factors may generate problems within the family, and these have serious implications for each family member's well-being. Illnesses, for example, are part of life, and people may face not only their own ailments but also the ailments of family members and other loved ones. Thus, a person's well-being is expected to be affected by illnesses other family members face. The main purpose of this chapter is to study this issue in Mexico.

In 2012, Mexico's National Statistical Office administered a representative survey to gather information about the subjective well-being of citizens. The survey also inquired about possible grave ailments and addictions (alcohol or drug) within the family. This data is leveraged to learn how the health and addiction problems of family members affect the subjective well-being of the interviewed person.

M. Rojas (✉)
FLACSO-México and UPAEP, Carretera al Ajusco 377, Colonia Héroes de Padierna, Delegación Tlalpan, Mexico, D.F. C.P. 14200, Mexico
e-mail: mariano.rojas.h@gmail.com

© Springer Science+Business Media Dordrecht 2015
R.E. Anderson (ed.), *World Suffering and Quality of Life*,
Social Indicators Research Series 56, DOI 10.1007/978-94-017-9670-5_16

16.2 Well-Being and the Family

16.2.1 The Family: A Central Human Institution

The family is an ancient institution and almost universally recognized as a pillar of society. Most children grow up within families, and the majority of adults live in families. Human beings are familiar with words such as mom, dad, brother, sister, son, daughter, wife, and husband. Words for more distant relations, such as grandpa, grandma, uncle, aunt, and cousin, are also common. Though most people are well-acquainted with the concept of the family, its nature and understanding is highly diverse across cultures (Zimmerman and Frampton 1935).

Most understandings of the family make reference to close emotional and economic ties among family members. Emotional ties are expected to be mostly positive, while economic ties emphasize cooperation and even altruism. The list of qualities associated with the family vary but, in general, it is common to think about love, respect, caring, understanding, acceptance, encouragement, guidance, security, recognition, nurturing, empathy, reciprocity, and long-run commitment (Becker 1981, 1991; Lowman 1987). Negative aspects such as abuse, dispute, control, fear, fighting, anxiety, burden, and conflict may also come to mind when thinking about the family (Palomar 1999).

Joaquim Vogel points towards the important role the family plays in providing the conditions in which people's well-being emerges. Vogel states:

> In the case of the labour market the distribution of resources is based on competition and individual performance. The welfare states' redistribution is focused at solidarity between citizens. In the case of the family the principle is reciprocity and an informal contract between family members concerning responsibilities for the welfare of family members. There is a contract between spouses, between parents and their children, between adults and their elderly parents, and between adults and further relatives (Vogel 2003: 393).

It is clear that the family implies a long-run shared project for all family members, in which commitment, formal or informal, plays an important role. A "family is more than just a collection of people who might expose each other to infections and pollutants" by inhabiting the same house (Ross et al. 1990: 1059). The family is expected to make an important contribution to the satisfaction of each member's material and psychological needs (Antonucci 1990; Demo and Acock 1996; Evans and Kelley 2004; Kim and Kim 2003).

The literature on family structure, family arrangements, and intra-family arrangements discusses such important topics through the existence of size economies within the family, the economic and emotional costs and benefits from additional members, and the intra-family distribution of the benefits from living in family arrangements (Rojas 2007a; Yang 2003). Censuses commonly define the family as "*two or more individuals related by blood, marriage, or adoption who reside in the same household*" (Cherlin 1981). Different family typologies may be advanced within this definition, such as nuclear two-parent family, nuclear one-parent family, extended family, and three-generation extended family. Still, this definition may neglect important emotional and economic links that prevail among people who do not reside in the same household. The concept of extended family helps us reference those who understand themselves as emotionally linked, either because they grew up together, share the same progenitors, or share a special, stable bond (Murtan and Reitzes 1984; Ofstedal et al. 1999; Schwarze and Winkelmann 2011).

Each person defines the boundaries of his or her own family on the basis of his or her own understandings and expectations. For some, and in some countries, the family does not go beyond spouse and parental links, while for others it includes uncles, aunts, grandparents, cousins, and even close friends. Caring about those considered "part of the group" is an important feature in all families (Altonji et al. 1992; Rossi and Rossi 1990).

16.2.2 Well-Being and the Subjective Well-Being Approach

16.2.2.1 The Experience of Being Well

The subjective well-being approach understands well-being as the experience people have of being well. Well-being happens in the realm of the person, not in objects. And even though the experience of being well can be analytically separated from the person for academic purposes, it is a subjective experience that does not exist without the person who is experiencing it.

It is in the human condition to be able to recognize different types of well-being experiences, such as: first, sensorial experiences associated to pain and pleasure; second, affective experiences related to emotions and moods which are usually classified as positive and negative affects and understood in terms of enjoyment and distress; third, evaluative experiences assessed on the basis of the attainment of goals and aspirations individuals hold and are usually termed as achievements and failures in life; fourth, very intense, short, and global experiences of being well which are usually classified as flow states. Thus, when talking about well-being, it is common to make reference to affective, sensorial, evaluative and even mystical experiences (Argyle 2002; Csikszentmihalyi 2008; Rojas and Veenhoven 2013; Veenhoven 1991).

16.2.2.2 A Synthesis: Life Satisfaction

The subjective well-being approach also recognizes that people are able to synthesize their essential experiences into a measure of how well life is going. For example, it is very likely for people experiencing pleasure, joy, and achievement to make a synthesis in terms of their life going great or being highly satisfied with their life. In other cases, when there are conflicting experiences, people are challenged to come up with a synthesis. They may end up reporting being modestly satisfied or unsatisfied with their life, depending on the weight or personal importance they give to the conflicting experiences.

A crucial feature in the subjective well-being approach is the recognition that every person is in a privileged position to judge and report his or her well-being. The best way to learn about people's well-being is to ask them. One common question is, "Taking everything in your life into consideration, how satisfied are you with your life?" The incorporation of this approach into academic studies of well-being is relatively new; some sociologists, psychologists, and economists started using subjective well-being information in the 1970s and 1980s (Andrews and Withey 1976; Argyle 1987; Campbell 1976; Campbell et al. 1976; Diener 1984; Easterlin 1973, 1974; Michalos 1985; van Praag 1971; Veenhoven 1984). While still new, this is now a well-accepted approach, included in the OECD guidelines for measuring subjective well-being (OECD 2013) and used by national statistical offices around the world, including Mexico.

16.2.2.3 Understanding People's Well-Being: Domains of Life

Life satisfaction can be understood on the basis of people's essential sensorial, affective, and evaluative experiences. The domains-of-life literature states that a person's life can be approached as a general construct of many specific domains and that life satisfaction can be understood as the result of satisfaction in the domains of life (Cummins 1996; Headey et al. 1984, 1985; Headey and Wearing 1992; Rojas 2006, 2007b; van Praag and Ferrer-i-Carbonell 2004; Veenhoven 1996). The approach attempts to understand a general appraisal of life as a whole on the basis of a vector of specific appraisals in more concrete spheres of being.

The enumeration and demarcation of the domains of life is arbitrary; it can range from a small number to an almost infinite recounting of all imaginable human activities and spheres of being. Thus, there are many possible partitions of a human life, and the selected partition depends on the research's objectives. Nevertheless, any partition must value parsimony, meaning, and usefulness. Van Praag et al. (2003) studied the relationship of satisfaction in different domains of life (health, financial situation, job, housing, leisure, and environment) and satisfaction with life as a whole. They state that "satisfaction with life as a whole can be seen as an aggregate concept, which can be unfolded into its domain components" (van Praag et al. 2003: 3). A similar approach is followed by Rojas (2006), who argues for a non-linear relationship between satisfaction in *domains* of life and *overall* life satisfaction.

16.2.3 Ailments and Addiction Problems in the Family and People's Well-Being

Researchers have stated that the family constitutes a first-level human ecosystem in the generation and sustainability of individuals' well-being (Bronfenbrenner 1979). Following this human ecosystem approach, whatever happens to one family member will affect others' well-being (Ross et al. 1990; Winkelmann 2005). The strength of links, which can be thought of as both economic and emotional, between a person's well-being and the events that take place in his or her family may depend on the specific event under consideration.

Economic links refer to the generation and allocation of scarce resources used to satisfy material needs. The family can be understood as a production unit in which many resources need to be efficiently allocated in order to generate and distribute well-being across all members. Many such economic decisions are made within the family. For example, there is an intra-household division of labor that requires family members to perform specific tasks; the benefits from the total goods and services generated by the household resources then have to be allocated among household members on the basis of some norms. Because of specialization and division of labor, sharing and reciprocity rules may emerge within the family (Rojas 2009). It is expected that these within-family decisions will make an important contribution to the well-being of all family members; any disruption within the family may be detrimental to people's well-being.

To return, however, to the earlier metaphor, a family is not only a production unit but also an ecosystem in which people grow up and develop as persons. Strong and close emotional links emerge in this process. Within the family, regard for others, nurturing, and care allow members to satisfy psychological needs and develop identity. Affection is expected, and emotions play a crucial role in generating long-run stable bonds (Olson and Barnes 1987; Rettig and Leichtentritt 1999; Stevens 1992). Any problem within the family can impact all family members' well-being to differing degrees. In this chapter, two specific kinds of problems are studied: grave ailments and addiction problems, both of which are generally associated with suffering.

16.3 Database and Variables

16.3.1 The Survey

Mexico's National Statistical Office (INEGI) ran its first subjective well-being survey in 2012. The Self-Reported Well-Being Survey (BIARE, for its name in Spanish) is representative at the country level and included 10,654 observations of respondents aged 18–70 years old. This is the first survey done by a Latin American National Statistical Office to gather subjective well-being information. Due to its experimental nature, the survey is rich in subjective well-being variables as well as in information about life events. The database incorporates expansion factors, which are used in this study.

16.3.2 Variables in the Survey

16.3.2.1 Subjective Well-Being Variables

The following variables are used to represent the subjective well-being situation of the population of adults:

– Life satisfaction: How satisfied are you with your life?
– Satisfaction with affective life: How satisfied are you with your affective life?

Table 16.1 Subjective
well-being situation
Mexico 2012

Variable	Mean	Std. Dev.
Life satisfaction	8.04	1.94
Satisfaction with		
Life achievements	7.55	2.13
Affective life	8.20	1.99
Free time	6.86	2.68
Job	7.78	2.33
Economic	6.50	2.32
Family	8.53	1.76
Health	8.22	1.91

Source: BIARE 2012, INEGI

- Satisfaction with life achievements: How satisfied are you with your achievements in life?
- Domain satisfaction: Availability of free time, economic situation, job, family relations, and health.

The response scale for these variables goes from 0 to 10, implying that it is reasonable to treat these variables as cardinal or interval measures.

Table 16.1 presents the subjective well-being reported by Mexicans. Life satisfaction is relatively high, with an average value above 8. The affective situation (satisfaction with affective life) is higher than the evaluative situation (satisfaction with achievements in life). This is common in Latin America, and points toward the importance of the effects in generating Latin Americans' well-being and toward their relatively poor situation regarding access to those goods and services considered as necessary for high standards of living. Another constant in Latin American studies is the relatively high satisfaction with family relations and the relatively low satisfaction with their economic situation.

16.3.2.2 Grave Ailments and Addiction Problems in the Family

The survey also gathered information about whether a relative was experiencing a grave ailment. The questionnaire accounted for different kinds of affinity: spouse or partner, mother or father, sister or brother, daughter or son. The response scale was dichotomous: yes (1) or no (0). Unfortunately, the survey does not provide in-depth data about the nature of the ailments family members are experiencing.

There is also information about somebody at home (presumably a relative) facing alcoholism or drug addiction problems (again, the response scale is dichotomous). Table 16.2 shows the situation in Mexico; approximately 15 % reported that their mother or father had a grave ailment, and more than 7 % reported a grave ailment affecting a sister or brother. The situation is similar in the case of the spouse or stable partner. Only about 4 % of people in the survey reported that at least one of their children had a grave ailment. Almost 9 % reported facing alcoholism in their home, with drug addiction at 2.5 %.

Table 16.2 Grave ailment and addiction in the family

Variable	Percentage
Grave ailment of	
Spouse or partner	5.89
Mother or father	15.59
Sister or brother	7.48
Daughter or son	3.82
Addiction problems at home	
Alcoholism	8.95
Drug addiction	2.58
Number of observations	10,649

Source: BIARE 2012, INEGI, Mexico

Table 16.3 Descriptive statistics – subjective well-being by problems in the family

	Satisfaction with					
	Life as a whole		Achievements in life		Affective life	
Grave ailment of	**Yes**	**No**	**Yes**	**No**	**Yes**	**No**
Spouse or partner	8.06	7.39	7.56	7.36	8.21	8.04
Mother or father	8.08	7.82	7.57	7.43	8.24	7.99
Sister or brother	8.06	7.84	7.56	7.41	8.22	7.97
Daughter or son	8.06	7.43	7.56	7.27	8.22	7.63
Addiction problems at home	**Yes**	**No**	**Yes**	**No**	**Yes**	**No**
Alcoholism	8.10	7.47	7.59	7.12	8.24	7.78
Drug addiction	8.06	7.32	7.56	6.95	8.22	7.43

Source: BIARE 2012, INEGI, Mexico

16.3.3 Some Descriptive Statistics

My main objective is to understand how experiencing ailments and addiction problems in the family affect personal well-being. Table 16.3 presents the situation for some subjective well-being indicators (life satisfaction, satisfaction with life achievements, and satisfaction with affective life) for people who report having a family member with grave health problems or an addiction problem. As expected, people who have a relative with a grave ailment or other problem at home had, on average, lower life satisfaction as well as lower affective and achievement satisfactions.

In the case of grave ailments, the difference in life satisfaction between those who had a relative with a serious illness and those who did not was greater when the relative was a spouse or a child. The pattern repeats in the case of the satisfaction with achievements in life. However, in the case of satisfaction with affective life, the impact was larger in the case of a daughter or son having a grave ailment.

Alcoholism and drug addiction seem to be associated with lower life satisfaction as well as lower satisfaction with life achievements and with affective life; the impact is larger in the case of drug addiction than in alcoholism.

16.4   The Impact of Grave Ailments in the Family

Regression analyses were used to further explore the well-being impact of ailments in the family. This allowed me to control for other variables that may play a role in people's well-being and helps show the net impact of grave ailments in the family.

The following regression specification was estimated:

$$SWB_i = \propto_0 + \propto_1 A_{Spouse} + \propto_2 A_{Parent} + \propto_3 A_{SisterBrother} + \propto_4 A_{DaugtherSon} + \phi \log Y_{hpc\_i} \quad (16.1)$$

$$+ \beta_1 Age_i + \beta_2 Age_i^2 + \beta_3 Gender_i + \sum_{j=1}^{6} \gamma_j Edu_{ij} + \sum_{k=1}^{5} \delta_k MS_{ik}$$

Where:

SWB_i: Proxy for subjective well-being of person i.
A_{Spouse}: Dummy variable with value of 1 if spouse or partner has grave ailment.
A_{Parent}: Dummy variable with value of 1 if father or mother has grave ailment.
$A_{SisterBrother}$: Dummy variable with value of 1 if sister or brother has grave ailment.
$A_{DaughterSon}$: Dummy variable with value of 1 if daughter or son has grave ailment.
Y_{hpc}: Total household current expenditure
Age: age in years
Gender: gender
Edu: vector of dichotomous variables for schooling level
MS: vector of dichotomous variables for marital status

Table 16.4 presents the results from the econometric exercise regarding the coefficients for grave ailments in the family. It also shows the estimated coefficient for household total current expenditure. Regarding people's life satisfaction, there was a substantial well-being cost when a child had a grave ailment (a decline of 0.4 on a scale of 0–10). For perspective, it is handy to compare this to the estimated coefficient for household current expenditure. An increase of 100 % in household per capita expenditure raises reported well-being by 0.3. It is possible to monetize the well-being impact of having a daughter or a son with a grave ailment; this cost is about 125 % of household per capita expenditure.

The life satisfaction cost of the spouse having a grave ailment is also large, about 0.3 points in life satisfaction. The cost of a father or mother having a grave ailment is 0.24 points and statistically significant.

Table 16.4 allows for further understanding of the impact of grave ailments in the family. The evaluative well-being experience associated with "achievements in life" was impacted by grave ailments in the family; especially those ailments of or sibling. Notably, ailments of a son or daughter have a non-significant impact in

Table 16.4 Regression analyses of subjective well-being and grave ailments in the family, Mexico 2012

| | Satisfaction with | | | | | | | |
Grave ailment of	Life	Affect	Achievement	Free time	Job	Economic	Family	Health
Spouse or partner	−0.303***	−0.202**	−0.176**	−0.246**	−0.278**	−0.504***	−0.179**	−0.354***
Mother or father	−0.238***	−0.134**	−0.260***	−0.396***	−0.136*	−0.390***	−0.111**	−0.395***
Sister or brother	−0.108	−0.188**	−0.166**	−0.101	0.076	−0.113	−0.145**	−0.318***
Daughter or son	−0.409***	−0.140	−0.412***	−0.621***	−0.254*	−0.502***	−0.271***	−0.434***
Log Yhpc	0.304***	0.368***	0.287***	0.220***	0.392***	0.701***	0.203***	0.174***

Source: Own estimations based on information from BIARE-INEGI 2012
Notes:
Yhpc stands for household per capita total expenditure
Regressions do also include the following control variables: age and age squared, gender, schooling, marital status
Significance levels at 0.01 (***), 0.05 (**), and 0.10 (*)

satisfaction with the evaluative situation. On the other hand, the affective situation is highly impacted by a grave ailment of a child or parent.

Satisfaction with free time is highly impacted by a grave ailment of a daughter or son, and to a lesser degree by an ailment of a parent. Satisfaction with the economic domain of life is strongly impacted by grave ailments of a spouse or children, while satisfaction with one's own health is impacted by any relative's ailment. In general, Table 16.4 shows that what happens to other members of the family ends up impacts everyone's well-being. The magnitude and nature of this impact depends on the relationship of the individual to the family member suffering.

16.5 The Impact of Alcoholism and Drug Addiction in the Family

A similar econometric exercise explored the impact of alcoholism or drug addiction in the family. Table 16.5 shows that addictions at home have a significant well-being cost. From a life-satisfaction perspective, the impact of alcoholism seems larger than the impact of drug addiction; however, drug addiction more strongly affects people's affective situation. Alcoholism has a larger impact on family and health satisfaction.

From a monetary perspective, the life satisfaction cost of alcoholism in the family is a reduction of 0.5, while a 100 % raise in household per capita expenditure increases life satisfaction by 0.2. Thus, having alcoholism at home implies a well-being burden that can be valued at about 166 % of household per capita expenditure. Following the same methodology, it is possible to observe that a drug addiction problem at home implies a burden that can be valued at about 130 % of household per capita income.

16.6 Final Comments

The experience of being well is personal; it is never accurate to generalize the well-being of groups such as the family or society. Yet, it would also be incorrect to understand the experience of being well as an individual phenomenon, devoid of context. Well-being depends on what happens in individuals' surrounding relational and physical context. The family constitutes a first-level human ecosystem and, as such, a full understanding of well-being requires knowing what happens at the family level.

This chapter discovered the well-being effects of problems taking place at the family level. As expected, it is shown that people significantly suffer as a consequence of ailments and addictions in their family. Overall assessments of life (life satisfaction) as well as evaluative and affective assessments are largely impacted by these family-related problems. The well-being impact of these problems depends

Table 16.5 Regression analyses subjective well-being and addictions in the family, Mexico 2012

Addictions in the family	Satisfaction with							
	Life	Life achievements	Affective situation	Time	Job	Economic	Family	Health
Alcoholism	−0.509***	−0.329***	−0.323***	−0.196**	−0.320**	−0.351***	−0.445***	−0.329***
Drug addiction	−0.391***	−0.302*	−0.537***	−0.205	−0.297*	−0.357***	−0.380***	−0.210*
Log Yhpc	0.299***	0.363***	0.285***	0.222***	0.390***	0.698***	0.199***	0.170***

Source: Own estimations based on information from BIARE-INEGI 2012

Notes:

Yhpc stands for household per capita total expenditure

Regressions do also include the following control variables: age and age squared, gender, schooling, marital status

Significance levels at 0.01 (***), 0.05 (**), and 0.10 (*)

on the kinship role of the person directly suffering. Disruptions within the family due to grave ailments and addictions also affect the well-being of other members of the family.

Though well-being is a personal experience, its understanding requires moving beyond individualistic perspectives. The concept of the person as somebody who has attributes associated with their family and social context has been validated by this study. Given the emotional and economic links that predominate within families, it is necessary to emphasize the "we" rather than the "I" in the study of people's well-being. It is possible to understand statements like "we are suffering an illness" rather than "I am suffering an illness."

Finally, while this study did not ask persons they were personally suffering, the observed drops in well-being suggest that suffering is contagious within families. While we can only infer that a decrease in well-being represents an increase in suffering, the study may have shown a direct connection between the suffering of family members. Several chapters in this volume, as well as an extensive literature on caregiver burden, suggest that some family caregivers suffer from that role. While the burden of caregiving may be one significant route by which suffering spreads, this chapter shows that many other routes exist, particularly when close emotional and economic links prevail, such as in the case of the family.

References

Altonji, J. G., Hayashi, F., & Kotliko, L. J. (1992). Is the extended family altruistically linked? Direct tests using micro data. *American Economic Review, 82*, 1177–1198.

Andrews, F. M., & Withey, S. B. (1976). *Social indicators of well-being, American's perception of life quality*. New-York: Plenum Press.

Antonucci, T. C. (1990). Social supports and social relationships. In R. H. Binstock & L. K. George (Eds.), *Handbook of aging and social sciences*. New York: Academic.

Argyle, M. (1987). *The psychology of happiness* (1st ed.). London: Methuen.

Argyle, M. (2002). *The psychology of happiness* (2nd ed.). New York: Routledge.

Becker, G. S. (1981). Altruism in the family and selfishness in the market place. *Economica, 48*, 1–15.

Becker, G. S. (1991). *A treatise on the family*. Cambridge, MA: Harvard University Press.

Bronfenbrenner, U. (1979). *The ecology of human development: Experiments by nature and design*. Cambridge, MA: Harvard University Press.

Campbell, A. (1976). Subjective measures of well-being. *American Psychologist, 31*, 117–124.

Campbell, A., Converse, P. E., & Rodgers, W. L. (1976). *The quality of American life. Perceptions, evaluations and satisfactions*. New York: Russell Sage.

Cherlin, A. J. (1981). *Marriage, divorce, remarriage*. Cambridge, MA: Harvard University Press.

Csikszentmihalyi, M. (2008). *Flow: The psychology of optimal experience*. New York: Harper Perennial Modern Classics.

Cummins, R. A. (1996). The domains of life satisfaction: An attempt to order chaos. *Social Indicators Research, 38*, 303–332.

Demo, D. H., & Acock, A. C. (1996). Family structure, family process, and adolescent well-being. *Journal of Research on Adolescence, 6*, 457–488.

Diener, E. (1984). Subjective well-being. *Psychological Bulletin, 95*, 542–575.

Easterlin, R. (1973). Does money buy happiness? *The Public Interest, 30*, 3–10.

Easterlin, R. (1974). Does economic growth enhance the human lot? Some empirical evidence. In P. A. David & M. Reder (Eds.), *Nations and households in economic growth: Essays in honour of Moses Abramovitz* (pp. 89–125). Palo Alto: Stanford University Press.

Evans, M. D. R., & Kelley, J. (2004). Effect of family structure on life satisfaction: Australian evidence? *Social Indicators Research, 69*, 303–349.

Headey, B., & Wearing, A. J. (1992). *Understanding happiness: A theory of subjective well-being*. Melbourne: Longman Cheshire.

Headey, B., Holmström, E., & Wearing, A. J. (1984). The impact of life events and changes in domain satisfactions on well-being. *Social Indicators Research, 15*, 203–227.

Headey, B., Holmström, E., & Wearing, A. J. (1985). Models of well-being and Ill-being. *Social Indicators Research, 17*, 211–234.

Kim, I. K., & Kim, C.-S. (2003). Patterns of family support and the quality of life of the elderly. *Social Indicators Research, 63*, 437–454.

Lowman, J. C. (1987). Inventory of family feelings. In N. Fredman & R. Sherman (Eds.), *Handbook of measurement for marriage and family therapy* (pp. 91–99). New York: Brunner/Mazel.

Michalos, A. (1985). Multiple discrepancy theory. *Social Indicators Research, 16*, 347–413.

Murtan, E., & Reitzes, D. C. (1984). Intergenerational support activities and well-being among the elderly: A converge of exchange theory and symbolic interaction perspectives. *American Sociological Review, 49*, 117–130.

OECD. (2013). *OECD guidelines on measuring subjective well-being*. Paris: OECD Publishing.

Ofstedal, M. B., Knodel, J., & Chayovan, A. (1999). *Intergenerational support and gender: A comparison of four Asian countries* (Elderly in Asian research report no. 99–54). Ann Arbor: University of Michigan Population Studies Center.

Olson, D. H., & Barnes, H. L. (1987). Family quality of life. In N. Fredman & R. Sherman (Eds.), *Handbook of measurement for marriage and family therapy* (pp. 186–190). New York: Brunner/Mazel.

Palomar, J. (1999). The relationship between family functioning and quality of life in families with an alcoholic member. *Salud Mental, 22*(6), 13–21.

Rettig, K. D., & Leichtentritt, R. D. (1999). A general theory for perceptual indicators of family life quality. *Social Indicators Research, 47*(3), 307–342.

Rojas, M. (2006). Life satisfaction and satisfaction in domains of life: Is it a simple relationship? *Journal of Happiness Studies, 7*(4), 467–497.

Rojas, M. (2007a). Communitarian versus individualistic arrangements in the family: What and whose income matters for happiness? In R. J. Estes (Ed.), *Advancing quality of life in a turbulent world* (pp. 153–167). Dordrecht: Springer.

Rojas, M. (2007b). The complexity of well-being: A life-satisfaction conception and a domains-of-life approach. In I. Gough & A. McGregor (Eds.), *Researching well-being in developing countries: From theory to research* (pp. 259–280). Cambridge: Cambridge University Press.

Rojas, M. (2009). A monetary appraisal of some illnesses in Costa Rica: A subjective well-being approach. *Pan American Journal of Public Health, 26*(3), 255–265.

Rojas, M., & Veenhoven, R. (2013). Contentment and affect in the estimation of happiness. *Social Indicators Research, 110*(2), 415–431.

Ross, C., Mirowsky, J., & Goldsteen, K. (1990). The impact of the family on health: The decade in review. *Journal of Marriage and the Family, 52*, 1059–1078.

Rossi, A. S., & Rossi, P. H. (1990). *Of human bonding: Parent-child relations across the life course*. New York: Aldine DeGruyter.

Schwarze, J., & Winkelmann, R. (2011). Happiness and altruism within the extended family. *Journal of Population Economics, 24*, 1033–1051.

Stevens, E. S. (1992). Reciprocity in social support: An advantage for the aging family. *Families in Society, 73*, 533–541.

van Praag, B. M. S. (1971). The welfare function of income in Belgium: An empirical investigation. *European Economic Review, 2*, 337–369.

van Praag, B. M. S., & Ferrer-i-Carbonell, A. (2004). *Happiness quantified: A satisfaction calculus approach*. Oxford: Oxford University Press.

van Praag, B. M. S., Frijters, P., & Ferrer-i-Carbonell, A. (2003). The anatomy of subjective well-being. *Journal of Economic Behaviour and Organization, 51*, 29–49.

Veenhoven, R. (1984). *Conditions of happiness*. Dordrecht: Kluwer.

Veenhoven, R. (1991). Questions on happiness: Classical topics, modern answers, blind spots. In F. Strack, M. Argyle, & Y. N. Schwarz (Eds.), *Subjective well-being. An inter-disciplinary perspective* (pp. 7–26). London: Pergamon Press.

Veenhoven, R. (1996). Developments in satisfaction research. *Social Indicators Research, 37*, 1–45.

Vogel, J. (2003). The family. *Social Indicators Research, 64*, 393–435.

Winkelmann, R. (2005). Subjective well-being and the family: Results from an ordered probit model with multiple random effects. *Empirical Economics, 30*, 749–761.

Yang, O. K. (2003). Family structure and relations. *Social Indicators Research, 63*, 121–148.

Zimmerman, C., & Frampton, M. (1935). *Family and society: A study of the sociology of reconstruction*. New York: Van Nostrand.

Chapter 17
Suffering and Good Society Analysis Across African Countries

Ferdi Botha

17.1 Introduction

Within the context of research on societal quality of life (QOL), the concept of the Good Society (GS) has emerged as a paradigm or framework for formulating how a public can create and maintain a well-functioning society. Many different intellectual communities have focused on the concept of the Good Society. The first book called *The Good Society* (Lippmann 1937) was written by a journalist and public opinion researcher, but another came 60 years later and was written by several philosophers and sociologists (Bellah et al. 1991). Many social scientists have been interested in the challenge of defining the key elements of the Good Society but referred to it as the Civil Society (Ehrenberg 1999); others referred to it as Social Capital (Bourdieu 1983; Coleman 1988). Political scientists focused on democratic processes in society (Draper and Ramsay 2011), while economists evaluated societal well-being in terms of a combination of economic and socio-political goals (Schiller 2013). A group of political scientists, economists, and philosophers launched a scholarly journal in 2002 titled "The Good Society"; it is still published twice a year by Penn State University Press.

Jordan (2012) discusses the GS primarily in psychological terms and provides some insight into contextual aspects of good societies for the individual. Using the GS framework as an overarching foundation, Holmberg (2007) and Anderson (2012a) developed quite different Good Society indexes. A society is considered "good" if the combination of qualities and factors incorporated improves the lives of all citizens. For the 20 richest societies, Anderson's (2011a) Good Society Index

I am grateful to Ron Anderson for valuable comments and suggestions. This research was partly supported by Rhodes University (Grant #RC2013).

F. Botha (✉)
Department of Economics and Economic History, Rhodes University,
Grahamstown, South Africa
e-mail: F.Botha@ru.ac.za

© Springer Science+Business Media Dordrecht 2015
R.E. Anderson (ed.), *World Suffering and Quality of Life*,
Social Indicators Research Series 56, DOI 10.1007/978-94-017-9670-5_17

(GSI) includes "Compassion" as one of the sub-indexes. Three Nordic countries (Sweden, Norway, and Denmark) topped the index and the United States scored very low. An important conclusion from Anderson's (2011a) research was that countries' wealth explained very little of the differences in QOL across countries, and that only a very few countries managed to score high on the GSI, suggesting that being a good society is challenging. Using the same 20 developed nations, Anderson (2012a) later expanded his original GSI to include a total of 48 indicators based on 12 main components, with additional focus on the issues of social cohesion and factors such as social and environmental sustainability.

One important area that has not been studied sufficiently within the GS framework is the African continent. The African continent is home to some of the poorest countries in the world which, coupled with political and economic strife, is detrimental to the well-being of African citizens and cause substantial suffering (Guest 2006; Meredith 2006; Mills 2011). Moreover, in constructing a multidimensional index of global suffering, Anderson (2012b) found that of the ten countries with the highest levels of suffering, nine are in Africa. Holmberg (2007) constructed a GSI with three components (life expectancy, infant mortality, and life satisfaction) for 71 countries, eight of which were African: Algeria, Egypt, Morocco, Nigeria, South Africa, Tanzania, Uganda, and Zimbabwe. Among these, Algeria ranked highest on the GSI, but was only ranked 55th overall. Tanzania and Zimbabwe took the lowest spots on the list. Democratic countries scored higher on the GSI, as did countries with attributes such as low corruption and a high gross national income per capita.

Concurrently, literature is addressing the concept of suffering and its various dimensions (Anderson 2014). Knowing which factors positively affect the overall well-being of countries and how this relates to suffering is important for understanding how countries can help their citizens flourish.

Using a Good African Society Index (GASI), this study aims to examine the association between the GASI and some of its selected sub-components (the latter serve as indicators or likely causes of suffering). This allows for an investigation into how suffering differs across African countries at various points on the GASI and whether pursuit of GASI criteria could pave the way for reducing suffering. The better a country manages to attain the various elements contained in the GASI, the closer that country moves towards being a "good society". The traits of such a society in broad terms include, for example, genuine caring for others, sensible policy, and the state pursuit of improving citizen well-being (DeLeon and Longobardi 2002; Holmberg 2007; Tronto 2007; Anderson 2012a; Jordan 2012). Possessing the traits of a good society, and thereby obtaining a high GASI score, could contribute substantially to the reduction of suffering in a variety of domains.

17.2   The Good African Society Index

Originally developed and reported in Botha (2014), the Good African Society Index (GASI) was constructed for 46 African countries. Countries excluded due to data unavailability were Eritrea, Equatorial Guinea, Libya, Mauritius, Sao Tome and

Principe, Seychelles, Somalia, and South Sudan. The GASI has nine sub-indices or components and each sub-index has four indicators, for a total of 36 indicators. The nine sub-indices and their indicators are[1]:

17.2.1 Economic Performance

- *Population living below poverty line of $2 a day* (UNDP 2007; World Bank 2013b): Good societies have appropriate poverty alleviation programs and have low proportions of the population living in poverty.
- *Real GDP per capita growth, 2010–2011 (in 2000 $)* (World Bank 2013b): High levels of growth in real GDP per capita generally signify an improvement in overall living standards.
- *Export diversification* (World Bank 2013b): The more diversified a country's exports, the higher the GASI score is expected to be, since countries are not vulnerable to global demand shocks. Ranges from 0 (low diversification) to 1 (high diversification).
- *Income inequality* (UNDP 2013): In good societies, income is relatively evenly spread across the population. The Gini Index ranges from 0 (perfect equality) to 1 (perfect inequality).

17.2.2 Democracy, Freedom and Governance

- *Democracy index* (EIU 2012): More democratic societies allow citizens to voice their opinions and have freedom of choice, among other things. The democracy index falls between 0 (no democracy) and 10 (full democracy).
- *Freedom of the press* (RWB 2012): In good societies, there is freedom of expression and freedom of the press. This indicator is based on the 2011–2012 World Press Freedom Index, with a higher score denoting less press freedom.
- *Proportion of female parliamentary members* (UNDP 2013): Good societies are focused on achieving greater gender equality.
- *Government effectiveness* (World Bank 2013a): Good societies have effective governments that provide for the needs of their citizens. The index used ranges from −2.5 (weak performance) to 2.5 (very high performance), and measures issues such as the quality of public services, the quality of policy formulation and implementation, and the credibility of government commitment to such policies.

---

[1] Though some components are based on intuitive and theoretical reasoning, the various sub-components and how they relate to the relevant primary component are also supported by existing research. Due to space constraints, the various studies are not listed here but can be found in Botha (2013). In the current study, the various GASI components are only briefly summarized. Refer to Botha (2013) for a more detailed discussion of and motivation for the respective components.

17.2.3   Child Well-Being

- *Child mortality* (World Bank 2013a): Good societies have low rates of child mortality. Measured as the probability per 1,000 that a newborn baby will die before reaching age five, if subject to current age-specific mortality rates.
- *Immunization against measles* (World Bank 2013a): Coverage of treatments for immunization against various diseases is broad in good societies. Measured as the child immunization rate against measles for children ages 12–23 months.
- *Teen fertility rate* (UNDP 2013): Good societies have fewer teen pregnancies. Measure relates to teen (age 15–19) fertility rate per 1,000 women.
- *Child nutrition* (AfDB 2013; WHO 2013): In good societies, very few children are underweight and malnutritioned. Measured as the percentage of underweight children younger than 5 years.

17.2.4   Environment and Infrastructure

- *CO$_2$emissions* (AfDB et al. 2011): Good societies have relatively low carbon dioxide emissions, measured as CO_2 emissions per capita.
- *Forest area lost* (UNDP 2013): Good societies look after the environment, including their forests. Denotes the percentage change in forest area between 1990 and 2010.
- *Percentage of roads paved* (AfDB et al. 2013): The more comprehensive the road transport infrastructure of the country, the better a society. Measured as the percentage of paved roads relative to total roads.
- *Communication networks* (World Bank 2013a): Good societies have well-established networks that foster efficient communication between citizens and businesses. Measured as total main line and mobile telephone subscribers per 100 people.

17.2.5   Safety and Security

- *Homicide rate* (UNDP 2013): Good societies have low rates of intentional murder. Measured in this study as the number of intentional homicides per 100,000 population.
- *Road fatalities* (World Life Expectancy 2012): In good societies, there are few road accidents and, more important, few fatalities from the road accidents that do occur. Measured as road traffic deaths per 100,000 population.
- *Political stability and absence of violence* (World Bank 2013a): Good societies have stable political systems, and low political violence. Ranges from −2.5 (weak performance) to 2.5 (very high performance) and relates to perceptions of the likelihood that the government will be destabilized or overthrown by unconstitutional or violent means.

• *Security apparatus* (FFP 2013): Good societies do not have severe security issues such as protests, rebel activities, and riots. Indicator relates to the prevalence of security issues such as internal conflict, riots, protests, military coups, rebel activity, and bombings.

17.2.6   Health and Health Systems

• *Life expectancy* (UNDP 2013): In good societies, people have the opportunity to live long lives. Denotes life expectancy at birth, in years.
• *Infant mortality rate* (AfDB et al. 2011): Infant mortality is low in good societies. Measured as infant mortality rate per 1,000 births.
• *Obesity levels* (WHO 2013): High levels of obesity are detrimental to the health of citizens and thus less prevalent in good societies. Measured as the prevalence of population (age 15+) that is obese, i.e. BMI >30.
• *Doctors per 100,000 population* (AfDB et al. 2011): Indicates the availability of essential health care to citizens. The greater the density of doctors, the better the society.

17.2.7   Integrity and Justice

• *Corruption* (Transparency International 2012): Indicates perceived levels of corruption, expected to be lower in better societies. Measured by the 2012 Corruption Perception Index, ranging from 0 (highly corrupt) to 100 (very clean).
• *Enforcement of contracts* (World Bank 2013a): Contracts are easier to enforce in good societies. Indicated by the number of days from the filing of a lawsuit in court until the final determination and payment.
• *Prison population* (ICPS 2011): Good societies have low prison populations. Measured as number of people incarcerated per 100,000 persons.
• *Rule of law* (World Bank 2013a): Good societies manage to uphold the prevailing rule of law. Indicator ranges from −2.5 (weak performance) to 2.5 (very high performance), and measures the extent to which agents have confidence in and abide by the rules of society, specifically issues such as the quality of contract enforcement, police, and the courts, as well as the likelihood of crime and violence.

17.2.8   Education

• *Combined gross enrolment ratio in education* (UNDP 2011): Higher enrolment ratios are found in better societies. Measured as the number of students enrolled in primary, secondary and tertiary education, regardless of age, expressed as a percentage of the population of theoretical school age for the three levels.

- *Expected years of schooling* (UNDP 2013): In good societies, people can expect to attain reasonably high levels of education. Measured as the years of schooling a child of school entrance age can expect to receive if prevailing patterns of age-specific enrolment rates persist throughout the child's life.
- *Youth literacy rate* (CIA 2013): Good societies place emphasis on improving literacy levels. Measured as proportion of people aged 15–24 who can read and write.
- *Pupil/teacher ratio* (AfDB et al. 2011): A proxy for educational quality. Good societies have lower primary school pupil/teacher ratios.

17.2.9 Social Sustainability and Social Cohesion

- *Group grievance* (FFP 2013): Lower levels of group grievance are associated with better societies. Indicates tension and violence among particular groups, including factors such as discrimination, powerlessness, ethnic violence, and religious violence.
- *Human flight and brain drain* (FFP 2013): Better societies have less human flight and brain drain. The indicator relates to migration and human capital flight given lack of sufficient opportunities and includes factors such as migration per capita and emigration of educated population.
- *Stock of immigrants* (UNDP 2013): Great numbers of immigrants are associated with poorer societies, based on the assumption that more immigrants make group conflict more likely. Measured as the stock of immigrants as proportion of population.
- *Uneven economic development* (FFP 2013): More equal economic development is associated with better societies. Indicator is related to issues such as income inequality, urban-rural service distribution, access to improved services, and slum population.

Standardized scores of each indicator were calculated and re-standardized to a mean of 100 and standard deviation of 15: A GASI score of 100 implies that a country is ranked as average, while a GASI score above (below) 100 would imply an above-average (below-average) score. The overall GASI is obtained by summing the mean index scores of all nine components. Where necessary, index scores were reversed prior to summation. Cronbach's alpha for the overall index is 0.82, while sub-component alphas range from 0.78 to 0.84.

17.3 Indicators of Suffering

For the purpose of this paper, the overall GASI is compared to the following indicators of suffering. Note that each is a reverse-scored sub-index of the GASI, except for Poverty, which is the first indicator of the first sub-index above labeled Economic Performance.

- *Poverty.* "Population living below poverty line of $2 a day" (an indicator of Economic Performance). This component serves as a proxy for personal suffering including food deprivation and psychological strive associated with being poor. This indicator is used separately from the overall economics sub-index, as there is virtually no correlation between the overall GASI and the remaining three economics indicators.
- *Child Ill-Being* (reverse-scored sub-index). The purpose of this measure is to provide an indication of the suffering of children, and covers areas such as child mortality and malnutrition. The better the well-being of a country's children, the lower the suffering of those children.
- *Insecurity* (reverse-scored sub-index). This measure is deemed an indicator of suffering due to violence and fear for safety. In countries with very little safety, severe violence, and fear of such violence, suffering is a major outcome.
- *Poor Health* (reverse-scored sub-index). People who are exposed to poor health and health services will experience greater levels of suffering, as poor health or a lack of medical facilities are important factors that negatively affect the quality of life.
- *Low Cohesion and Social Sustainability* (reverse-scored sub-index). This measure serves as a proxy for the social suffering of individuals.

17.4   The Results

Table 17.1 contains the GASI's sub-index scores, the overall GASI score, and countries' GASI rankings. Tunisia ranks highest, followed by Cape Verde and Botswana. Chad fares worst on the GASI, followed by the Central African Republic (CAR), Cote d'Ivoire, and the Democratic Republic of the Congo (DRC). Countries prone to conflict and civil war score lowest on the GASI, which implies high levels of suffering. The suffering of children is particularly high in countries such as Chad, Mali, and Niger. Citizens in countries such as Cote d'Ivoire and Sudan experience constant suffering due to lack of safety and security (it is well known, of course, that Sudan has seen ongoing civil war and genocide for over a decade), whereas Botswana and Djibouti do particularly well in this domain. Health-related suffering is rife in countries such as Chad, Lesotho, and Sierra Leone, whereas social suffering is a problem in areas such as Cote d'Ivoire, Nigeria, and Sudan. In general, the picture emerging from Table 17.1 is that suffering is not high in countries due to a single indicator. Rather, on average countries that fare badly do so across most, if not all, suffering measures.

Table 17.2 presents correlation coefficients between the overall GASI and the five indicators of suffering. All suffering indicators negatively correlate with the GASI, with the GASI's correlation with Child Ill-Being as the being the strongest. The proportion of people living below $2 a day and all of the four additional indicators of suffering are negatively associated with the GASI. Of additional interest in Table 17.2 are the positive associations among all of the indicators of suffering.

Table 17.1 The GASI and its sub-indices

	Economic performance	Democracy, freedom and governance	Child well-being	Environment and infrastructure	Safety and security	Health and health systems	Integrity and justice	Education	Social sustainability and social cohesion	Good African Society Index	Rank
Algeria	110.05	92.22	119.45	108.06	92.01	114.79	98.49	114.65	106.89	106.29	6
Angola	101.92	100.41	90.70	97.17	106.53	90.69	99.79	103.73	97.65	98.73	25
Benin	97.84	102.70	96.09	100.89	106.81	96.18	104.91	93.28	109.90	100.96	15
Botswana	100.69	115.51	114.99	109.98	115.86	100.42	112.79	113.81	107.39	110.16	3
Burkina Faso	100.60	99.31	89.60	95.24	101.17	98.88	103.65	80.25	97.86	96.28	36
Burundi	101.73	99.98	97.90	90.54	88.92	94.18	95.28	98.51	100.74	96.42	35
Cameroon	105.89	96.19	89.75	95.52	95.18	92.19	97.53	101.63	96.90	96.75	34
Cape Verde	104.34	119.32	111.57	119.65	106.75	114.33	108.05	114.68	102.83	111.28	2
Central African Republic	86.59	89.56	92.61	96.16	84.64	92.99	97.21	75.39	92.95	89.79	45
Chad	93.39	87.60	74.25	94.54	93.32	89.50	94.82	81.45	85.65	88.28	46
Comoros	90.31	89.67	98.08	94.05	100.77	104.69	97.07	102.59	106.65	98.21	27
Congo	101.90	91.61	93.52	99.97	96.34	99.65	96.41	99.60	99.88	97.65	30
Cote d'Ivoire	91.84	84.50	90.47	101.81	76.83	97.77	98.96	88.93	85.00	90.68	44
Democratic Republic of Congo	96.59	81.71	89.34	94.96	86.09	91.61	91.85	97.50	90.29	91.10	43
Djibouti	103.93	87.10	100.28	96.62	110.51	99.36	111.64	88.94	98.21	99.62	19
Egypt	104.97	87.72	117.57	119.48	109.18	115.27	110.15	112.76	104.97	109.12	4
Ethiopia	107.57	100.39	99.48	93.01	91.88	101.29	99.54	88.63	98.11	97.77	28
Gabon	114.31	97.49	101.44	103.19	104.56	103.14	105.45	116.33	97.84	104.86	8
Gambia	87.28	90.31	105.83	107.13	111.12	100.20	101.16	94.76	95.63	99.27	22
Ghana	114.64	109.08	107.96	95.79	108.85	102.25	106.94	105.43	101.73	105.85	7

Guinea	100.61	94.13	86.81	99.65	88.93	95.22	89.18	91.67	91.53	93.08	42
Guinea-Bissau	111.43	91.09	93.89	100.93	94.51	90.91	103.03	87.98	97.11	96.76	33
Kenya	93.25	99.11	100.53	99.63	95.97	102.47	92.87	105.87	89.54	97.69	29
Lesotho	98.38	110.83	106.04	101.47	100.29	88.60	108.14	107.60	109.56	103.43	11
Liberia	102.36	96.65	94.35	94.76	103.39	93.69	112.23	104.31	98.28	100.00	17
Madagascar	85.11	98.75	89.25	98.42	102.31	106.57	103.69	100.71	108.91	99.30	21
Malawi	98.58	101.20	104.00	96.18	97.94	97.75	100.58	92.72	96.63	98.40	26
Mali	103.07	106.47	81.47	99.47	102.27	92.13	103.68	84.94	99.05	96.95	32
Mauritania	104.32	100.86	96.64	101.77	98.62	94.52	96.76	94.65	106.66	99.42	20
Morocco	105.75	95.06	121.19	109.86	105.40	111.22	101.32	103.60	104.51	106.43	5
Mozambique	101.34	113.04	95.88	95.60	109.34	95.25	102.75	92.02	101.23	100.72	16
Namibia	91.41	117.64	106.58	96.65	108.61	109.62	102.81	112.18	96.09	104.62	10
Niger	97.37	102.15	79.17	92.26	103.16	97.03	101.39	79.05	99.29	94.54	40
Nigeria	104.39	89.44	84.33	100.31	91.15	93.76	95.05	96.29	87.21	93.55	41
Rwanda	96.78	105.56	112.83	104.46	105.43	96.48	86.08	95.88	94.37	99.76	18
Senegal	97.88	109.92	101.82	100.14	105.98	100.66	107.03	90.13	104.74	102.03	13
Sierra Leone	97.95	97.92	88.62	94.81	104.11	87.95	98.12	87.27	94.58	94.59	39
South Africa	92.14	126.98	106.97	92.89	102.10	97.31	100.70	116.22	107.82	104.79	9
Sudan	112.55	85.05	98.90	102.91	85.10	103.42	94.63	88.54	84.94	95.12	38
Swaziland	91.86	94.68	108.64	106.68	102.74	94.17	103.34	107.51	107.57	101.91	14
Tanzania	96.20	115.17	102.13	96.05	104.91	101.62	100.38	97.77	108.38	102.51	12
Togo	102.45	92.54	101.72	92.53	100.98	99.38	98.80	100.25	103.65	99.14	23
Tunisia	99.11	107.98	122.95	120.32	109.44	114.80	100.71	118.48	112.11	111.77	1
Uganda	97.03	105.08	95.58	94.07	85.37	99.76	98.91	100.20	97.38	97.04	31
Zambia	97.79	103.79	99.35	97.90	98.66	94.97	99.70	98.79	98.39	98.82	24
Zimbabwe	97.51	97.54	107.56	93.44	90.53	97.72	85.12	105.77	86.06	95.69	37

Table 17.2 Correlation coefficients

	GASI	Poverty	Child ill-being	Insecurity	Poor health	Low social cohesion
GASI	1.000					
Poverty	−0.622***	1.000				
Child ill-being	−0.822***	0.597***	1.000			
Insecurity	−0.731***	0.293**	0.545***	1.000		
Poor health	−0.677***	0.632***	0.674***	0.329**	1.000	
Low social cohesion	−0.723***	0.336**	0.493***	0.602***	0.359**	1.000

Note: p <0.01***, p <0.05**

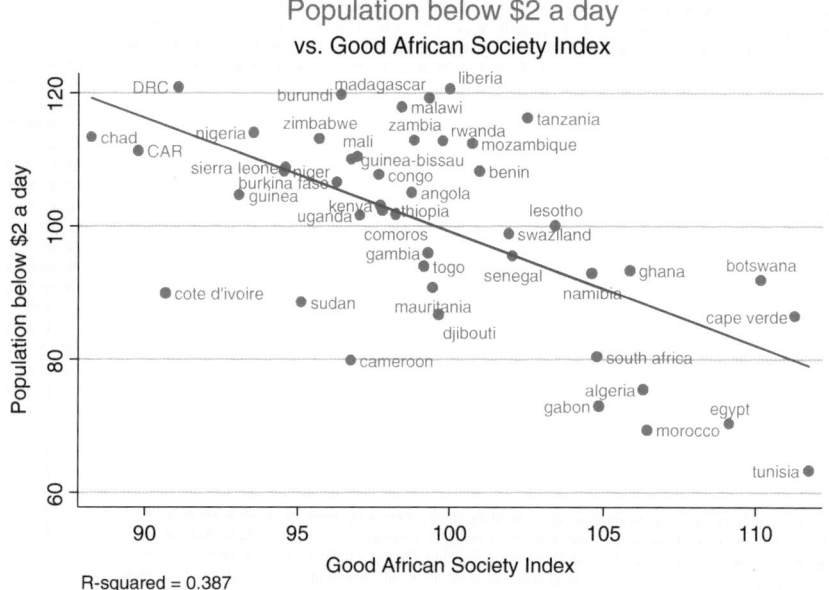

Fig. 17.1 Poverty and the GASI

In plotting poverty prevalence with the GASI in Fig. 17.1, an R^2 of 0.39 suggests that the GASI explains only a moderate proportion of the variation in the population living below $2 a day. Keep in mind that a huge difference exists among African countries in the percent living on less than $2 a day. In the DRC, 95 % live on less than $2 a day; only 8 % of Tunisians do the same.

Nations that meet more GASI criteria on average have fewer people living below the $2 a day poverty line. The scatterplot in Fig. 17.1 reveals some interesting patterns. Despite the DRC and Cote d'Ivoire having roughly similar GASI scores, in the DRC a much higher proportion of people live below $2 a day than in Cote d'Ivoire. A similar case is found, for example, between Cameroon (lower poverty) and Burundi (greater poverty), with a possible explanation being Burundi's higher incidence of long-term civil war, which had negative and long-lasting effects on the poor (Guest 2006). Tanzania scored above-average on the GASI yet has very high poverty. One likely explanation for Tanzania's relatively high poverty can be the "supertax" previously levied on its poorest communities, which were forced to sell grain to the government far below its true value (Guest 2006). This policy further entrenched poverty among the already poor.

Significantly, a clustering of countries occurs around a GASI slightly below the average, all of which mean high percentages of people living below the $2 a day poverty line. While getting high scores on the GASI will to some extent help in reducing the incidence of poverty, it does not guarantee lower poverty nor insulate the poor from suffering.

Shown in Fig. 17.2, the GASI is associated closely with Child Ill-Being ($R^2 = 0.68$). While there are few outliers in this case, partly because of high child mortality rates, Chad by far is the worst in terms of both Child Ill-Being and the GASI. Tunisia, in contrast, has the highest GASI score and also does best in limiting the suffering of its children, for which one likely explanation is a low teen fertility rate relative to other nations. The results for Rwanda show that while this country only ranks average on the GASI, it does very well in enhancing the well-being of its

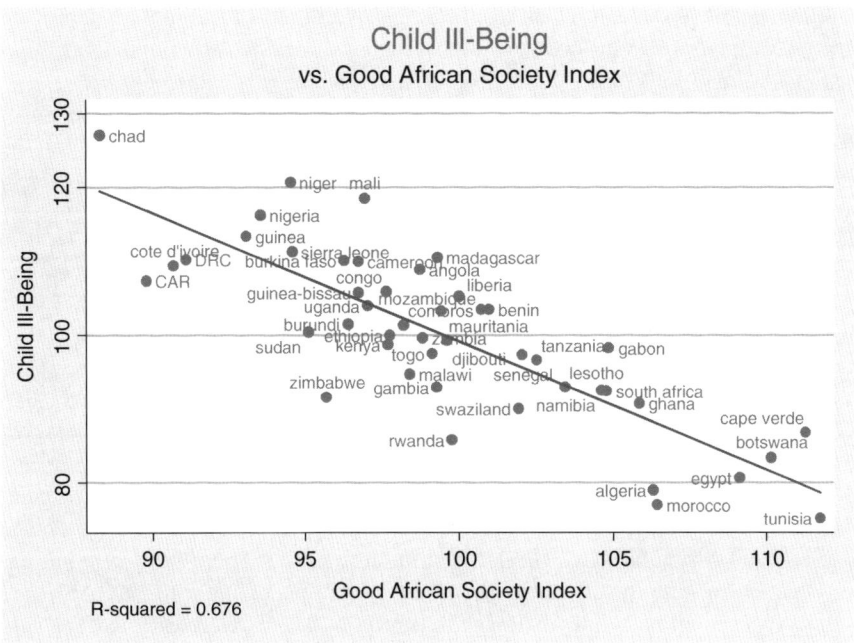

Fig. 17.2 Child ill-being and the GASI

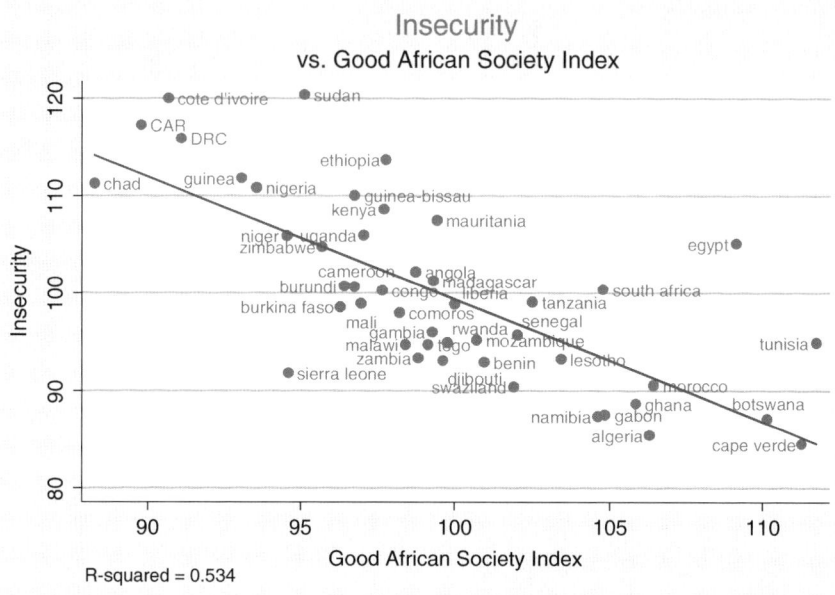

Fig. 17.3 Insecurity and the GASI

children. While Rwanda has had a long history of attending to child well-being, the large-scale genocide in the country in 1994 demonstrated that without paying attention to all dimensions of the Good Society, a nation remains vulnerable.

Regarding Insecurity (Fig. 17.3), nations with high GASI also have lower Insecurity for their citizens, which may explain much of the variation in the Insecurity sub-index. Cote d'Ivoire owes most of its high ranking on Insecurity to an extremely high homicide rate relative to other countries. Levels of suffering are adversely affected by such violence. One notable outlier in the present case is Algeria, scoring below-average on Insecurity despite faring quite well on the GASI. One potential reason for Algeria's high level of violence-based suffering is its long history of serious, internal political and religious conflict (Meredith 2006). High levels of violence and their psychological impact produce severe suffering.

GASI scores are also related to quality of health, as is evident in Fig. 17.4. Chad scores lowest on the GASI and third-lowest in Poor Health, with Sierra Leone scoring highest on the Poor Health sub-index. Although Madagascar is average on the GASI score, it is substantially above average on Health. Lesotho, on the other hand, performs poorly in Health even though the country scores above-average on the GASI. South Africa falls in a similar position to Lesotho. There are two main reasons that scores on the health sub-index are sometimes out of line with the GASI. One is that Africa's public health challenge is enormous because of Neglected Tropical Diseases (NTDs) and highly infectious diseases like *E. coli*. The health systems are uneven in part because both private and governmental intervention programs often focus on specific countries rather than all of Africa. For example, the HIV/AIDS

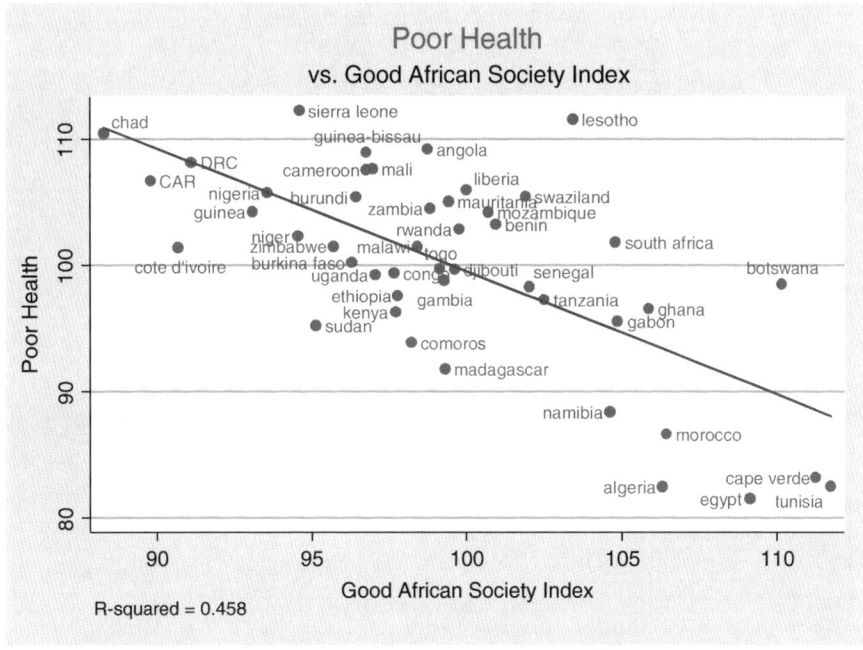

Fig. 17.4 Poor health and the GASI

prevalence rates in South Africa and Botswana are high, despite their relatively strong economic progress. Second, none of the African countries has a sufficiently advanced healthcare system, despite both NGO and governmental aid, to administer the high quality health care needed to cope with epidemics like HIV/AIDS.

The Low Cohesion/Sustainability sub-index, as shown in relation to the GASI in Fig. 17.5, generated numerous outlier countries. Countries prone to civil war or other violent conflict are low in societal cohesion and sustainability. People in these nations are highly prone to extreme social suffering because of the race/ethnicity aspect of much of the conflict in Africa. Namibia and Gabon have relatively good GASI scores, yet both nations score high in Low Cohesion. Guest (2006) notes that Namibia has experienced constant ethnic violence, eroding almost all public and community trust. In contrast to the Child Ill-Being case, Rwanda scores very highly on the Low Cohesion and Social Sustainability component, likely due to the legacy of its 1994 genocide, which continues to cause massive social suffering. Madagascar, an opposite type of outlier to Rwanda, shows outstanding Cohesion and Social Sustainability, but only has an average GASI score. In general, having a high place on the GS scale provides some social protection in that the GASI represents activities intended to benefit the common good of the society as a whole. However, a moderate or moderately high GASI does not insulate a society from attack by either a deadly virus or deadly civil war. Once such an outbreak becomes widespread it may take decades, if not generations, to return to normal civility and practices that minimize pain, mental suffering, and social suffering.

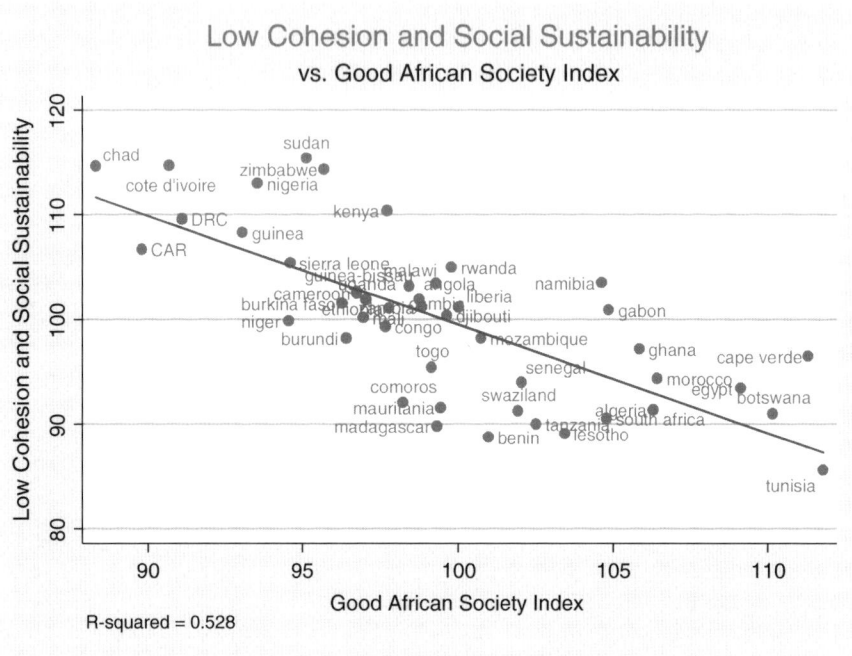

Fig. 17.5 Low cohesion and social sustainability and the GASI

17.5   Conclusion

This study makes the case for African countries to focus on policy consistent with the Good Society concept by either focusing on the common good or reducing suffering. The results suggest that improvements in the GASI ranking are likely to be associated with lower child suffering especially. Social suffering and violence-based suffering may also decline as a country attains a higher GASI score.

On all indicators examined, CAR, Chad, Cote d'Ivoire, and DRC fare worst and have the most devastating social problems (including widespread suffering). These are the so-called "failed states," which are plagued by continued civil war, famine, and internal conflict. The finding that the DRC is among those countries with the worst suffering is consistent with the Anderson (2012b) study finding that this nation has the greatest suffering among those analysed. In addition, while Anderson (2011b, 2012b) reports that most countries with severe suffering are in Africa, this study shows significant variation in the degree of suffering across African countries.

Many countries do consistently poorly on most of the suffering indicators. This suggests that in countries with the greatest suffering, the types of suffering may be diverse, rather than limited to suffering in only one domain. When there is suffering in these countries, people experience a range of sufferings rather than only a few.

The measures used as indicators of suffering are preliminary, indirect measures, and they are certainly not exhaustive. This study provides some idea as to how factors that may cause suffering differ across African nations. One potential policy implication is that while indicators of economic development are potentially important deterrents of suffering, it is generally non-economic factors that are most useful in reducing suffering. African societies that focus on attaining the various GASI components are likely to see improvements in many important areas that may substantially reduce the overall degree of suffering. However, none of the African countries may be sufficiently high on a large number of Good Society indicators to make them resilient to civil wars, health epidemics, or other major disasters.

References

African Development Bank (AfDB). (2013). *Gender, poverty and environmental indicators on African countries* (Vol. XIV). Tunis: African Development Bank.

African Development Bank (AfDB), Organization for Economic Cooperation and Development (OECD), United Nations Development Programme (UNDP), & United Nations Economic Commission for Africa (UNECA). (2011). *African economic outlook 2011*. Paris: OECD.

African Development Bank (AfDB), African Union Commission (AUC), & United Nations Economic Commission for Africa (UNECA). (2013). *African statistical yearbook, 2013*. Tunis: African Development Bank.

Anderson, R. E. (2011a). *Good societies index for the 20 richest societies*. Paper presented at the conference of the International Society for Quality of Life Studies, 23 July 2009, Florence, Italy.

Anderson, R. E. (2011b). *World suffering: Conceptualization, measurement, and findings*. Paper presented at the 2011 annual meetings of the American Association for Public Opinion Research (AAPOR), 13 May 2011, Phoenix, Arizona.

Anderson, R. E. (2012a). *Good societies index 2012: Comparing quality of life in relatively wealthy societies*. Paper presented at the conference of the International Society for Quality of Life Studies, 1–4 November 2012, Venice, Italy.

Anderson, R. E. (2012b). *Human suffering and measures of human progress*. Paper presented at the International Sociological Association Forum, 1–4 August 2012, Buenos Aires, Argentina.

Anderson, R. E. (2014). *Human suffering and quality of life: Conceptualizing stories and statistics* (SpringerBriefs in well-being and quality of life research). Dordrecht: Springer.

Bellah, R. N., Madsen, R., Sullivan, W. M., Swidler, A., & Tipton, S. M. (1991). *The good society*. New York: Knopf.

Botha, F. (2014). *The good African society index*. (ERSA Working Paper No. 441). Cape Town: Economic Research Southern Africa.

Bourdieu, P. (1983). Forms of capital. In J. C. Richards (Ed.), *Handbook of theory and research for the sociology of education*. New York: Greenwood Press.

Central Intelligence Agency (CIA). (2013). *The world factbook*. Available from: https://www.cia.gov/library/publications/the-world-factbook/. Accessed 18 Feb 2013.

Coleman, J. C. (1988). Social capital in the creation of human capital. *American Journal of Sociology, 94*, 95–120.

DeLeon, P., & Longobardi, R. C. (2002). Policy analysis in the good society. *The Good Society, 11*(1), 37–41.

Draper, A., & Ramsay, A. (2011). *The good society: An introduction to comparative politics* (2nd ed.). New York: Pearson.

Economist Intelligence Unit (EIU). (2012). *Democracy index 2012: Democracy at a standstill.* London: Economist Intelligence Unit.

Ehrenberg, J. R. (1999). *Civil society: The critical history of an idea.* New York: New York University Press.

Fund for Peace (FFP). (2013). *Failed states index 2013.* Washington, DC: Fund for Peace.

Guest, R. (2006). *The shackled continent: Africa's past, present and future.* London: Pan Macmillan.

Holmberg, S. (2007). *The good society index* (QoG Working Paper No. 6). Göteborg: Göteborg University.

International Centre for Prison Studies (ICPS). (2011). *World prison population list* (9th ed.). London: ICPS.

Jordan, P. W. (2012). The good society framework: Psychosocial ergonomics and quality of life. In M. Anderson (Ed.), *Contemporary ergonomics 2012.* London: Taylor and Francis.

Lippmann, W. (1937). *The good society.* Boston: Little, Brown.

Meredith, M. (2006). *The state of Africa: A history of fifty years of independence.* London: The Free Press.

Mills, G. (2011). *Why Africa is poor and what Africans can do about it.* Johannesburg: Penguin.

Reporters Without Borders (RWB). (2012). *World press freedom Index, 2012.* Paris: Reporters Without Borders.

Schiller, R. (2013). *Finance and the good society.* Princeton: Princeton University Press.

Transparency International. (2012). *Corruption perceptions index 2012.* Berlin: Transparency International.

Tronto, J. (2007). Human rights, democracy and care. *The Good Society, 16*(2), 38–40.

United Nations Development Programme (UNDP). (2007). *Human development report 2007/2008.* New York: Oxford University Press.

United Nations Development Programme (UNDP). (2011). *Human development report 2011.* New York: Oxford University Press.

United Nations Development Programme (UNDP). (2013). *Human development report 2013.* New York: Oxford University Press.

World Bank. (2013a). *Africa development indicators 2012/13.* Washington, DC: World Bank.

World Bank. (2013b). *World development indicators 2013.* Washington, DC: World Bank.

World Health Organization (WHO). (2013). *WHO global infobase.* Available from: https://apps.who.int/infobase/. Accessed 20 Feb 2013.

World Life Expectancy. (2012). *Road traffic accidents, by country.* Available from: http://www.worldlifeexpectancy.com/cause-of-death/road-traffic-accidents/by-country/. Accessed 12 Dec 2012

Chapter 18
Lifetime Suffering and Capabilities in Chile

Francisca Dussaillant and Pablo A. González

18.1 Introduction

This chapter analyzes the determinants of lifetime suffering in Chile. A key contribution is that, in addition to the standard variables considered in the literature, the chapter explores the relationship between suffering and individual capabilities. As the audience of this book might not be familiar with the capability approach, it is worthwhile to start with a brief summary of its basic concepts before explaining how this chapter attempts to bridge a gap between this approach and human suffering.

Amartya Sen and Martha Nussbaum pioneered the capabilities approach that draws attention to what human beings can do and be, instead of looking at the resources they have or their subjective wellbeing. Sen and Nussbaum defined functionings as "beings and doings that people value and have reason to value" (Alkire 2008: 5) and capabilities as "the various combinations of functionings (beings and doings) that the person can achieve. Capability is, thus, a set of vectors [or n-tuples] of functionings, reflecting the person's freedom to lead one type of life or another… to choose from possible livings" (Sen 1992: 40).

Most traditional statistical indicators measure functionings (e.g. number of years of education or level of education attained, body-mass, etc.). However, both functionings and capabilities are necessary to assess a person's wellbeing. For instance, the functioning "being hungry" might be experienced by a person who is well off in

F. Dussaillant (✉)
School of Government, Universidad del Desarrollo, Avenida Plaza 700, Las Condes, Santiago, Chile
e-mail: mfdussaillant@udd.cl

P.A. González
Department of Industrial Engineering, Faculty of Physical and Mathematical Sciences, Universidad de Chile, República 701, Santiago, Chile
e-mail: pgonzale@dii.uchile.cl

© Springer Science+Business Media Dordrecht 2015   233
R.E. Anderson (ed.), *World Suffering and Quality of Life*,
Social Indicators Research Series 56, DOI 10.1007/978-94-017-9670-5_18

terms of wellbeing if this functioning is a consequence of fasting for religious or other personal reasons or by a person who has a very low wellbeing when a person lacks access to food. What differs between the two persons is the capability set, not the observed functioning.

However, there are only a few attempts to measure capabilities (Anand and van Hees 2006; Robeyns 2005; Alkire 2008). Moreover, standard surveys only record what might be called *"traditional" functionings*. These are the variables typically considered relevant by public policies and that can be measured with some objectivity, such as health, nutrition, housing and education. In our case, we also have non-traditional dimensions (both as capabilities and functionings) such as respect and human security. More importantly, the survey included a direct measure of lifetime suffering as well as most independent variables usually included in subjective wellbeing studies. In this sense, the survey we conducted with UNDP Chile in 2011 for its 2012 Human Development Report is unique due its design, scope and sample size.

Using these measures, in this chapter we analyze which capabilities are more associated with lifetime suffering. Our key research question is therefore: from the list of capabilities selected by Chileans for a good life, which ones are related to lifetime suffering? To check the robustness of this association, we control for different variables usually related to subjective wellbeing in the empirical literature. The question is relevant both to achieve a deeper understanding of the relationship of suffering and capabilities as well as to get a first approximation to the policy question of which capabilities should be strengthened to reduce suffering in Chile.

The article is organized as follows. The relationship between the capability approach and suffering is briefly discussed from a theoretical point of view in Sect. 18.2. Section 18.3 discusses the less-than-perfect association of positive and negative measures of wellbeing in the literature. Our capability indicators are introduced in Sect. 18.4. Our measure of lifetime suffering is introduced and compared with life satisfaction in Sect. 18.5. Section 18.6 presents the empirical association between suffering and capabilities and summarizes our main findings. Section 18.7 concludes.

18.2 Suffering from a Capabilities Perspective

Subjective wellbeing and capabilities have been proposed as different approaches to development that concentrate on what happens to people's lives, questioning the dominant focus on economic growth (Alkire 2002; Comim 2005; Frey and Stutzer 2010). However, both approaches have for the most part drifted along diverging paths except for a few exceptions, such as Comin (2005), UNDP (2012) and Binder (2014). These authors build bridges for a reconciliation of both approaches suggesting a focus on *capabilities to produce subjective wellbeing*. In particular, in UNDP (2012) we suggested that governments must act building capabilities to advance valued human objectives such as subjective wellbeing. Acting directly on subjective wellbeing is not morally legitimate, as illustrated by Nozik's happiness machine or Huxley's soma.

It is less clear that this moral objection against acting directly on happiness carries over to suffering. Even soma might be more acceptable for relieving pain rather than boosting happiness, as the discussion regarding the medical use of marihuana illustrates. Moreover, it can be argued that concern for suffering is an implicit concept in champions of capability theory, especially suffering produced by lack of access to rights and freedoms (see for instance, Nussbaum 2001; Sen 2009). The concept of moral obligation of power in Sen's work (which can be traced back to the concept of compromise in Sen 1977) is particularly attractive to reflect on the place of suffering in capability theory. It is tempting to argue that what is at the basis of this moral obligation is the possibility to avoid or lessen human suffering.

If the later is true, then suffering deserves much more attention from capability theorists than it has received so far. In particular, capability theory has been silent, to our knowledge, on the question of evil, so clearly stated by Hutcheson (2002): "Evil is proportionate to the number of people made to suffer." This argument would imply that suffering could not be treated only as another functioning as Sen himself has suggested for happiness (Sen 1992: 39).

Nonetheless, it would be true that suffering, as happiness or other measures of subjective wellbeing are outcomes, is the combined realization of capabilities, decisions and social events that lead human beings on a particular path and not on others that were also possible. However, if our interpretation is correct, then it is a functioning that deserves particular attention as the key source of moral obligation and therefore of concern for justice.

Hence, from the perspective of justice within the capability framework, the distribution of suffering should be of interest on its own, much more than the distribution of happiness. In addition, a key question of interest is what capabilities are more related with suffering, as these would be the capabilities that might be targeted when the purpose is to reduce suffering. This is our key research question and is also a question of interest to the wider audience of this book, more concerned with the determinants and distribution of suffering, as it adds a new set of variables to care about.

A priori, one would expect that an expansion of the capability set might reduce suffering, but this effect would be higher for certain capabilities and functionings than others. For instance, an improvement in the access to health care is likely to reduce suffering. Similarly, an increase in the chance of finding a partner might make life more enjoyable and relieve the suffering of loneliness and boredom. Other capabilities might not be related to suffering. For instance, the effect of education opportunities on wellbeing seems to occur mostly through income and health. This might be also true for the case of suffering.

18.3 Subjective Wellbeing and Suffering

Table 18.1 presents a list of the different measures of subjective wellbeing available in international surveys. In the second column, the ranking of Chile based on the average value of each indicator is reported (strictly speaking, it is misleading to

Table 18.1 International
indicators of subjective
wellbeing

Indicator	Rank of Chile/ No. of countries
Life satisfaction[a]	36/99
Life satisfaction[b]	55/129
General happiness[a]	69/100
Happiness yesterday[c]	52/148
Positive emotions (affect)[d]	41/156
Negative emotions[d]	134/156
Affect balance[d]	73/156
Best possible life[d]	43/156

Source: First World Happiness Report (2012)
[a]World Values Survey and European Values Study (1999–2008)
[b]World Gallup Survey (2007–2010)
[c]World Gallup Survey (2008–2011)
[d]World Gallup Survey (2005–2011): countries were ordered from low to high frequency of negative emotions. Therefore, being in the first places of the ranking implies a better outcome (and vice versa) for all indicators reported in the Table

speak of a "ranking of countries" because sample sizes were small), as well as the number of countries included in the survey. As judged by these international survey measures, Chile is a country with above average life satisfaction, happiness, and positive affect while at the same time a high frequency of negative affect, i.e., Chileans report to be angry, stressed, worried, bored, and sad with a higher frequency than inhabitants of most other countries covered in the survey.

Most scholars use in their analyses measures of life satisfaction or happiness while neglecting the negative side of the equation. This may be founded, at least somehow, on the influence of utilitarianism, which through neoclassical economics extended well beyond the realms of political philosophy. Its recognized father, Jeremiah Bentham (1789), suggested that the objective of good government should be to maximize aggregate happiness or the happiness of the greatest number, and most utilitarian scholars follow his lead, in general replacing the word happiness by the concept of utility. For Bentham, both individual and societal objectives are to maximize the difference between pleasure and pain, what is called hedonic calculus. Mainstream modern economics still sticks to this assumption, both as the sole driver of human behavior and as the measure for efficiency of allocation and use of scarce resources.

Popper (1956) suggested that from the moral point of view, pain could not be offset by pleasure, and "especially not one person's pain by another person's pleasure. Instead of asking for the greatest happiness for the greatest number, one should demand, more modestly, the least amount of avoidable suffering for all; and further, that unavoidable suffering – such as hunger in times of food shortage – should be distributed as equally as possible" (Kadlec 2007). Furthermore, there is a moral appeal in human suffering: the appeal for help. There is no similar moral appeal to increase happiness when the person is doing fine anyway. Anderson (2014) also made a compelling argument in favor of putting the reduction of suffering as the center of humanitarian action.

A key problem to operationalize this approach is the lack of indicators. For instance, some scholars have dealt with the lack of available measures of suffering by simply working with the lower end of standard subjective wellbeing indicators, which might be considered a measure of dissatisfaction rather than suffering. Leikes (2013), for instance, considers dissatisfied those responding between 0 and 3 in the life satisfaction scale.

However, negative aspects of human subjectivity are not just the opposite of positive states, as Bentham's hedonic calculus – questioned by Popper – seems to suggest. Even when analyzing affect balance, it is clear that the frequency of negative moods or emotions is not just the reverse of positive ones. The case of Chile in Table 18.1 illustrates this: while it ranks in the first third of positive emotions it is at the same time classified in the worst 20 % of negative emotions (i.e. has a high frequency of both positive and negative emotions, for international standards). In Sect. 18.6 we will see that our data confirms the less-than-perfect correlation between positive emotions and lifetime suffering in Chile.

18.4 Capabilities to Reduce Suffering: Data

In UNDP (2012) a list of basic capabilities was elaborated on the basis of the proposals of various authors (Alkire 2002; Nussbaum 2001) and various focus groups. This list was discussed with different socioeconomic and demographic groups. The result, a list of capabilities considered valuable for "having a good life" by Chileans, was measured with different indicators. The final UNDP (2012) list includes: being healthy (hereafter health); fulfilling basic physical and material needs (basic needs); self-knowledge and inner life (self-knowledge); feeling secure and free from threats (human security); participation and influence in society (participation); experiencing pleasure and emotions (pleasure); enjoying relationships and social bonds with others (social bonds); being recognized and respected in dignity and rights (respect); comprehension of the world we live in (education); enjoying and being part of nature (nature); and being able to develop a life project (project). It is possible that the deliberation exercise might have produced a slightly different list had the question been posed referred to suffering, but we still believe this is a complete list of capabilities because it is consistent with most lists proposed in the literature, and it is also one of the most complete lists ever measured.

Although capabilities have a social component, measurement requires assessing each individual's perception, experience, or appropriation. All these capabilities were measured in a survey along two dimensions: entitlement and evaluation. Our entitlement indexes summarize information obtained from questions like "If you wanted/needed more... how hard it would be to...?" or "Do you have the alternative of...?" On the other hand, our evaluation indexes summarize the individual's subjective assessment of their capability endowment, with questions such as, "Do you feel that it is enough/adequate to your needs or expectations?" or "Do you have all what you need?"

Information relative to the "functionings" for each capability, which go over the actual realization or attainment in each dimension, was also gathered. In this sense, entitlements and evaluations are proxies of the opportunity sets of individuals, while functionings measure the realization, which depends on the opportunity set, actual decisions (partly dependent on preferences), and social circumstances (including luck).

The relationship between suffering, on the one hand, and capability and functioning indicators on the other, is the subject of Sect. 18.6. The theory would predict that smaller and restricted opportunity sets would lead to constrained choices that will in many cases lie far away from the optimal unconstrained choices the individuals would have made if they had the chance and opportunity. It is possible that this distance from the unconstrained optimum should be associated with levels of suffering. In addition, as suggested in the last Section, there might be some capabilities that are more related to suffering than others are, and there might be some that are not even related at all. It is also possible that our sample size is too small for discovering the true relationship, especially if the effect is small.

18.5   Lifetime Suffering Index and Positive Affect in Chile

We use a direct scale of self-reported lifetime suffering similar to the life satisfaction scale. The survey asks, "Taking into account that all persons sometimes in their lives must face pain and suffering, could you tell me how much suffering you have experienced in your life?" The respondent answered using a 10 point scale where 1 means "no suffering" and 10 "a lot of suffering." Mean lifetime suffering in our data is 6.23, and standard deviation 2.51.

We can examine how the lifetime suffering index correlates with positive measures by studying its relation to two alternative measures of positive affect. These arise from the answers to the questions: a. (Have a good life) "Overall, how satisfied are you with your life as a whole these days?" (1 to 10 scale where 1 means "completely unsatisfied" and 10 means "completely satisfied"); and b. (Satisfied these days) "In a 0 to 10 scale, where 0 means the worst possible life and 10 the best possible life, where would you locate yourself?"

The correlation between our two measures of positive affect is positive and high (0.63), meaning that people who are "satisfied these days" tend to report to "have had a good life" and vice versa. On the other hand, correlations of lifetime suffering with each of our positive affect measures have the expected negative sign (the more satisfied tend to report, on average, less suffering), but they are low (coincidentally, the correlation is −0.20 in both cases).

Table 18.2 Bivariate distributions of wellbeing and suffering indexes[a]

		(a) "Have a good life" index					(b) Lifetime suffering index				
		1–2	3–4	5–6	7–8	9–10	1–2	3–4	5–6	7–8	9–10
"Satisfied these days" index	1–2	0.95	0.56	0.91	0.2	0.28	0.28	0.12	0.44	0.6	1.47
	3–4	0.99	2.42	2.1	0.6	0.24	0.16	0.68	1.03	1.67	2.82
	5–6	0.64	1.87	14.81	5.68	1.03	1.19	3.34	8.07	5.68	5.6
	7–8	0.4	0.95	8.66	20.41	4.73	2.46	6.04	11.08	9.77	5.8
	9–10	0.04	0.48	3.65	9.81	17.59	4.25	5.8	8.78	7.19	5.68

[a]Each cell displays percentage of population that reports the combined index values. Percentages in Table 18.2a add to 100; percentages in Table 18.2b add to 100

Table 18.2a, b show the bivariate distribution of combinations of the three variables mentioned above. Each cell in Table 18.2a represents the percentage of the population that ascribes to a certain combination of levels in the "Have a good life" index and the "Satisfied these days" index. Similarly, cells in Table 18.2b represent proportions of the sample ascribing to each combination of levels in the "Satisfied these days" and lifetime suffering indexes. For the sake of space, we collapse index categories into five (remember that each of the indexes has ten distinct values).

We observe the high correlation between our positive affect measures in Table 18.2a. In this case, 56.2 % of the occurrences lie on the dark grey diagonal line, and almost all 90.6 % lie on the diagonal or its immediate neighbors (dark and light gray cells). In other words, each respondent reporting a high/low value in one measure also displays a high/low value on the other, with few exceptions.

On the other hand, in Table 18.2b there is less correspondence between indexes. Gray categories represent cases where reported lifetime suffering is, as one would expect, inversely related to reports of having had a "good life." This time, only 54.3 % fall in any of the gray categories. Actually, we see a large concentration of cases in the lower right corner of Table 18.2b. One possible source of this is that respondents really recall a very hard lifetime with a lot of suffering, even though at the moment "these days" they are satisfied. Nevertheless, the bivariate distribution of "Have a good life" (which does not have the temporary component of the "satisfied these days" index) and lifetime suffering is qualitatively similar to Table 18.2b, with only 58.8 % of the responses lying in the would-be gray cells. This low correlation is not new in the literature. For example, Helliwell et al. (2012) show that Chile ranks relatively high in the positive affect scale, and at the same time it ranks high in the negative affect scale (see Table 18.1 in this chapter). Chile is not the only country displaying these counterintuitive results: Our neighbors Peru and Bolivia, among others, seem to be quite similar.

This may be read as confirmation of Popper's argument quoted in Sect. 18.3 so that pain couldn't be offset by pleasure. Although Popper's argument is moral and applies especially to the aggregation of different people ("especially not one person's pain by another person's pleasure"), it seems verified on empirical grounds for the case of Chile even at the individual level, in the sense that suffering is not simply the reverse of positive affect.

It also stands out from Table 18.2b that both having had a good life and lifetime suffering are represented by remarkably skewed distributions. Very few respondents (9.3 %) rated themselves with less than a 5 in the "Have a good life" scale, and only 24,3 % report as having minimal suffering (scores 1–4) in their lifetimes. Thus the estimations of effects on suffering that we present in the following sections are discriminating between those who have had a huge amount of suffering and those who have had a moderate amount of suffering.

18.6 Suffering and Capabilities: An Empirical Inquiry

In the analyses that follow we seek to get a deeper understanding of the associations among suffering, capabilities and *functionings*. As explained previously, UNDP (2012) characterized capabilities with indexes of *entitlement* and indexes of *evaluation*. It also included measures of corresponding functionings. Entitlements and evaluations intend to describe the opportunity or choice set the individual faces, regarding a certain scope of her life (education, health, basic needs among other). Functionings refer to the actual attainments or realizations of the individual (educational level, health service usage, income) given opportunity constraints.

We estimate standard regression analyses to look, among other things, for an association between size of the opportunity sets, represented by the evaluations, and lifetime suffering levels. This is of great interest because there is scarcely any research that considers this type of index in the prediction of either wellbeing or suffering. We also report results on the much widely studied association of what we call *functionings* (achieved levels of a certain dimension) on lifetime suffering. We next describe the variables used in the empirical analyses.

18.6.1 Description of Variables

The dependent variable we used in the empirical analysis of the following sections is the 10 point scale index of lifetime suffering described in detail in Sect. 18.5. The independent variables can be grouped in two main categories: basic controls and variables associated with capabilities. Both are described next.

18.6.1.1 Basic Controls

Our data set is rich, so we were able to control for several basic characteristics of individuals that might be good predictors of lifetime suffering. In our model, we control by sex, age (and its square), indexes associated with personality traits (extraversion, emotional stability, neuroticism, conscientiousness and openness) and measures of recent positive and negative exogenous events in the past 6 months. We also include a variable associated to religion and/or spirituality.

Our indexes of extraversion, emotional stability, neuroticism, conscientiousness and openness were drawn from a 10-question personality inventory included in the survey. Nine of the questions are very similar to the TIPI (Ten Item Personality Inventory) proposed by Gosling et al. (2003), but with different scales. The scales range from −1 to 1 and take five possible and equidistant values each. More on the inventory used can be found in UNDP (2012).

Positive events include whether the interviewee got married, was part of a couple or fell in love, whether there was a planned pregnancy of self or partner, birth of a child, a wage increase or work promotion, a housing acquisition, or any other positive event. Negative events in the last 6 months include deaths, severe illness (own or a relative), breakup of relationship or divorce, severe family problem or breakup within the family, job loss (own or someone in the household), unplanned pregnancy (self or partner) or any other negative event. The number of positive events, by construction, has a minimum of 0 and a maximum of 5. The number of negative events has a minimum of 0 and a maximum of 8.

The variable "spirituality" is a categorical variable that indicates frequency of prayer or meditation. In the sample we analyzed, 52.8 % report praying or meditating frequently, 34.5 % say they do sometimes and 12.7 % never.

18.6.1.2 Variables Thought to Be Associated With Capabilities

Although in UNDP (2012) we characterized eleven different capabilities (see Sect. 18.4 above), after many trials we realized that six of them were redundant or definitely not relevant in the prediction of lifetime suffering. Thus, these were excluded from our final analysis: "self-knowledge," "nature," "participation," "project," and "human security." The capability "basic needs" was simplified from its original specification since the questions related to housing were redundant to income. The capability "understanding the world we live in," mostly related to educational levels, was also found redundant to income and therefore also excluded. *Entitlement indexes* were also less related to lifetime suffering than their *evaluation* or *functioning* counterparts; therefore entitlements were omitted from the analysis.

The capabilities we maintained were Health, Income, Pleasure, Social Bonds and Respect. In our empirical analysis, each of them is represented by an *evaluation index* that represents the individual's subjective assessment of her capability endowment, summarizing answers to questions like "Do you feel that it is enough/adequate to your needs or expectations?" or "Do you have all that you need?" Evaluations are constructed as continuous indexes with 0 as a minimum and 1 as a maximum value, where higher levels of the index represent the more desirable outcomes. Details on index construction can be found in UNDP (2012). The characterization also includes variables related to *functionings*, or the actual realization or attainment for each dimension.

18.6.1.2.1   Functionings

A description of each of the functionings included in our analyses follows.

In Health, the functioning variable is a binary indicator of the presence of an ill-ness or health problem of the respondent in the last year. About 23 % of the popula-tion reports a health issue in the past 12 months.

In Income, the functioning is a categorical variable containing seven income slots. Respondents were asked to classify their household monthly income in one of the categories. The slots were designed to be representative of Chilean income lev-els. Each of the five lower slots comprise between 14 and 22 % of the sample. The higher income slots are smaller in size and comprise about 8 % for the second high-est and 5 % for the highest.

In Social Bonds, we include three functionings, each of them a binary variable indicating whether the respondent is a parent (80.7 %), has a partner (66.9 %) or is a widower (8.3 %). We decided to include widowhood when we realized that, unlike other civil statuses, being a widow did relate to increased lifetime suffering even after taking into account the existence of a living partner.

In Pleasure, we include two indexes of pleasurable activities, each taking values from 0 to 1. The *monthly index* gathers information as to whether, in the past month, the respondent read a book, listened to music, took a nap, danced, practiced a hobby or played sports. The *yearly index* gathers information of whether, in the last year, the respondent went out to the cinema or theater, to concerts or to the stadium. In both cases a value of 0 means that the respondent did not perform any of the activi-ties (4.3 % in the monthly index, 57.8 % in the yearly index), and a value of 1 means that all the activities mentioned in the list were carried out (6.7 % in the monthly index, 6.0 % in the yearly index). Values in between reflect that respondents carried out only some of the activities.

In Respect, we include two categorical variables as functionings. One represents the respondent's report of the frequency with which she experienced situations of maltreatment (never: 64.6 %; very small/small frequency: 29.2 %; some/high fre-quency: 6.2 %). The other represents the respondent's report of the frequency with which she experienced situations of discrimination (never: 61.3 %: very small/small frequency: 31.7 %: some/high frequency: 7.0 %). When considering these variables as functionings we are assuming that they are objective measures of maltreatment or discrimination. It can be argued that these are subjective measures, since the respondent is not given a definition of maltreatment or discrimination, and the meaning of high/low frequency is also subject to interpretation. We are, neverthe-less, comfortable with this assumption. Note that the question requests the report of maltreatment or discrimination *situations* (not feelings), facilitating a more objec-tive answer. Also note that the percentage of people reporting these events is rela-tively low, especially for those reporting some or high frequency, which, as we will see later, is the category that correlates significantly with lifetime suffering. We think these low percentages are reflecting a correct and more objective reading (from the respondent) of what a maltreatment or discrimination event is. On the other hand, since we have no means to prove our previous statements, the interpreta-tion of the coefficients associated to this variable should be cautious.

18.6.1.2.2   Evaluations

As explained in Sect. 18.4, evaluation indexes summarize the individual's subjective assessment of her capability endowment, with questions such as "Do you feel
that it is enough/adequate to your needs or expectations?" or "Do you have all that
you need?" As just stated, in the present analysis the five categories of capabilities
we included are Health, Income, Pleasure, Social Bonds and Respect. Each category is represented with one evaluation index. These indexes are all on a continuous
scale, with a minimum of 0 and a maximum of 1, where 0 is the most undesirable
outcome and 1 the most desirable.

The Health evaluation index arises from a survey item that asks the respondent
how she perceives her health overall on a five-point scale from very good to very
bad. The respondents with value 0 (very bad) amount to 1.6 % of the sample; those
with value 1 (very good) amount to 10.9 % of the sample.

The Income evaluation index is built using a question about sufficiency of total
family income. Answers come in a four-point scale (not sufficient, experiences
great difficulties to cover basic needs: 7 %; not sufficient, experiences difficulties to
cover basic needs: 27 %; just adequate: 51 %; more than enough, can save 15 %).

The Social Bonds evaluation index is constructed using two questions that ask
about agreement (in a four-point scale from "strongly agree" to "strongly disagree")
with the sentences "I think I am a loved and valued person" and "I frequently feel
lonely." A value of zero in the overall Social Bonds evaluation index means that the
person strongly disagrees with the first and strongly agrees with the second (0.5 %)
sentence. A value of 1 in the index means that she strongly agrees with the first
sentence and strongly disagrees with the second (10.8 %). Values in between correspond to intermediate combinations, with both questions having equal weights.

The Pleasure evaluation index relates to the subjective perception of the respondent about whether she carried out in sufficient amount the activities she reports
enjoying the most (as much as you like, almost as much as you like, less than you
would like, much less than you would like). Of the sample, 9 % report carrying out
pleasurable activities as much as they like, therefore obtaining a value of 1 in the
index; 19 % report carrying them out much less than they would like, obtaining a
0 in the index.

The Respect evaluation index relates to how fully the respondent perceives dignity and rights of persons like her are respected in society. In this sample, 5 % get a
1 in this variable, 15 % get a 0, and the rest obtain values in between.

18.6.2   Estimation and Results

We estimate four standard regression models with lifetime suffering as the dependent variable. The results are provided in Table 18.3. The original database had
2,526 cases, but some cases were lost in the analysis due to missing values. In the
worst case (or column 4 in Table 18.3), we are able to keep 78 % of the original
sample.

Table 18.3 Linear regression analysis. Dependent variable: lifetime suffering

	Model 1: Base model†	Model 2: Base plus functionings†	Model 3: Base plus evaluations†	Model 4: All†
Female	0.402***	0.228	0.335**	0.229
	(0.105)	(0.117)	(0.105)	(0.118)
Age	0.068***	0.059**	0.046**	0.049**
	(0.015)	(0.018)	(0.015)	(0.019)
Age squared	−0.000**	−0.000*	−0.000	−0.000*
	(0.000)	(0.000)	(0.000)	(0.000)
Positive events in last 6 months (number)	0.004	0.020	0.074	0.048
	(0.073)	(0.078)	(0.072)	(0.078)
Negative events in the last 6 months (number)	0.307***	0.197***	0.225***	0.166***
	(0.040)	(0.044)	(0.040)	(0.044)
Personality (Big Five)				
Extraversion	−0.254***	−0.174*	−0.118	−0.119
	(0.073)	(0.080)	(0.074)	(0.081)
Openness	−0.196*	−0.104	−0.131	−0.111
	(0.083)	(0.090)	(0.083)	(0.090)
Neuroticism	0.429***	0.343***	0.226**	0.270**
	(0.084)	(0.089)	(0.085)	(0.092)
Agreeableness	0.098	0.083	0.025	0.055
	(0.059)	(0.064)	(0.059)	(0.064)
Conscientiousness	0.066	0.218	0.164	0.219
	(0.133)	(0.146)	(0.134)	(0.147)
Spirituality				
Sometimes prays or meditates[a]	−0.011	0.021	−0.097	−0.030
	(0.109)	(0.117)	(0.109)	(0.119)
Never prays or meditates[a]	−0.365*	−0.351*	−0.419**	−0.382*
	(0.159)	(0.172)	(0.159)	(0.174)
Health				
Subjective evaluation index			−1.355***	−0.906**
			(0.255)	(0.288)
Health problem in last 12 months		0.318*		0.206
		(0.125)		(0.130)
Income				
Subjective evaluation index			−0.875***	−0.180
			(0.262)	(0.311)
Household monthly income[b]: U$301 to U$440		−0.265		−0.215
		(0.175)		(0.178)
U$440 to U$600		−0.537**		−0.432*
		(0.189)		(0.194)
U$600 to U$920		−0.762***		−0.670***
		(0.183)		(0.191)
U$921 to U$1,460		−0.989***		−0.885***
		(0.202)		(0.211)

(continued)

Table 18.3 (continued)

	Model 1: Base model†	Model 2: Base plus functionings†	Model 3: Base plus evaluations†	Model 4: All†
U$1,461 to U$3,000		−1.193***		−1.025***
		(0.239)		(0.252)
More than U$3,000		−1.263***		−1.060***
		(0.276)		(0.291)
Pleasure				
Subjective evaluation index			−0.381*	−0.374*
			(0.169)	(0.185)
Index of monthly pleasurable activities		0.016		0.199
		(0.233)		(0.237)
Index of yearly pleasurable activities		0.001		0.098
		(0.201)		(0.203)
Social Bonds				
Subjective evaluation index			−1.468***	−0.660*
			(0.271)	(0.306)
Has a partner		−0.327*		−0.359**
		(0.127)		(0.128)
Is a widower		0.557*		0.464*
		(0.227)		(0.229)
Is a parent		0.348*		0.368*
		(0.166)		(0.167)
Respect				
Subjective evaluation index			−0.238	−0.156
			(0.184)	(0.202)
Experience situations of abuse: very small/small frequency[c]		0.097		0.032
		(0.122)		(0.123)
Experience situations of abuse: some/high frequency[c]		0.822***		0.727**
		(0.230)		(0.233)
Experience situations of discrimination: very small/small freq[c]		0.214		0.161
		(0.119)		(0.120)
Experience situations of discrimination: some/high frequency[c]		0.932***		0.792***
		(0.215)		(0.219)
Constant	3.794***	4.502***	7.160***	6.106***
	(0.378)	(0.474)	(0.493)	(0.589)
R-squared	0.096	0.153	0.134	0.164
N	2,522	2,022	2,453	1,979

†Unstandardized coefficients, standard errors between parentheses. *$p<0.05$; **$p<0.01$; ***$p<0.001$
[a]Reference category: frequently prays or meditates
[b]Reference category: less than U$300
[c]Reference category: no experience of abuse/no experience of discrimination

Our base specification (model 1) includes the control variables described in Sect. 18.6.1.1. These are variables that (with the exception of spirituality) are exogenous and not modifiable. Although their coefficients are helpful to the characterization of lifetime suffering, what we mostly want to know is how suffering is determined *with these as a given*. Therefore, our second specification (model 2) includes the variables from the previous model adding the functionings that we characterized in Sect. 18.6.1.2.1. The third specification (model 3) also includes the controls and adds the evaluation indexes depicted in Sect. 18.6.1.2.2. We end with model 4, that includes basic traits, functionings, and evaluation indexes altogether.

Results from the estimation must be read carefully: A significant coefficient does not necessarily imply causation. In addition, we are estimating a model with a large number of independent variables so there are potential problems of multi-collinearity. Therefore, ours must be understood as an initial effort to analyze the rich data that is available. Several specification refinements can be tried in subsequent research, in order to answer the specific questions that arise from this general overview.

The parameters in the different models seem relatively stable (with few exceptions). Results from the complete model (model 4 in Table 18.3) show that some capabilities predict suffering mainly through their subjective evaluations (Pleasure and Health) while others are predictive through their functionings (Respect and Income). The capability related to Social Bonds is significant both through its evaluation index and through its functionings. Its subjective evaluation is especially significant when the corresponding functionings (being a parent, having a partner, being a widower) are excluded. We will later analyze results capability by capability.

The number of negative events in the past 6 months is a very significant predictor of increased suffering, while positive events do not seem to decrease its level. Older individuals evaluate their life's suffering higher. These results are consistent through the four models. Personality traits do not seem to predict significantly the lifetime suffering levels with the exception of *neuroticism*, which is significantly related to suffering throughout models. People with more neurotic traits seem to suffer more. Extraversion has a loosely significant effect (the more extroverted suffer less) only in the base model, and the model that excludes evaluations (models 1 and 2, in Table 18.3). Significance disappears in the complete specification. Gender shows a loose relation to lifetime suffering in two of the models but sign praying or meditating (lower spirituality) seem to suffer less. This outcome may be the result of reverse causality, meaning that people that suffer less have a lower urge recur to spiritual practices. Nonetheless, the significance of the coefficient is loose ($p < 0.05$ in three of the models, $p < 0.01$ in model 3). Given the size of the sample it might be premature to draw definitive conclusions regarding this result.

Next, we will discuss the estimation's results capability by capability,

18.6.2.1 Health

In the health dimension, the subjective evaluation of health is more predictive of lifetime suffering than the report of a health problem in the past 12 months (functioning). Estimations from the complete model (model 4, Table 18.3) show that people who consider themselves very healthy (with the highest value in the health evaluation index) place themselves 0.906 points lower in the 1–10 suffering scale than those who evaluate their health as very bad. On the other hand, having had a health problem in the past 12 months has some significance only in the model where the evaluation indexes are absent and the coefficient amounts to less than a third of a point in the 1–10 lifetime suffering scale.

18.6.2.2   Income

The income dimension exhibits a behavior that is opposite to that observed with the health capability. In this case, the functioning (i.e. household monthly income) is a better predictor of suffering than the subjective evaluation index (that relates to survey items asking about sufficiency of reported income). Subjective evaluation of income is significant only in the model specification where actual income is absent (model 3, Table 18.3). When income is included, its significance vanishes. Coefficients show that increased income is related to decreased lifetime suffering by an amount that is quite stable when moving from one income step to the neighboring one (about 0.25 suffering points per step). Nevertheless, additional tests showed that coefficients for adjacent income categories do not significantly differ from one another probably due to the restricted sample size. On the other hand, differences between any two coefficients on income categories that are not adjacent are always significant.

18.6.2.3   Pleasure

Neither of the functionings associated with this capacity appear related to lifetime suffering in any model specification. However, the evaluation does relate to lifetime suffering in a slightly significant way ($p < 0.05$). Those who report carrying out pleasurable activities as much as they would like score between 0.37 and 0.4 less suffering points than those who report carrying out these activities with a frequency that is much lower than preferred.

18.6.2.4   Social Bonds

This capability is important in the prediction of lifetime suffering, both through the subjective evaluation index and the functioning. Our results indicate that she who feels loneliest and least loved (as indicated by the evaluation index), suffers more. Regarding the functionings, we observe that having a partner is inversely related to suffering, and that being a parent or being a widow is predictive of increased lifetime suffering. Overall, from the complete model (model 4 in Table 18.3) we extract that a person who feels very lonely (and not loved or valued), does not have a partner, is a widower and a parent scores 1.85 more points in the suffering scale than another who never feels lonely (and feels loved and valued), has a partner, and is neither a widower nor a parent. This amounts to three quarters of a standard deviation of lifetime suffering.

18.6.2.5 Respect

This capability is one in which the subjective evaluation index does not show significant relation to lifetime suffering. Nevertheless, the functionings that we associate to it throw very significant coefficients, regardless of the model specification. Reports of frequent discrimination events and frequent abuse events are related to lifetime suffering quite strongly, though lower frequencies do not. Someone who reports frequent abuse and discrimination scores between 1.52 and 1.75 (depending on the model) more points in the lifetime suffering scale than she who reports never having been subject to a maltreatment or discrimination situation.

18.7   Conclusions

This chapter explores the relationship between capabilities and suffering from a theoretical and mostly empirical point of view using a unique data set for Chile. Theoretically, we would expect that the larger the capability set, the lower the level of lifetime suffering. Of course, the relationship is imperfect, as long as outcomes depend on multiple sources aside capabilities, such as actual decisions and social circumstances, including luck, as well as on adaptive preferences. Capabilities and functionings are additional (and sometimes novel) determinants of lifetime suffering. On this basis, we advanced in the answer of which capabilities and functionings are more associated to lifetime suffering in Chile.

The first part of the empirical analysis reports evidence of a less-than-perfect correlation between positive emotions and lifetime suffering in Chile. We find that suffering seems not to be simply the reverse of positive affect. This corroborates previous data on Chile from international surveys.

Several standard regression analyses gave us opportunity to study the associations among several variables and lifetime suffering. Among the results, we found that Social Bonds, both as evaluations and as functionings, have a relationship to lifetime suffering. Feeling lonely, not having a partner and being a widow or widower increases lifetime suffering. However, having children also increases suffering. This might be related to the fact that having children yields more concern and responsibility for others' wellbeing and the fact that our child's suffering may be experienced as suffering as well by parents.

In the case of Pleasure and Health capabilities, the variables significantly associated to lifetime suffering correspond to their evaluations rather than their functionings. This means that, in the second case, it is not medical events but the evaluation of one's own health that matters for the experience of suffering. Similarly, it is the feeling of not having enough opportunities for pleasure that affects lifetime suffering rather than its actual frequency. It is of course possible to have reverse causality: More lifetime suffering might reduce our possibilities for pleasure.

On the contrary, it is actual income and the experience of being respected in rights and dignity that are associated to lifetime suffering and not their corresponding subjective evaluation. In the former case, moving two income brackets (considering 7 groups) is linked to a significant reduction in lifetime suffering. Finally, it is noteworthy that the actual experience of repeated discrimination and maltreatment is one of the most important predictors of lifetime suffering.

Regarding the other variables included in the analysis we found, as expected, that age and negative recent events are positively associated with lifetime suffering. Of the Big Five personality traits, only neuroticism is positively related to suffering.

Our analyses must be understood as an initial effort to study a rich data set that permits us to generate unique variables that allow an empirical study of suffering using a framework based on the capability approach. This is novel in that empirical indexes related to capabilities have seldom been used in the literature of subjective wellbeing. We were able, therefore, to check whether the inclusion of these atypical variables improves our understanding of lifetime suffering. The drawback is that in this initial stage of research, when trying to respond to general questions, our models come with a large number of independent variables, generating the potential of multi-collinearity. For instance, it is well known that education influences the dependent variable through the enlargement of other capabilities, especially income, and both are highly correlated in the case of Chile. We nonetheless provide the reader with results from traditional model specifications to make the study comparable with other mainstream investigations of suffering from other countries.

On the other hand, the fact that only five out of eleven capabilities considered valuable by Chileans were relevant predictors of suffering, suggests focusing policies on the enlargement of these capabilities if the objective is in reducing suffering. Of course, this proposal requires more evidence to be safely sustained.

This is only a beginning. Several specification refinements should be tried in subsequent research in order to answer the specific questions that arise from this general overview. Of interest are possible modeling and data improvements to allow identification of causality.

References

Alkire, S. (2002). *Valuing freedoms. Sen's capability approach and poverty reduction.* Oxford: Oxford University Press.

Alkire, S. (2008). *Choosing dimensions: The capability approach and multidimensional poverty,* Munich Personal RePec Archive, Paper 8.862.

Anand, P., & van Hees, M. (2006). Capabilities and achievements: An empirical study. *The Journal of Socio-Economics, 35*, 268–284.

Anderson, R. (2014). *Human suffering and quality of life: conceptualizing stories and statistics,* New York, NY: Springer.

Bentham, J. (1789). *Introduction to the principles of moral and legislation*. Oxford: Clarendon Press, 1907.

Binder, M. (2014). Subjective well-being capabilities: Bridging the gap between the capability approach and subjective well-being research. *Journal of Happiness Studies, 15*(5) 1197–1217.

Comim, F. (2005). Capabilities and happiness: Potential synergies. *Review of Social Economy, 63*(2), 161–176.

Frey, B., & Stutzer, A. (2010). Happiness and public choice. *Public Choice, 14*, 557–573.

Gosling, S. D., Rentfrow, P. J., & Swann, W. B., Jr. (2003). A very brief measure of the big five personality domains. *Journal of Research in Personality, 37*, 504–528.

Helliwell, J., Layard, R., & Sachs, J. (2012). *World happiness report*. New York: The Earth Institute, Columbia University.

Hutcheson, F. (2002). The original of our ideas of beauty and virtue. In J. B. Schneewind (Ed.), *Moral philosophy from Montaigne to Kant* (p. 515). Cambridge: Cambridge University Press.

Kadlec, E. (2007). *Popper's "Negative Utilitarianism"*. From Utopia to Reality.

Leikes, O. (2013). Minimising misery: A new strategy for public policies instead of maximizing happiness? *Social Indicators Research, 114*, 121–137.

Nussbaum, M. (2001). *Women and human development: The capability approach*. Cambridge: Cambridge University Press.

Popper, K. (1956). *The open society and its enemies*. Princeton: Princeton University Press.

Robeyns, I. (2005). The capability approach: A theoretical survey. *Journal of Human Development, 6*, 93–114.

Sen, A. (1977, Summer). Rational fools: A critique of the behavioral foundations of economic theory. *Philosophy & Public Affairs, 6*(4), 317–344.

Sen, A. (1992). *Inequality reexamined*. New York/Cambridge, MA: Russell Sage Foundation/ Harvard University Press.

Sen, A. (2009). *The idea of justice*. Cambridge, MA: Harvard University Press.

UNDP. (2012). *Subjective wellbeing: The challenge of rethinking development*. Santiago: Chile Human Development Report.

Chapter 19
Shame, Humiliation and Social Isolation: Missing Dimensions of Poverty and Suffering Analysis

China Mills and Diego Zavaleta

19.1 Introduction

While 'suffering is a problem in life that affects everyone' (Schulz et al. 2010: 782), "not all suffering is equal" (Farmer 2005: 279). Like poverty, suffering – the distress resulting from threat or damage to one's body or self-identity (Anderson in this same volume) – is multi-dimensional; it is imperative to understand how its various dimensions interact and interconnect: their dynamics, intensities and types, and their implications on wellbeing and quality of life. Little current information exists on the extent, distribution, quality or quantity of suffering internationally, largely due to lack of refined measures (Anderson 2014).

In an attempt to overcome this lack of information, Anderson (2014) has proposed using a series of indicators of both objective and subjective suffering to assess its prevalence on a global scale. One of the key indicators used (and one of two defined to assess *social* suffering) is that of poverty, and, in particular, poverty measured in a multidimensional way. Multidimensional poverty differs from traditional measures of poverty in income space and aims at measuring several deprivations that a person suffers at the same time (e.g. the situation of that person in terms of health, education, and living standards and not only through income level). One specific way of measuring this is the Multidimensional Poverty Index (MPI) used by the United

C. Mills (✉)
Faculty of Education, University of Sheffield,
388 Glossop Road, Rm 8.04, Sheffield S10 2JA, UK
e-mail: china.mills@qeh.ox.ac.uk

D. Zavaleta
Oxford Poverty and Human Development Initiative, Queen Elizabeth House,
University of Oxford, Mansfield Road, Oxford, UK
e-mail: diego.zavaleta@qeh.ox.ac.uk

© Springer Science+Business Media Dordrecht 2015
R.E. Anderson (ed.), *World Suffering and Quality of Life*,
Social Indicators Research Series 56, DOI 10.1007/978-94-017-9670-5_19

Nations Development Programme to calculate worldwide multidimensional acute poverty (Alkire and Santos 2010, 2013), and used by Anderson (2014) with data on corruption as a proxy of social suffering. In this same work, Anderson suggests two ways to continue the quest for more accurately estimating global suffering. One is to limit the estimates of suffering to indicators of severe suffering, and the second is to expand the number of indicators in order to be more inclusive.

We suggest that a key obstacle in the refinement of the measurement of suffering is the assumption that poverty equals suffering, and thus the use of poverty as a proxy for suffering within the literature. We argue that the use of this proxy conceals the multidimensional nature of poverty and the differential distributions of suffering among the poor, overlooking the fact that some people in poverty suffer more than others. Therefore, this chapter aims to begin addressing the challenge of refining measurement of suffering by focussing on specific and concrete aspects of poverty that poor people report are important in their lives, and by exploring how these aspects may relate to suffering. We will argue that drawing upon research into multidimensional poverty and focusing attention on concrete aspects of suffering is fruitful as it enables more precise conceptualisation of differential experiences of suffering. Specifically, this chapter will outline the importance of social connectedness in the lives of the poor, and discuss findings in relation to deprivations in this connectedness – social isolation, shame, and humiliation – as concrete dimensions of poverty.

19.2   The Multidimensionality of Poverty and Suffering

A growing number of local and global initiatives (spanning the developing and developed world) attest to the importance that human beings place on social relations in the evaluation of their wellbeing, alongside other dimensions of life (see Zavaleta et al. 2014 for an outline of a number of initiatives exploring aspects of social connectedness.) They reflect the acknowledged gap between what people value and the dimensions currently used for assessing the wellbeing of people. An example of this attention to the importance of social connectedness is provided by the commission established by former French President, Nicholas Sarkozy, to identify the limits of current indicators of economic performance and social progress. It also suggests how to improve indicators for all countries, with a primary focus on Europe. The commission, led by Joseph Stiglitz, Amartya Sen, and Jean-Paul Fitoussi, concluded that "social connections and relationships" should be among the dimensions taken into account for measurement of quality of life globally. Moreover, they argue that social connections should be considered *simultaneously* alongside other dimensions, such as material living standards (income, consumption, and wealth) and health (Stiglitz et al. 2009). The report emphasises the need to document the diversity of people's experiences, the linkages across different dimensions of wellbeing, and the need to look across different types and domains of inequalities (for example, being both poor and female, or being disabled and poor) "to see how these can compound one another and are combined in both experience and affect" (White et al. 2012: 770).

The research outlined in this chapter is part of the work currently being undertaken by the Oxford Poverty and Human Development Initiative (OPHI) to examine those aspects of life that people living in poverty often state are important to them and yet on which there is little to no international data – the "missing dimensions" of poverty analysis. In particular, OPHI explores aspects of quality of work, empowerment, physical safety, psychological and subjective well-being, and social connectedness (for further details, see: www.ophi.org.uk/research/missing-dimensions/).

The development of indicators that measure these dimensions, and the inclusion of these indicators as short modules on household surveys, allows not only for different aspects of one dimension to be explored (for example, different experiences of social isolation) but furthermore enables exploration of the connections between different dimensions (for example, between empowerment and shame, or between income and social isolation). Highlighting the multidimensional nature of both suffering and poverty is important because

> The predicaments of people below the poverty line are not by means homogenous even when their respective abilities to convert commodities into capabilities are identical, since they differ from each other in the size of their respective shortfalls of income from the poverty line (Sen 1983: 165).

Because few attempts have been made to quantify the distribution of suffering on a global scale, and due to the need to refine measures of suffering, some early research views poverty as an indicator of suffering (see Anderson 2014). While these early attempts are admirable and welcome, it may be problematic to assume that all poor people suffer, and that poor people suffer equally or homogenously. Thus, Sen's call for "distribution-sensitive measures of poverty" (Sen 1983: 165) may also be useful for attempts to measure differential distribution of suffering, both between and within communities.

Furthermore, Anderson (2014: 54) points out that "when multiple types of suffering occur together, their individual effect may multiply rather than add to one another". In Anderson's (2014) research into the global distribution of suffering, he found that major types of suffering often co-existed. This is particularly significant when looking at suffering in contexts of poverty because developing countries with high rates of (income) poverty are likely to have higher co-existence of all three major types of suffering; mental, physical, and social. Through understanding poverty and suffering as multidimensional, we can explore how people experience deprivations and suffering in some dimensions and not in others, and the ways these dimensions may interact. We can also identify those who may be experiencing deprivations in all dimensions, and thus those who's suffering (or poverty) may be most acute or chronic.

19.3 What Matters Most: The Intrinsic and Instrumental Importance of Social Connectedness

"Social connections…. are among the most robust correlates of subjective wellbeing" and indeed, people place such high value in this aspect that they "report that good relationships with family members, friends or romantic partners – far more than money or fame – are prerequisites for their own happiness" (Helliwell and Putnam 2004: 1437). Many people attach high intrinsic value to social contacts: they value the sense of belonging to a community, having friends and emotional attachments, and being able to participate in society. This is evident in a quote from Voices of the Poor, participatory research into poverty conducted in 60 developing countries, where a woman living in poverty in Bulgaria states that, "I like money and nice things, but it's not money that makes me happy. It's people that make me happy" (cited in Narayan and Petesch 2002: 258).

Research consistently shows that social support is a key factor in the relationship between poverty (low income) and wellbeing (Biswas-Diener and Diener 2001). Helliwell et al. (2012) found that when social support was taken into account, the explanatory value of income fell dramatically. This implies that psychological well-being may result from a "horizontal" interaction between physical, social, and psychological needs, with some of the negative effects of material deprivation counterbalanced by positive social relationships (Biswas-Diener and Diener 2001, 2006: 201). This aligns with Anderson's findings of a stronger association between higher social support and lower suffering, where "social support networks play a very large role in diminishing suffering" (2014: 85). This may provide a more nuanced framework for understanding how poverty (or low income) may relate to suffering. For example, while social connectedness may help mitigate the negative relationship between income and life satisfaction, low income may result in people being unable to engage in the reciprocal exchanges that often constitute community participation (e.g. poor people may not be able to afford food to share at communal gatherings). This means that the chronic poor may remain so because of their inability to reciprocate in terms of material resources (Gonzalez 2007).

Through the lens of Sen's capability approach, it seems that people, and perhaps especially poor people, have "good reason to value not being excluded from social relations", and thus social isolation (and social exclusion) would seem to be direct elements of capability poverty and of suffering (Sen 2000: 4). Adam Smith makes the point that "the inability to interact freely with others is an important deprivation in itself (like being undernourished or homeless)" (Sen 2000: 5). This makes a strong case for understanding social isolation (and shame and humiliation) as constitutive components of poverty and suffering. For Sen, absolute deprivation also includes being ashamed to appear in public and not being able to participate in the life of the community (1985). Social isolation and shame can lead to other deprivations and limit other freedoms. For example, being isolated may exclude a person from job opportunities, which can in turn lead to deprivations in being able to purchase food; feeling discriminated against within the health system may lead to deprivations in health.

There is plentiful literature on the deleterious effects of social isolation on both psychological and physical health – where it is related to feelings of loneliness and despair (Biordi and Nicholson 2013), along with research into the affective responses to social exclusion, including social anxiety, jealousy, loneliness, and depression (Baumeister and Tice 1990; Leary 1990). Like social exclusion and rejection, social isolation can have "intense and often disruptive effects…on individual cognitive, motivational, and emotional functioning" (Brewer 2005: 344–45). This is something that poor people seem painfully aware of. An interviewee from Bangladesh in the Voices of the Poor study explained that being too poor to participate in community gatherings, and thus having to remain isolated in the house, is when a "person goes mad and wishes to commit suicide" (cited in Narayan et al. 2000: 258).

The *pain* of subjective isolation – or "social pain" – is a deeply disruptive hurt that also has striking effects on physical health (See Cassidy and Asher 1992; Cole et al. 2007; Eisenberger et al. 2003; Gustafsson et al. 2012; Hawkley and Cacioppo 2010; MacDonald and Leary 2005; Stranahan et al. 2006; Westerlund et al. 2012; Wilson et al. 2007). Furthermore, Eisenberger et al. (2003) have tested the neural correlates of social exclusion through neuroimaging studies and concluded that the brain bases of social pain are similar to those of physical pain. The quality and quantity of individuals' social relationships has been linked not only to mental health but also to both morbidity and mortality. The magnitude of risk to health is comparable to the effect of high blood pressure, lack of exercise, obesity, or smoking (Cacioppo and Patrick 2008; House et al. 1988) and is a predictor of functional decline and death among individuals older than 60 years (Perissinotto et al. 2012). The *distress* produced by subjective social isolation is a serious and common problem and the effects can be considerable, especially if it becomes chronic. While all individuals are prone to feel loneliness at several points in their lives, this becomes "an issue of serious concern only when it settles in long enough to create a persistent, self-reinforcing loop of negative thoughts, sensations, and behaviors" (Cacioppo and Patrick 2008: 7).

Social isolation, shame, and humiliation, could be "constitutively a part of capability deprivation as well as instrumentally a cause of diverse capability failures" (2000: 5). Despite what poor people say about the intrinsic importance of social connectedness, and a growing literature on social support as playing a mediating role between income and low subjective wellbeing, little policy exists to develop and strengthen support networks, especially in developing countries. It is important for research to take seriously the need to expand people's relational capabilities and the real freedoms that people value.

19.4 Shame, Humiliation and Isolation – Unpacking the Terms

Shame and humiliation are affective states that define distinct yet related aspects of human psychology. Shame is a

"global, painful, and devastating experience in which the self, not just behaviour, is painfully scrutinized and negatively evaluated...This global, negative affect is often accompanied by a sense of shrinking and being small, and by a sense of worthlessness and powerlessness" (Tangney 2003). "Shame is likely to be accompanied by a desire to hide or escape from the interpersonal situation in question..." (Tagney quoted in Sabini and Silver 1997).

Shame is both a moral emotion (in the sense that it acts as an evaluator of self) and is linked to the self in relation to others (as actions by others or our perception of their judgement may affect our sense of shame). Humiliation refers to both an act – to humiliate someone or feeling humiliated – or to a feeling. In reference to an act (an *external* event), it is commonly linked to the feeling or condition of being lessened in dignity or pride and associated with unequal power relations (Lindner 2007). In terms of the feeling (an *internal* event), humiliation is "the deep dysphoric feeling associated with being, or perceiving oneself as being, unjustly degraded, ridiculed, or put down—in particular, one's identity has been demeaned or devalued" (Hartling and Luchetta 1999: 7).

Although both are negative emotions that refer to the self, and although these terms are frequently used interchangeably as synonymous in common language, there are several important differences between shame and humiliation. Shame emphasises an individualistic evaluation; humiliation is inherently interactional. They may occur simultaneously, as suffering from a humiliating act may entail feeling ashamed; yet one emotion does not result ipso facto in the other (e.g. one can have the feeling of being humiliated without the sensation that one has failed one's own standards). While shame is the result of a personal judgment of failure (and thus involves the belief that one deserves the shame), humiliation tends to involve the belief by the target that he or she does not deserve the treatment he or she is getting (Jackson 1999; Hartling and Luchetta 1999). The response to both experiences is quite different. While shame can result in withdrawal, humiliation typically arouses hostility (Jackson 1999).

Social isolation is the inadequate quality and quantity of social relations with other people at the different levels where human interaction takes place (individual, group, community and the larger social environment) (Zavaleta et al. 2014). This implies that the social isolation of a person has both quantitative and qualitative aspects, such as the number or frequency of interactions with other people (e.g. the social networks we belong to, the number of groups in which we participate, or the frequency with which we meet friends and family), and how *meaningful* these relations are (e.g. if they satisfy a person's expectations or standards). Both quantitative and qualitative aspects of deprivations in connectedness contribute in a myriad of ways to the social isolation of a human being, yet the relationship between these aspects is not direct. For example, being alone (lack of or inadequate number of relations) may trigger feelings of loneliness (a qualitative aspect), and feeling isolated may result in being alone. One may feel lonely while being surrounded by people, family or friends, and people with few social contacts may not feel isolated at all (indeed, many individuals enjoy their solitude and value it) (see, for example, Fromm 1942/2001; Hawkley and Cacioppo 2009).

The importance of social connectedness has been documented both conceptually and empirically in the rich and overlapping literatures on social capital, social cohesion, and social exclusion. (While there is not space here to elaborate on these theories, see Zavaleta et al. (2014) for a more detailed discussion of how the research outlined in this chapter connects to, and diverges from, the wider literature). This literature has contributed enormously to increasing focus on, and developing measures of, aspects of social connectedness. However, along with problems in defining and operationalizing concepts, research into the measurement of social capital, social cohesion, and social exclusion has tended to concentrate mainly on the instrumentality of social connections – the positive impact they can have on key aspects of life, such as a person's health, well-being, or job opportunities, and how they may enable people to gain access to resources (Berkman and Glass 2000; Coleman 1988; Easterly et al. 2006; Grootaert 1998; Putnam 2000; Woolcock 1998, 2001). While the instrumental importance of social connectedness is important, much of this research overlooks the intrinsic value that many people attach to having social connections.

The point of this research lies in the emphasis placed on the intrinsic *and* instrumental importance of social connectedness, specifically for those living in poverty. It aims to develop indicators that measure both external and internal (objective and subjective) aspects of deprivations in social connectedness. The inclusion of internal characteristics follows an increasing number of studies that use data reflecting people's perceptions of their own life (Hawthorne 2006; Hortulanus et al. 2006; WHO-QoL Group 1993). Anderson (2014) highlights a similar need for the combination of subjective and objective indictors in the conceptualisation and measurement of suffering as multidimensional.

19.5   Data Resources

In this chapter, we use two specific indicators – discrimination and loneliness – to explore their intensity and relationship with other variables in two different countries: Chile and Chad. These two indicators are part of a series of concrete indicators proposed to collect data on shame, humiliation and isolation (Zavaleta 2007; Zavaleta et al. 2014). The analysis draws on two datasets collected by the Oxford Poverty and Human Development Initiative (OPHI). The first dataset was collected in Chile using a nationally representative subsample of Chile's national household survey (CASEN) in 2009. A total of 1,432 households were interviewed using several modules of traditional socio-economic variables available in the CASEN 2006, alongside five modules on "missing dimensions of poverty data" developed by OPHI and collected in 2009.

The second dataset comes from the Multidimensional Poverty and Vulnerability in Chad (EPMVT) household survey. This survey was designed and collected by the Institute of National Statistics of the Government of Chad (INSEED), the Oxford Poverty and Human Development Initiative (OPHI) and UNICEF-Chad. Data collection took place in 2012 and gathered information from a nationally representative sample of 4,426 households. As with the Chilean exercise, the dataset contains a rich array of traditional socio-economic variables alongside modules on quality of employment, empowerment, shame, humiliation, isolation, psychological well-being, and physical safety.

The datasets drawn upon here allow preliminary exploration of these diverse variables within two extremely divergent realities. Chile is a high-income country with low levels of poverty (with 2.7 % of its population living under less than US $2 a day in 2009), and high levels of human development (it ranks 40 of 186 in the Human Development Index). Chad is a low-income country and one of the poorest in the world by any standard: 83.3 % of its population lived with less than US $2 a day by 2003; 62.9 % of the population is multidimensionally poor (OPHI 2013); and the country ranks 184 of 186 in the Human Development Index (all income poverty data from The World Bank Databank 2014, The World Bank, accessed 25-02-2014, http://data.worldbank.org/topic/poverty; Human Development data from UNDP dataset, United Nations Development Program, accessed 25-02-2014, https://data.undp.org/dataset/Table-1-Human-Development-Index-and-its-components/wxub-qc5k).

We use data on discrimination from the Chilean dataset here to exhibit some basic results. Discrimination has been characterized as the "most overt form of ascriptive humiliation" (Lukes 1997: 44) and is characterized by unequal power relations and actions that affect the dignity and pride of individuals and result in feelings of being degraded. This affective state has been associated with numerous psychosocial maladies, such as low self-esteem, school-related difficulties, pernicious child-rearing practices, delinquency, poverty, social phobia, anxiety, depression, paranoia, marital discord, domestic violence, sexual aggression, rape, serial murder, torture, and suicide (Hartling and Luchetta 1999).

Data on discrimination is obtained on the basis of responses to three questions:

1. Have you been treated in a way that you felt was prejudiced during the past 3 months? (Response alternatives: Yes, always; Yes, often; Yes, occasionally; No, never; Don't Know or No answer)
2. Who treated you in a way that you felt was prejudiced? (the response alternatives included a series of institutions, people, situations or places);
3. Why were you treated in a way that you felt was prejudiced? (Response alternatives: Ethnic or racial background, Gender, Sexual orientation, Age, Disability, Religion, Other – open question, Don't know).

19.6   Results from Chile

The general results for this set of questions in Chile are as following: up to 16.6 % of the population claims to have been treated with prejudice either "always", "often" or "occasionally" in the last 3 months, while 82.2 % claimed to have never been treated with prejudice, and 1.3 % did not know or did not respond. As can be observed in Table 19.1., of the people who claimed to have been the subject of a discriminatory act, a large majority stated that these acts took place either in the health services (26.3 %), at work (21.1 %), in the street by an unknown person (11.4 %), or by a close relative (9.1 %). Finally, the alleged reason for this act of prejudice can be seen in Table 19.2. The most often cited reason in the experience of prejudice is the socio-economic condition of the respondent (40 %), followed by

Table 19.1 Who treated you in a prejudiced way?

Category of prejudice location	Percent
Health care services	26.3
School	1.5
Work	21.1
Police/judicial system	3.5
Social services	5.4
Shops/restaurants	2.7
Bank/insurance company	3.8
Government housing office	2.4
Close relative	9.1
Unknown person in a public place	11.4
Other	6.4
DK/NA	6.3

Source: own estimates using OPHI-CASEN survey

Table 19.2 Why were you treated in a prejudiced way?

Location prejudicial exposure	Percent
Ethnic, racial or cultural background	7.7
Gender	2.5
Sexual orientation	1.2
Age	5.4
Disability	1.9
Religion	3.0
Socio-economic group	40.0
Education	8.7
Other	3.2
DK/NA	26.5

Source: own estimates using OPHI-CASEN survey

an unknown reason or refusal to answer (26.5 %), the level of education of the respondent (8.7 %), or his or her ethnic, racial, or cultural background (7.7 %). The large percentage of respondents who do not know or refuse to answer why they perceive they have been subject to a prejudicial act is telling, as it is possible that a portion of these respondents refuse to provide a concrete answer due to the shame of exposing a particular background.

However, these general results conceal important sub-group realities, including differences by income level, gender, age, and ethnic, racial or cultural background. As can be observed in Fig. 19.1, the sense of discrimination varies significantly. We find a negative, significant relationship between the income group of the respondent and discrimination, varying from 24.2 % in the poorest 20 % of the population to

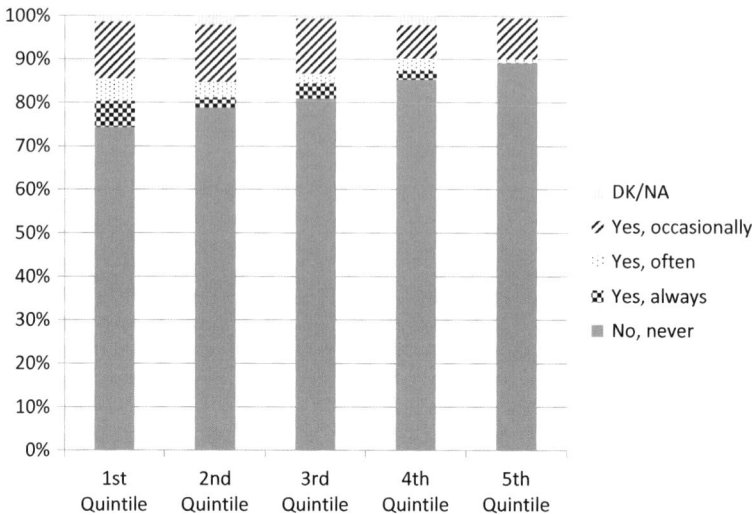

Fig. 19.1 Percentage of respondent being treated with prejudice by income group (Source: own estimates using OPHI-CASEN survey)

10.3 % in the highest income-earning group. How regularly the respondent feels treated with prejudice also tends to decrease the higher the income group. Similarly, we observe significant differences between the poor and non-poor populations in being the subject of a prejudicial act (14.5 % versus 21 %) [The income cut-offs are those used by the Ministry of Planning of Chile (MIDEPLAN) for the official poverty estimates of 2009]. The result of the main perceived cause for the discriminatory act being the socio-economic background of the respondent remains the highest perceived cause for each income group.

Where the discrimination takes place also has important variations, with respondents in the first two quintiles claiming it takes place predominately in the health services (39.4 and 31.1 %, respectively), while respondents in the higher three quintiles claiming that it takes place at work (36, 29.3 and 24.9 %, respectively). Gender differences are also evident in these two spaces of discrimination, with women feeling significantly more discrimination in the health care system (30.9 versus 19.8 %), while men tend to experience more at work (28.8 versus 15.7 %). Finally, differences due to ethnic background exhibit the largest variations. For example, the Aymara group – the second largest ethnic group, based in the less populated northern part of Chile – identifies the main source of discrimination as coming from an unknown person in a public place (42.5 %) with the perceived reason for discrimination given being due to their ethnic background (51.9 %). Space limitation does not allow for a comparison between countries, which add examples of the variety and magnitude of discriminatory acts. In Chad, for example, the main source of discrimination by far comes from a close relative, showing important intra-household dynamics of discrimination (Fig. 19.2).

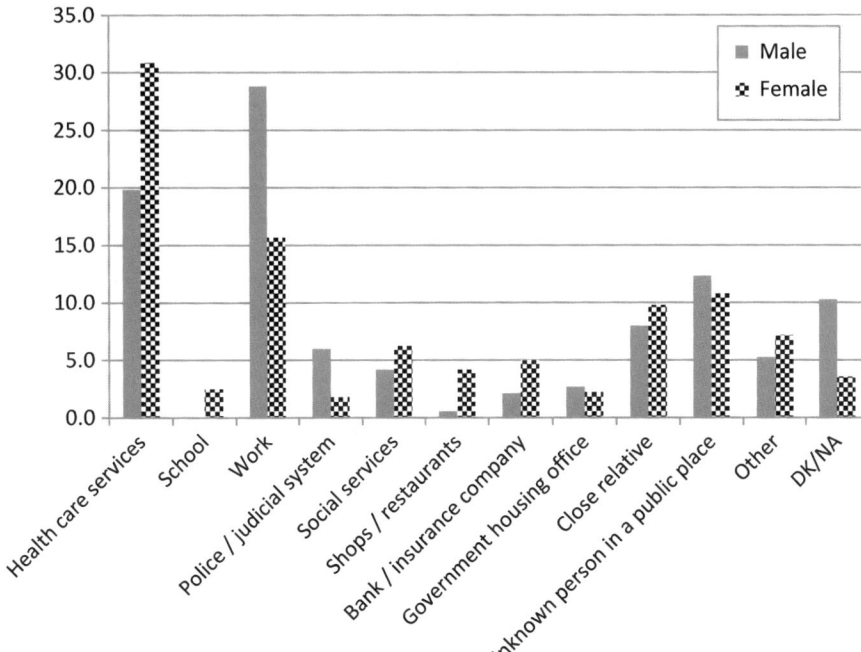

Fig. 19.2 Gender differences in where discrimination took place (% of female and male respondents per each category) (Source: own estimates using OPHI-CASEN survey)

19.7 Results from Chad

Results from Chad show relevant insights for poverty analysis by introducing information on loneliness. Loneliness is "the distress that results from discrepancies between ideal and perceived social relationships" (Hawkley and Cacioppo 2009). Loneliness is relevant because it can be argued that, in its chronic form, it is one of the most extreme forms of social disconnection, carrying deleterious effects on physical and psychological health (as discussed earlier). Information for this variable was obtained from specific statements from version III of the UCLA Loneliness scale (Russell 1996). Respondents were requested to indicate how often they feel they can find companionship when they want it. The response structure is a 4-point scale ranging from "never" to "often".

Results from the Chad survey show that 20.2 % of the population claimed they "never" or "rarely" find companionship when they want it, while 25.6 % find companionship only "sometimes", and 53.7 % claimed they can "often" find companionship. These general results hide important sub-group differences. For example, gender differences show the strongest size effect found in the loneliness data with women on average reporting 0.16 points higher on the score than men (see Fig. 19.3). The worse the results, the more skewed the gender difference, with women reporting over 70 % of the entire results of people not being able ("never") to find companionship when they want it.

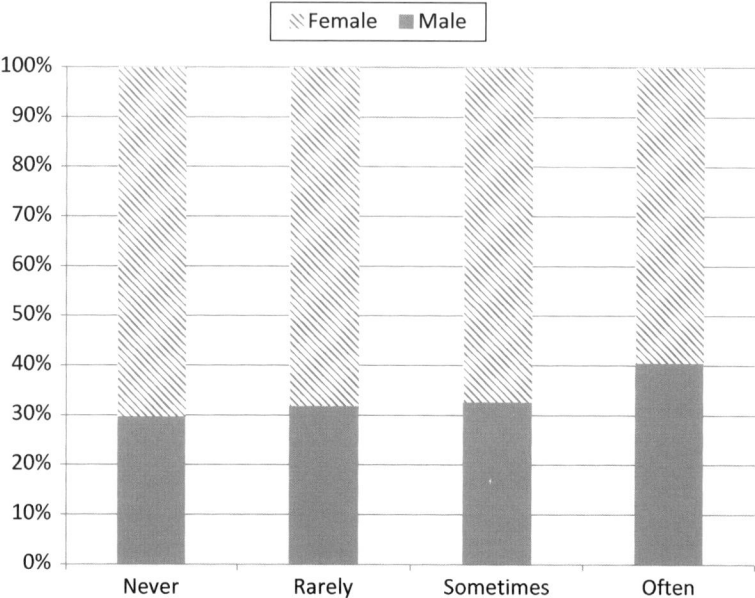

Fig. 19.3 Gender differences in perceptions of how often can respondents find companionship when they want it (% of female and male respondents per each category) (Source: own estimates using OPHI-CASEN survey)

Being able to find companionship when you want it is negatively and significantly correlated with per capita household expenditure and education level. The higher their per capita household expenditure (per quintile), or level of education (by category, e.g. from primary completed to secondary completed), the less lonely people are compared to their counterparts in lower levels. Urban dwellers also feel less lonely than their rural counterparts.

19.8   Conclusions

This chapter has argued that focusing attention on concrete and poignant aspects that affect people's lives – namely shame, humiliation, and social isolation – can help refine the measurement of both poverty and social suffering. The motivation behind moving to measure poverty in a multidimensional way is rooted in people's lived realities of experiencing multiple forms of deprivations simultaneously. Although income is a crucial aspect for understanding poverty, it is insufficient in capturing this diversity, leading to important shortcomings in poverty measurement. Measuring poverty in a multidimensional way can enrich the understanding about this social malady. In this respect, using multidimensional poverty as a proxy to social suffering is a sensible move. Yet, data on the crucial aspects for people living in poverty are still missing. This includes the lack of agency to live a life in the way that one values, or the demeaning of one's identity due to the stigma of poverty, discrimination or social isolation. These aspects, we argue, are intrinsically linked to potential, perceived, or actual damage to one's body or self-identity, and thus need to be developed and incorporated to refine the measurement of both poverty and suffering.

The basic results shown in this chapter provide a glimpse into the reality of discrimination: its magnitude, its sub-group differences, the links between the income level of a person and how often she or he suffers from discriminatory acts, and the areas of life most affected by it. Group-based discrimination (ethnic, racial, cultural, or religious) is especially relevant as it can lead to important political instability and even violent conflict (see Stewart 2001). It can also result in important negative psychological and sociological phenomena linked to the concealment of identities in order to avoid discrimination.

It is important to note that the answer of the respondent refers to an actual act, and not simply to a perception of the existence of situations involving discrimination. This act may indeed be due to a reason different to what the respondent perceives it to be (e.g. a personal problem between a person performing the act and the subject of the act, rather than due to her ethnic background or gender). Yet, there are still a significant number of people in the sample claiming to having been subject of prejudice, so it is highly unlikely that such a large number of the population simply perceive this as real. And even then – if that was the case – it would still be telling that such a number of people feel that the cause of the act was due to prejudice.

The results also provide a glimpse into the diversity of how discrimination is suffered in different contexts. The data on loneliness (though limited) points to the existence of this condition in a significant portion of the population of Chad and confirms previous qualitative analysis in different contexts showing its links to poverty (see De Jong Gierveld and Van Tilburg 2010). As in the case of data on discrimination, quantitative information on loneliness will advance our understanding of the characteristics of the population who suffer from this malady and its relationship with other dimensions of wellbeing and suffering.

The use of particular indicators of shame, humiliation, and social isolation can better indicate differential distributions of suffering and help identify individuals and sub-groups within people living in poverty that are affected by concrete and particularly hurtful situations. Consequently, they can help to identify levels of suffering which are higher within a specific population. These types of indicators could form the basis of more refined measures that help generate more concise data on suffering. Most importantly, better data on who is suffering and how they are suffering paves the way for the development of interventions that are sensitive to people's lived realities of suffering, and thus better able to provide the conditions for people to live the lives they value.

References

Alkire, S., & Santos, M. E. (2010). *Acute multidimensional poverty: A new index for developing countries* (OPHI Working Paper 38). Oxford: Oxford Poverty & Human Development Initiative.

Alkire, S., & Santos, M. E. (2013). *Measuring acute poverty in the developing world: Robustness and scope of the multidimensional poverty index* (OPHI Working Paper 59). Oxford: Oxford University.

Anderson, R. E. (2014). *Human suffering and quality of life -conceptualizing stories and statistics*. New York: Springer.

Baumeister, R. F., & Tice, D. M. (1990). Point-counterpoints: Anxiety and social exclusion. *Journal of Social and Clinical Psychology, 9*(2), 165–195.

Berkman, L. F., & Glass, T. (2000). Social integration, social networks, social support, and health. In L. F. Berkman & I. Kawachi (Eds.), *Social epidemiology* (pp. 137–173). New York: Oxford University Press.

Biordi, D. L., & Nicholson, N. R. (2013). Social isolation. In I. M. A. L. Lubkin & P. D. Burlington (Eds.), *Chronic illness: Impact and intervention*. Boston: Jones and Bartlett.

Biswas-Diener, R., & Diener, E. (2001). Making the best of a bad situation: Satisfaction in the slums of Calcutta'. *Social Indicators Research, 55*(3), 329–352.

Biswas-Diener, R., & Diener, E. (2006). The subjective well-being of the homeless, and lessons for happiness. *Social Indicators Research, 76*, 185–205.

Brewer, M. B. (2005). The psychological impact of social isolation: Discussion and commentary. In K. D. Williams, J. P. Fogas, & W. Hippell (Eds.), *The social outcast: Ostracism, social exclusion, rejection and bullying*. New York/London: Taylor and Francis.

Cacioppo, J. T., & Patrick, W. (2008). *Loneliness*. New York/London: W.W. Norton & Company.

Cassidy, J., & Asher, S. (1992). Loneliness and peer relations in young children. *Child Development, 63*(2), 350–365.

Cole, S. W., Hawkley, L. C., Arevalo, J. M., Sung, C. Y., Rose, R. M., & Cacioppo, J. T. (2007). Social regulation of gene expression in human leukocytes. *Genome Biology, 8*(9), 189–189.

Coleman, J. S. (1988). Social capital in the creation of human capital. *American Journal of Sociology, 94*(Suppl. Organizations and Institutions: Sociological and Economic Approaches to the Analysis of Social Structure), 95–120.

de Jong Gierveld, J., & Van Tilburg, T. (2010). The De Jong Gierveld short scales for emotional and social loneliness: Tested on data from seven countries in the UN generations and gender surveys. *European Journal of Ageing, 7*(2), 121–130.

Easterly, W., Ritzen, J., & Woolcock, M. (2006). Social cohesion, institutions and growth. *Economic and Politics, 18*(2), 103–120.

Eisenberger, N. I., Lieberman, M., & Williams, K. D. (2003). Does rejection hurt? An fMRI study of social exclusion. *Science, 302*, 290–292.

Farmer, P. (2005). *Pathologies of power: Health, human rights and the new war on the poor*. Berkeley: University of California Press.

Fromm, E. (1942/2001). *The fear of freedom*. London/New York: Routledge.

Gonzalez de la Rocha, M. (2007). The construction of the myth of survival. *Development and Change, 38*(1), 45–66.

Grootaert, C. (1998). *Social capital: The missing link?* (Social capital initiative). Washington, DC: The World Bank.

Gustafsson, P. E., Janlert, U., Theorell, T., Westerlund, H., & Hammarström, A. (2012). Do peer relations in adolescence influence health in adulthood? Peer problems in the school setting and the metabolic syndrome in middle-age. *PloS One, 7*(6), e39385.

Hartling, L. M., & Luchetta, T. (1999). Humiliation: Assessing the impact of derision, degradation, and debasement. *The Journal Primary Prevention, 19*(4), 259–278.

Hawkley, L. C., & Cacioppo, J. T. (2009). Loneliness. In H. R. S. Sprecher (Ed.), *Encyclopedia of human relationships* (pp. 985–990). Thousand Oaks: Sage.

Hawkley, L. C., & Cacioppo, J. T. (2010). Loneliness matters: A theoretical and empirical review of consequences and mechanisms. *Annals of Behavioral Medicine, 40*, 218–227.

Hawthorne, G. (2006). Measuring social isolation in older adults: Development and initial validation of the friendship scale. *Indicators Research, 77*, 521–548.

Helliwell, J. F., & Putnam, R. D. (2004). The social context of well-being. *Philosophical Transactions of the Royal Society of London. Series B, Biological Sciences, 359*(1449), 1435–1446.

Helliwell, J., Layard, R., & Sacks, J. (2012). *World happiness report*. New York: The Earth Institute, Colombia University.

Hortulanus, R., Machielse, A., & Meeuwesen, L. (2006). *Social isolation in modern society*. London/New York: Routledge.

House, J. S., Landis, K. R., & Umberson, D. (1988). Social relationships and health. *Science, 241*, 540–545.

Jackson, M. A. (1999). *Distinguishing shame and humiliation*. Doctoral dissertation, Department of Philosophy, University of Kentucky: Lexington, KY.

Leary, M. R. (1990). Responses to social exclusion: Social anxiety, jealousy, loneliness, depression, and low self-esteem. *Journal of Social and Clinical Psychology, 9*(2), 221–229.

Lindner, E. G. (2007). 'In times of globalization and human rights: Does humiliation become the most disruptive force?', *Journal of Human Dignity and Humiliation Studies*, http://www.humiliationstudies.upeace.org/article.cfm

Lukes, S. (1997). Humiliation and politics of identity. *Social Research, 64*(1), 36–51.

MacDonald, G., & Leary, M. R. (2005). Why does social exclusion hurt? The relationship between social and physical pain. *Psychological Bulletin, 131*(2), 202–223.

Narayan, D., & Petesch, P. (2002). *Voices of the poor: From many lands*. New York: Oxford University Press for The World Bank.

Narayan, D., Chambers, R., Shah, M. K., & Petesch, P. (2000). *Voices of the poor: Crying out for change*. New York: Oxford University Press for the World Bank.

Oxford Poverty and Human Development Initiative. (2013). *"Chad Country Briefing", Multidimensional Poverty Index Databank*. OPHI, University of Oxford. Available at http://www.ophi.org.uk/multidimensional-poverty-index/mpi-data-bank/mpi-country-briefings.

Perissinotto, C. M., Stijacic Cenzer, I., & Covinsky, K. E. (2012). Loneliness in older persons: A predictor of functional decline and death. *Archives of Internal Medicine, 172*(14), 1078–1084.

Putnam, R. (2000). *Bowling alone: The collapse and revival of American community*. New York: Simon & Schuster.

Russell, D. W. (1996). UCLA loneliness scale (version 3): Reliability, validity, and factor structure. *Journal of Personality Assessment, 66*(1), 20–40.

Sabini, J., & Silver, M. (1997). In defense of shame: Shame in the context of guilt and embarrassment. *Journal for the Theory of Social Behaviour, 27*(1), 1–15.

Schulz, R., Monin, J. K., Czaja, S. J., Lingler, J., Beach, S. R., Martire, L. M., Dodds, A., Hebert, R., Zdaniuk, B., & Cook, T. B. (2010). Measuring the experience and perception of suffering. *The Gerontologist, 50*(6), 774–784.

Sen, A. K. (1983). Poor, relatively speaking. *Economic Papers, 35*(2), 153–169.

Sen, A. K. (1985). A sociological approach to the measurement of poverty: A reply to Professor Peter Townsend. *Economic Papers, 37*(4), 669–676.

Sen, A. (2000). *Social exclusion: Concept, application, and scrutiny* (Social Development Papers Manila). Manila: Office of Environmental and Social Development. Asian Development Bank.

Stewart, F. (2001). 'Horizontal inequalities: A neglected dimension of development', paper given at WIDER 2001 Annual Development Lecture, 2001.

Stiglitz, J. E., Sen, A., & Fitoussi, J. P. (2009). *Report by the commission on the measurement of economic performance and social progress*. Paris: The Commission.

Stranahan, A. M., Khalil, D., & Gould, E. (2006). Social isolation delays the positive effects of running on adult neurogenesis. *Nature Neuroscience, 9*(4), 526–533.

Tangney, J. P. (2003). *Shame and guilt*. New York: The Guilford Press.

Westerlund, H., Gustafsson, P. E., Theorell, T., Janlert, U., & Hammarström, A. (2012). Social adversity in adolescence increases the physiological vulnerability to job strain in adulthood: A prospective population-based study. *PloS One, 7*(4), e35967.

White, S. C., Gaines, S. O., & Jha, S. (2012). Beyond subjective well-being: A critical review of the Stiglitz report approach to subjective perspectives on quality of life. *Journal of International Development, 24*, 763–776.

Wilson, R. S., Krueger, K. R., Arnold, S. E., Schneider, J. A., Kelly, J. F., Barnes, L. L., Tang, Y., & Bennett, D. A. (2007). Loneliness and risk of Alzheimer disease. *Archives of General Psychiatry, 64*, 234–240.

Woolcock, M. (1998). Social capital and economic development: Toward a theoretical synthesis and policy framework. *Theory and Society, 27*(2), 151–208.

Woolcock, M. (2001). The place of social capital in understanding social and economic outcomes. *Canadian Journal of Policy Research, 2*(1), 11–17.

World Bank Databank. http://data.worldbank.org/topic/poverty. Accessed 25 Feb 2014.

World-Health-Organization. (1993). *WHOQOL Study Protocol*. Geneva.

Zavaleta, D. (2007). The ability to go about without shame: A proposal for internationally comparable indicators of shame and humiliation. *Oxford Development Studies, 35*(4), 405–430.

Zavaleta, D., Samuel, K., & Mills, C. (2014). *Social isolation: A conceptual and measurement proposal* (OPHI Working Papers 67).

Part IV
Suffering and Community: Online and Offline Contexts

Chapter 20
The Cultural Geography of Community Suffering

Daina Cheyenne Harvey

20.1 Introduction

In their book on environmental justice, Roberts and Toffolon-Weiss (2001), who use Louisiana as a proxy for the rest of the country, ask the obvious question, "Why Louisiana?" The answer, which they provide in part, is that historically, and even today, Louisiana has had a troubled history filled with vast racial divides, one of the highest rates of economic inequality in the country, weak civil society, politicians that are supported by the petrochemical industry, and an abundance of available land adjacent to the most-used waterway and one of the most important ports in the country.

Because of the confluence of the political, economic, racial, cultural, and geographical conditions, the entire stretch of land along River Road, a road stretching from New Orleans to Baton Rouge, was eventually developed by the petrochemical industry. Today there are more than 150 plants along this 70-mile stretch of road. These plants are responsible for 129 million pounds of toxic releases each year. And this total does not take into account the fact that 88 % of all U.S. offshore oil rigs are located in Louisiana's Outer Continental Shelf. Additionally, this area is also home to more than 2,000 hazardous waste pits and toxic dump sites (Roberts and Toffolon-Weiss 2001) and has more oil spills than any other in the nation. Below, in Table 20.1, is an abbreviated list and description of oil spills and refinery accidents or violations in the area over the past several years.

Likewise, in New Orleans, because development radiated out from the French Quarter to the *battures* (back swamps), poor people were continually pushed to the less desirable and notably less protected areas. As Colten (2005) notes, extending infrastructure to these areas became problematic because poor blacks typically

D.C. Harvey (✉)
Department of Sociology and Anthropology, College of the Holy Cross,
1 College Street, Worcester, MA 01610, USA
e-mail: dharvey@holycross.edu

© Springer Science+Business Media Dordrecht 2015
R.E. Anderson (ed.), *World Suffering and Quality of Life*,
Social Indicators Research Series 56, DOI 10.1007/978-94-017-9670-5_20

Table 20.1 Notable oil spills and accidents in southeastern Louisiana since 2000[a]

Date	Site	Event
3/15/2000	Stiles	380 barrels of crude oil spills into Miller Branch and other creeks
6/2/2000	Norco	Louisiana DEQ notifies Shell/Motiva of thousands of emission violations of benzene and other chemicals
8/18/2000	Convent	Refinery explosion
11/28/2000	New Orleans	Oil tanker Westchester spills 567,000 gallons of crude oil
2/12/2002	Geismar	Explosion and fire at Shell Chemical
3/2002	Franklin	EPA begins cleanup of abandoned well leaking into Intercostal Canal
6/2002	Southeastern, LA	BP spills 90,000 gallons of crude oil
10/2/2002	Norco	Shell/Motiva spews oily substance over community
5/3/2002	Baton Rouge	US Kirby spills 20,000 gallons of diesel into Mississippi River
12/2/2003	Barataria Bay	Exxon/Mobil pipelines leak 15,400 gallons of oil
2/19/2004	New Orleans	Tanker Genar Alexanders spills 40,000 gallons of crude and No. 6 oil
8/29/2005	Southeastern, LA	More than 7 million gallons of oil spills during Hurricane Katrina
7/23/2008	New Orleans	A collision results in 400,000 gallons of heavy fuel spills at the port
4/7/2010	Venice	Cypress Pipeline (BP and Chevron) leaks 18,000 gallons of crude oil into Delta National Wildlife Refuge and Gulf
4/20/2010	Southeastern, LA	Deepwater Horizon explosion kills 11 and leaks 210 million gallons of oil
7/27/2010	Barataria Bay	A tugboat strikes an abandoned wellhead that then leaks 12,240 gallons of oil
5/8/2012	Norco	Shell-Motiva emits 648,733 pounds of toxic chemicals into air
2/22/2014	Vacherie	31,500 gallons of oil spills after a collision on the Mississippi River

[a]Compiled from http://www.labucketbrigade.org/

inhabited them. Additionally many of the battures became used as dumps and land-fills. After WWII many of these landfills became hazardous waste sites and created what Foote calls "landscapes of tragedy" (in Colten 2005: 13).

Robert Bullard calls this combination of industrial and ecological exposure "toxic terror" (in Lerner 2005). Living with this terror shapes the ways in which residents make sense of peril and how they deal with suffering. In this chapter I briefly focus on what I call the *culture of suffering* and a few of the cultural tools residents use to make life livable in a community where suffering is normative. In this community, the Lower Ninth Ward in New Orleans and ground zero for Hurricane Katrina and the federal levee failures, decades of dealing with disasters, toxic events, unemployment three times the national average, and one of the highest murder rates in the country, has made suffering the dominant framework for one's worldview and for interacting with others. Suffering creates the social order and permeates the culture. It is the warp and the woof of the community.

20.2   A Culture of Suffering

Traumas often produce a common culture (Erikson 1976). They have the potential to create particular communities, what Fritz has called "communities of sufferers" ([1961] 1996). In these communities, suffering marks the community in identifiable ways. In a more modern treatment, Auyero and Swistun highlighted particular cultural aspects of this type of community, including toxic uncertainty and confusion (2007, 2009). They importantly pointed out that while not everyone in the community suffered in the same way, their reactions to peril nonetheless constituted "a repertoire of subjective, but not individual, schemes of perception, appreciation, and action" (2009: 141). That is, their reaction to suffering was shaped by a collective and cultural response.

Cultural work is essential to understanding suffering (Janes 1999; Quesada 1999). Honkasalo (2009), for instance, shows that our understanding of suffering comes from highly detailed cultural scripts that are often told as narratives or have become part of the collective memory of the groups to which we belong (see also DeGloma 2009). While there are macro-orientations to suffering found in various cultures, Davies' (2011) work, for instance, on a "positive model" which structured suffering in the eighteenth and nineteenth centuries or Sullivan's (2011) work on poor women using religious culture to make sense of their suffering, there are also micro-orientations to suffering. Here, analyses of culture result in understandings of how groups articulate suffering in publicly recognizable and meaningful terms, turning suffering into a locally constructed process (Janes 1999: 392; Leavitt 1995: 134).

The work of culture in making sense of suffering, however, is often under- defined. My use of culture follows in the newer tradition of the dual-process model of understanding culture in action (see Vaisey 2008, 2009). This model sees culture as both a set of tools (Swidler 1986) we make use of to discursively explain or make sense of our actions after the fact, and more practical modes of culture that unconsciously guide our behavior. This model makes use of decades of research from cognitive science (Chaiken and Trope 1999; Schwarz 1998) that conclusively demonstrates that we the use two different systems of thought—one fast and automatic, the other slow and deliberate. These systems provide us with both culturally available schemas that structure our cognitive response to suffering, but also give us the socially and culturally appropriate ways of making sense of or explaining our suffering.

Residents of the Lower Ninth Ward used their cultural toolkits (Swidler 1986) to attend to their suffering. Decades of dealing with social disruption helped them establish strategies for dealing with disasters. Because of the history of the Lower Ninth Ward, the lines between settled and unsettled times (Swidler 1986) has become blurred. These tools have come from living in a geography of trouble (Harvey 2012); a place that is at constant threat of peril.

The Lower Ninth Ward was the poster child for Katrina and the federal levee failures. The EPA declared 100 % of homes there uninhabitable. Residents were not allowed to return for 3 months, and only then were allowed to observe the damage under a "look and leave" policy. Water and electricity remained unavailable to most for up to a year and half after Katrina, furthering the damage caused by flooding. Furthermore, residents were uncertain if they would be allowed to rebuild or what kind of federal, state, or local support they might be given. Initial plans called for the Lower Ninth Ward to be turned into a green space.

Those who have returned have had to deal with racially discriminatory allocations by government agencies, which use pre-Katrina values as the basis for aid rather than the cost to rebuild. Those residents who have rebuilt have had to do so in a piecemeal fashion, leaving them susceptible to thieves who steal copper wiring and metal fixtures to sell for scrap. The neighborhood remains in a state of flux due to these secondary traumas (Gill 2007).

When I arrived to do participant observation there was no library, no grocery store, no fire station, no community center, no police station (or sub-station). It is the most blighted neighborhood in the United States. The bulk of it, north of Claiborne Avenue, is abandoned, heavily blighted, with intermittent areas serving as dumping grounds. The neighborhood is only at 25 % of its pre-Katrina population. It has become a paradigmatic example of geography of trouble—a place of widespread suffering (Harvey 2012).

The Lower Ninth, and similar places, shows us that suffering is not distributed evenly across societies (Anderson 2014). It comes to dominate certain places. Here it becomes normative. It is a "characteristic rather than accidental" feature of the environment (Hewitt 1983: 25). And while vulnerability has long been associated with particular places, the idea that certain geographies are marked as places of violence (Parenti 2011) or trouble is fairly new.

And yet rather than a culture of silence (Beamish 2000) developing, where peril is treated as an open secret involving a style of mental focusing that relegates the potential for peril to the background, in places like the Lower Ninth Ward suffering becomes the dominant framework for making sense of life. And rather than seeing the Lower Ninth Ward as "an archipelago of isolated misfortunes" (Hewitt 1983: 12), suffering is seen as constituting the social order itself (Laska and Morrow 2006; Wisner et al. 1976).

An important note needs to be made here. To be sure, residents have been made to suffer. This has come at the hands of the state—either unintentionally through everyday bureaucratic structures (Das and Kleinman 2001; Kleinman 2000), what results in "lumpen-abuse" (Bourgois and Schonberg 2009). I am not blaming residents of New Orleans for their suffering. Rather, much like Scott's (1985) weapons of the weak, I simply argue that residents have specific cultural tools that are deployed as cultural acts of mitigating their suffering, but also as acceptance. While much work in the post-Katrina period has documented particular conditions that cause suffering, this chapter is an attempt to document how residents deal with their suffering. Below I describe, in brief, two of these cultural tools.

20.2.1 *Diffuse Empathy*

People who experience trauma are drawn to others who have had similar experiences (Erikson 1994). Disasters have a way of bringing people together and facilitating the formation of new groups. Fritz (1996) notes that these new groups are not limited by preexisting social or geographical constraints. The disaster experience is itself enough to form new bonds. In the aftermath of the BP catastrophe, residents of the Lower Ninth Ward sought out likeminded others to help them make sense of the outcomes for their community.

Sandy's description, immediately below, of the first community meeting after the BP oil spill is significant, as many of the communities she mentions competed for resources after Katrina. Residents of the Lower Ninth Ward think that others, such as those in the neighboring St. Bernard Parish, received far more aid than they. But in the BP disaster and subsequent environmental threats, different communities came together to disseminate information and compare notes.

> And I looked around that room and Cecil B. DeMille, Frank Capra, it was like a Frank Capra thing, Lisa Jackson is in the front of the room with some other folk, there were people from the neighborhood, people from the North Shore, people from the Parish, people from further over…people from Houma Nation, there were people in, umm, work clothes, people who were clearly, uhh, I don't know like for example if they were from Lafourche or Thibodaux, or New Orleans East, but there were representatives of the Vietnamese community, and you looked around that room and people that were gathered together, and they were like having a pretty civil conversation… and it was like yeah, we can do this, we've done this before. Everyone in this room is a survivor. (Sandy, white female, 50s)

Suffering in the Lower Ninth was also a way of bringing people into or back to the community.

> We didn't live here before Katrina, so I don't know what it was like. We lived all over New Orleans before, but after, we came here and decided to stay. There was just something about this place. Like it shouldn't exist or something. You just wanted to help out, to pull for it. We moved here to be part of something larger.... It was like I can live in the Marigny and worry about the color of my house or my car getting hit or I can move to the Lower Ninth and do something worthwhile. (Terri, white female, 30s).

> I don't think we would have come back. I mean we have rental property here, so we would still be invested in the community. But if this had been any other place we wouldn't be back. I wouldn't be at these meetings or doing the [block cleaning] sweeps or… I wouldn't care. There's just something about the place, it's like the underdog thing, this place keeps taking a beating, but it just gets right back up. (Tim, white male, 50s)

Several residents mentioned how they thought about moving before Katrina and now would never consider leaving. A chemical release at the Chalmette refinery, a few miles away from the community, visibly increased participation at the neighborhood association meeting for several weeks as members "welcomed back" residents who had stopped coming to the meetings.

Cognitive scientists have found that if we are in pain we are likely to give more attention to others in pain or to information representing a painful condition (Pincus and Morley 2001). In a culture of suffering we could expect that this bias towards others would be extreme. After the Japanese tsunami and nuclear disaster, many residents, assuming I would know, asked what they could do to help. Several Japanese flags were flown throughout the Ninth Ward and donations were collected at bars and cafes. Likewise, volunteer organizations and non-profits in the Lower Ninth Ward were regularly visited by international delegations, such as from Haiti and Africa. These groups were drawn to the community as they felt that residents could offer strategies for helping them work through their own suffering. In each case residents empathized with these groups and formed long distance relationships with them.

In the Lower Ninth, suffering is understood as something that happens to everyone. Members of the community make sense of the failing infrastructure, industrial accidents, or flooding as things that just happen.

> D.H.: Did you think about staying in Texas after Katrina?

> B.D.: Heck no! They got hurricanes there too. And tornadoes. We were in Dallas and turned on the TV and watched Rita. Those poor people. It's dangerous everywhere, baby. You got earthquakes in California…earth just opens up and swallows you. You don't recover from that…terrorists in New York. Everyday you got to worry about something. No, everybody got their problems…so why not come back? (Mary, black female, 50s)

Ms. Mary and several other residents envisioned people in other places as suffering as much as those in the Lower Ninth Ward. Their empathy for others' suffering let them see their experiences as normal. Residents sometimes looked for suffering elsewhere to confirm their worldview.

> Nah, they suffering in other Parishes too. It ain't just us. I went to a meeting uptown the other day at Loyola and they talked about the BP spill. It was mainly women and family members of shrimpers and other people. Lots of those folks just now got over Katrina, you know, got their, umm, business and stuff back to normal, and now, and with the recession, they got hit with that too. It's tough. So, no I wouldn't say we're any different. (Steven, white male, 40s)

> Japan, I mean that's tough. Compared to what we went through, no, it don't compare at all. I mean they got the nuclear thing to deal with. That makes it much worse. People will be sick with that for a long time. They can't just go to the next parish or, you know, to family, like in another part of the state. That whole place is gone. People just left [to] deal with [the] scraps. We were better off, most of us, afterward. But they'll be okay. Watch, they'll be back on their feet just like us. (Robert, black male, 50s)

Both Steven and Robert were responding to a query to compare the problems in the Lower Ninth to other communities. Despite neither being back in their homes, they both felt that others in similar situations were actually worse off. The suffering of others made them feel like their community was, as one resident said, "on the right track," Here the empathy is spread out or diffused over other communities to make the experiences of those who live in the Lower Ninth Ward normal.

One of last interviews I did in New Orleans was with a political activist who after 6 years was still struggling to get back into his home in the Lower Ninth. He had just moved from Houston and was living in an apartment in Metairie, just outside of the City, so he could be closer to contractors, volunteers, etc. When I went to his apartment to speak with him we spoke for several hours about disasters and suffering, but the disaster was a tornado and the suffering was in Joplin, Mo. The interview became unfeasible because he only wanted to watch and talk about the news coverage of Joplin. Parts of the conversation, however, are very illustrative of using diffuse empathy to understand one's own suffering.

> T.B.: This is crazy. It looks just like NOLA [New Orleans, La.]. I keep thinking I'm gonna see my house. These people, I feel sorry for these people because they don't know what's coming. They think this is bad...walking around looking for your stuff. That ain't nothing. Wait until they have to call insurance or wait until the government gets involved, because that's when it's gonna get bad. These people, my heart goes out to them because that was me.... But they'll do what they have to do.
>
> D.H.: You think the Lower Ninth was different because of race....
>
> T.B: No. I mean, I hear what you saying. No. It's bad all over. I know lots of white people that ain't made it home. They just like me. They struggling, they's trying. These people [on television] ain't black and look what happened to them.
>
> D.H.: But maybe they'll rebuild quicker or get more help...
>
> T.B.: Nah, it's just messed up. That's the way it is. Some of them might have more money or whatever and get back, but look, I mean, that's they [sic] whole place like that. It's just like everyone gotta deal with that at some time in they lives. (Tony, black male, 50s)

This tactic of making sense of suffering is similar to those found in other marginalized neighborhoods where residents believe that whites simply live in equally bad ghettos (Young 2006). Residents of the Lower Ninth see people in diverse contexts or places suffering just like them, even when they are not. This helps them make sense of and mitigate their suffering.

While residents engaged in a number of tactics to deal with their suffering, most were aimed at assuaging themselves and other community members that their experiences and the level of suffering present in the community would likely be similar in other communities. This helped them confirm their decision to return to and rebuild their community, but it also lessened the exceptionalism with which others talked about or approached the community. In order to move on from Hurricane Katrina (and also make sense of the socio-economic and political abandonment of their community) residents needed to believe that people elsewhere were dealing with similar problems.

20.2.2   Boundary Making

Separating society into "us versus them" allowed some residents to build a simple cognitive model of the neighborhood in a time when such models were in flux. It was a path to restoring one's ontological security that was familiar—as most residents had fought to integrate portions of the neighborhood in the 1960s and had thus already struggled with "us and them" categories, but it was also familiar in that it allowed residents to put people they were uncomfortable with or suspicious of outside of the bounds of their community. This process has much in common with Anderson's (1983) imagined communities in that it is based on the mental images that community members have of themselves and their community rather than the actual day-to-day interactions they might have had with community members.

The separation of individuals and groups in to "us" and "them" categories often came about as information was sought or shared. Answers to the question, what is to be done, were frequently regarded as coming from "outsiders" if the solutions were unpopular with some of the residents. At one community meeting a resident threw her hands up and bemoaned "outsiders" trying to fix her neighborhood. She stormed away, only to turn around and yell, "You get to go home at night!" Her point was difficult to ignore, as many of those attempting to solve the social ills of the neighborhood were not living in the neighborhood. Other residents would frequently ask the opinions of long-term volunteers, those of us who had been in the community for several months, only to disparage our responses by claiming insider knowledge of the community's problems. At several meetings I was asked to leave the room or a decision might be tabled until, as one president of a neighborhood association noted, "It's just *us* here". In asking people for interviews or talking with people about my research, I would regularly hear: "So you not from here"; "Oh, you moved before Katrina"; "You not really one of us"; or "You white, so I knew you wasn't from the Lower Nine." But this was not limited to newcomers. One couple, whom I visited with almost weekly for a few months, lamented that they had only been living in the neighborhood for 20–25 years and hence weren't really from there and thus couldn't tell me much about the Lower Ninth Ward.

Sue spoke of how difficult negotiating these boundaries were for her. "There are certain ways of thinking things that we just don't do, or don't know about. People here think and see things in New Orleans in a different light then they do in the neighborhood where we lived. If you don't, and we definitely don't most of the time, it marks you as not from here." Sue, who is on a number of committees, said that she has a tendency to "sit on her hands" in most meetings—depending on whether there is a majority of "outsiders" or not—as there often is. "It's difficult," she continued, "because I'm a talker, as you know, but early on I would just say things and later on be called for it, and I spent more time defending what I said than actually doing anything. I was told several times that I didn't get it because I was from Mid-City."

During times of uncertainty we tend to respond negatively to criticisms of people we see as being similar to us and to respond positively to criticisms of those who are not like us (Holbrook et al. 2011). In general, we become biased towards those groups we perceive being part of when we feel attacked or threatened. This response seems universal, as it ranges from 9/11 to more micro-events like bullying or scapegoating. The defense of our imagined communities fosters social support and reduces anxiety by allowing us to maintain our perceived cultural values. Here suffering is owned. Residents became experts on suffering by refusing the interrogation by outsiders of the conditions of their suffering.

Another way boundary maintenance resulted in "us" and "them" categories to help make sense of suffering was to see the neighborhood as being at odds with the rest of the city.

> They don't like us. Never have. I mean I don't know if they dynamited us or not, but look at us. The city done this to us one way or another. It looks like Beirut or Baghdad. This ain't America. And people drive by or come by on the tour buses and they think this happened

all at once, but this is years, man. I mean, come on. This don't happen all at once. It takes years of neglect for this to happen. And you drive around the city. We're the only ones like this. I don't know why. It ain't about race, most of New Orleans is black, was black, before you know, and it will be again, I don't care what they say. But I don't know why they city does this to us (Andy, white male 50s).

This act of boundary maintenance prevented some from leaving the neighborhood. Darren, with whom I worked for 14 months rebuilding houses, refused to go into certain neighborhoods in New Orleans. He explained it as "people knowing where I'm from" or "not being comfortable in those places." When he absolutely had to do so, to register for housing services or other mundane bureaucratic exercises, he would ask me to drive him. But he would still be apprehensive as we drove through "those" neighborhoods. It was not the case that the racial demographics or the socio-economic levels of the surrounding neighborhoods were that different from the Lower Ninth Ward, he simply felt uncomfortable being out of his neighborhood. For Darren being from the least recovered neighborhood made other places different—even though they seemed similar to outsiders. Despite having lived in New Orleans his entire life, these once familiar neighborhoods now seemed impossible for him to navigate. It was as if they were painful reminders of just how far the Lower Ninth had to go to recover.

Perhaps the most visible way that boundary maintenance was used to mitigate suffering was to cognitively separate those portions of the neighborhood that had not recovered from those that were doing well.

> This section is doing well. I mean we're not all back. We saw that yesterday working [when we boarded up some neighboring homes], but this part is good. It's kind of its own little, a little place of its own, separate from everything else, from what's going on out there. It affects us. But not as much as if we were in it. I mean you know it [the neighborhood's problems] is out there, but they don't affect us as much here. (Gloria, black female, 60s)

This also took the form of not wanting to know what was going on elsewhere in the community. When asked how the neighborhood was doing Henri spoke of his two neighbors and a house "over there." Commenting on the safety of the neighborhood, Henri said he knew there were some problems *somewhere* in the neighborhood, but that *this* street was fine. Likewise, a good friend of mine, Lee, who regularly rode his bicycle more than 30 miles a day through the city and surrounding parishes, admitted one day when his bike was broken and he was forced to walk through the neighborhood, that he had been consciously avoiding certain streets so that he could keep a positive attitude about the rebuilding process.

20.3   Conclusion

In this chapter I looked at a particular geography where suffering is, in the words of one resident, "something we do." Residents of the Lower Ninth Ward have become accustomed to living with catastrophe. The various mechanisms of urban marginality, the ecological harm that comes from living in an area known to environmentalists as Cancer Alley, the sordid history of race relations, and the disastrous conditions stemming from the long-term aftermath of Hurricane Katrina have produced a set of lived experiences where suffering is normative. While the Lower Ninth Ward is a unique place, we might expect to find similar strategies of suffering in communities caught in civil wars, in border towns or divided cities, or in any other highly marginalized neighborhoods.

The two cultural tools discussed in this chapter simultaneously highlight the geographical aspect of suffering. Diffuse empathy allowed residents to connect their suffering to others while maintaining distance from them. Boundary-making allowed residents to own their suffering. Both, however, allowed residents to make sense of the aftermath of Katrina. These tools represent part of a larger cultural framework that has grown out of adapting to the suffering produced by constant disruption.

The response to regular hazards is an adaptive tool kit (Dyer 2002). While Dyer and others argue against the ability to use adaptive strategies after events like Katrina, the cumulative effect of living in a geography of trouble is that suffering is expected. Residents build a collective toolkit that allows them to deal with myriad causes of suffering. Hoffman described recovery from disasters as a tram hurtling over the cultural landscape (1999: 142). In places like the Lower Ninth the tram has tracks.

References

Anderson, B. (1983). *Imagined communities: Reflections on the origin and spread of nationalism*. New York: Verso.

Anderson, R. E. (2014). *Human suffering and quality of life: Conceptualizing stories and statistics*. New York: Springer.

Auyero, J., & Swistun, D. (2007). Confused because exposed: Towards an ethnography of environmental suffering. *Ethnography, 8*, 123–144.

Auyero, J., & Swistun, D. (2009). *Flammable: Environmental suffering in an Argentine shantytown*. Oxford: University of Oxford Press.

Beamish, T. (2000). Accumulating trouble: Complex organization, a culture of silence, and a secret spill. *Social Problems, 47*, 473–498.

Bourgois, P., & Schonberg, J. (2009). *Righteous dopefiend*. Berkeley: University of California Press.

Chaiken, S., & Trope, Y. (1999). *Dual-process theories in social psychology*. New York: Guilford.

Colten, C. (2005). *An unnatural metropolis: Wrestling New Orleans from nature*. Baton Rouge: Louisiana State University Press.

Das, V., & Kleinman, A. (2001). Introduction. In V. Das, A. Kleinman, M. Lock, & P. Reynolds (Eds.), *Remaking a world: Violence, social suffering, and recovery* (pp. 1–30). Berkeley: University of California Press.

Davies, J. (2011). Positive and negative models of suffering: An anthropology of our shifting cultural consciousness of emotional discontent. *Anthropology of Consciousness, 22*, 188–208.

DeGloma, T. (2009). Expanding trauma through space and time: Mapping the rhetorical strategies of trauma carrier groups. *Social Psychology Quarterly, 72*, 105–122.

Dyer, C. L. (2002). Punctuated entropy as culture-induced change: The case of the Exxon Valdez oil spill. In S. Hoffman & A. Oliver-Smith (Eds.), *Catastrophe and culture: The anthropology of disaster* (pp. 159–186). Santa Fe: School of America Research Press.

Erikson, K. (1976). *Everything in its path: Destruction of community in the Buffalo Creek flood.* New York: Simon and Schuster.

Erikson, K. (1994). *A new species of trouble: The human experience of modern disasters.* New York: W.W. Norton & Company.

Fritz, C. (1996). *Disasters and mental health: Therapeutic principles drawn from disaster studies* (Historical and comparative disaster series no. 10). Newark: University of Delaware Research Center.

Gill, D. (2007). Secondary trauma or secondary disaster: Insights from Hurricane Katrina. *Sociological Spectrum, 27*, 613–632.

Harvey, D. C. (2012). A new geography of trouble. In L. A. Eargle & A. M. Esmail (Eds.), *Black beaches and bayous: The BP Deepwater Horizon oil spill disaster* (pp. 119–133). New York: University Press of America.

Hewitt, K. (1983). The idea of calamity in a technocratic age. In K. Hewitt (Ed.), *Interpretations of calamity* (pp. 3–32). Boston: Allen and Unwin Inc.

Hoffman, S. (1999). The worst of times, the best of times: Toward a model of cultural response to disaster. In A. Oliver-Smith & S. Hoffman (Eds.), *The angry earth: Disaster in anthropological perspective* (pp. 134–155). New York: Routledge.

Holbrook, C., Sousa, P., & Hahn-Holbrook, J. (2011). Unconscious vigilance: Worldview defense without adaptations for terror, coalition, or uncertainty management. *Journal of Personality and Social Psychology, 101*, 451–466.

Honkasalo, M. L. (2009). Grips and ties: Agency, uncertainty, and the problem of suffering in North Karelia. *Medical Anthropology Quarterly, 23*, 51–69.

Janes, C. R. (1999). Imagined lives, suffering, and the work of culture: The embodied discourses of conflict in modern Tibet. *Medical Anthropology Quarterly, 13*, 391–412.

Kleinman, A. (2000). The violences of everyday life: The multiple forms and dynamics of social violence. In V. Das, A. Kleinman, & M. Ramphele (Eds.), *Violence and subjectivity* (pp. 226–241). Berkeley: University of California Press.

Laska, S., & Morrow, B. H. (2006). Social vulnerabilities and Hurricane Katrina: An unnatural disaster in New Orleans. *Marine Technology Society Journal, 40*, 7–17.

Leavitt, S. (1995). Suppressed meanings in narratives about suffering: A case from Papua New Guinea. *Anthropology and Humanism Quarterly, 20*, 133–152.

Lerner, S. (2005). *Diamond: A struggle for environmental justice in Louisiana's chemical corridor.* Cambridge, MA: The MIT Press.

Parenti, C. (2011). *Tropics of chaos: Climate change and the new geography of violence.* New York: Nation Books.

Pincus, T., & Morley, S. (2001). Cognitive-processing bias in chronic pain: A review. *Psychological Bulletin, 127*, 599–617.

Quesada, J. (1999). From Central American warriors to San Francisco Latino day laborers: Suffering and exhaustion in a transnational context. *Transforming Anthropology, 8*, 162–185.

Roberts, J. T., & Toffolon-Weiss, M. (2001). *Chronicles from the environmental justice frontline.* New York: Cambridge University Press.

Schwarz, N. (1998). Accessible content and accessibility experiences: The interplay of declarative and experiential information in judgment. *Personality and Social Psychology Review, 2*, 87–99.

Scott, J. C. (1985). *Weapons of the weak: Everyday forms of peasant resistance.* New Haven: Yale University Press.

Sullivan, S. C. (2011). *Living faith: Everyday religion and mothers in poverty.* Chicago: The University of Chicago Press.

Swidler, A. (1986). Culture in action: Symbols and strategies. *American Sociological Review, 51*, 273–286.

Vaisey, S. (2008). Socrates, Skinner, and Aristotle: Three ways of thinking about culture in action. *Sociological Forum, 23*(3), 603–613.

Vaisey, S. (2009). Motivation and justification: A dual-process model of culture in action. *American Journal of Sociology, 114*, 1675–1715.

Wisner, B., O'Keefe, P., & Westgate, K. (1976). Poverty and disaster. *New Society, 9*, 546–548.

Young, A., Jr. (2006). *The minds of marginalized black men: Making sense of mobility, opportunity, and future life chances*. Princeton: Princeton University Press.

Chapter 21
Social Organization of Suffering and Justice-Seeking in a Tragic Day Care Fire Disaster

Eric C. Jones and Arthur D. Murphy

21.1 Introduction

On June 5, 2009, a fire in the ABC Day Care Center killed 49 of the approximately 162 children and left at least 40 others hospitalized for burns and smoke inhalation in Hermosillo, state of Sonora, Mexico. The tragic news swept the country like a shock wave. Within hours, people were demanding answers to questions including the cause of the fire, who was responsible, and how the disaster could have been avoided. The tragedy lingers in the minds of Hermosillo residents the way 9/11 does in the minds of New Yorkers. Losing a young child is an extraordinarily difficult experience for a parent (Murphy et al. 1999, 2002); losing many children in one community is devastating for many. The loss is made all the more intense when the deaths seem to have been human-caused (Wortman et al. 1997).

ABC Day Care was licensed by the Mexican Social Insurance System (*Instituto Mexicano de Seguro Social*, known in Mexico by its acronym "IMSS") but owned by family members of high-ranking political officials (common in many industries in Mexico). The tragedy and its links to ranking officials in the city, state, and nation resulted in calls for justice that continue to this day.

In the 5 years since the fire, marches, candlelight vigils, memorials, lawsuits, judicial inquiries, and arrests of minor officials have become more frequent. The ABC Day Care was located in the south eastern quadrant of Hermosillo, but drew

E.C. Jones (✉)
Faculty of School of Public Health, University of Texas-Houston,
El Paso, TX 79902, USA
e-mail: Eric.C.Jones@uth.tmc.edu

A.D. Murphy
Department of Anthropology, UNC Greensboro, Greensboro,
NC 27412-5001, USA
e-mail: admurphy@uncg.edu

© Springer Science+Business Media Dordrecht 2015
R.E. Anderson (ed.), *World Suffering and Quality of Life*,
Social Indicators Research Series 56, DOI 10.1007/978-94-017-9670-5_21

clients from the entire city. Consequently, most parents and caretakers from the ABC Day Care did not know each other before the fire. However, in the months and years since the event, an elaborate web of personal, political, commemorative, work, and even social media relationships has developed among parents and caretakers of the children who attended the day care. This is now a network connecting nearly three-quarters of the several hundred parents and caretakers together. Members are divided into four distinct, named groups or sub-networks, are aware of one another, like and dislike one another, rely on one another, fashion meaning out of their suffering, and seek justice in myriad ways.

The quest for meaning and justice in the context of bereavement and related suffering is a complex process (Neimeyer 2015). The concept of *justice* (justice) in Hermosillo is conceived and leveraged differently by members of each of several ABC community subgroups, the people who interact but are not members, and non-connected parents and caretakers. Our interviews with individuals in named subgroups indicate that each group uses the principle of *justicia* to organize their efforts, find meaning in the event, and redefine their relationships to family, other parents and caretakers, and the larger society. While there is some discussion in the disaster and environmental justice literature of how groups seek justice in the wake of disaster (sometimes referred to as reparative justice) there is little work on how these groups emerge, stay together, and transform one another in the grieving and justice-seeking process.

21.2   Methodology

With funding from the United States National Institute of Mental Health, our team carried out structured psychological and social network interviews with 226 parents and caretakers from 95 of the 134 families affected by the fire (related to 106 of the 162 children). We studied how grief varies among people involved (males/females, mothers/fathers, parents/caretakers, parents of deceased/ injured), and how individuals differed in their responses to intense grief that lasts longer than 6 months—referred to as complicated or prolonged grief (Prigerson et al. 2009). The full interviews were conducted from January to April 2010, and then January to April 2011 (8 and 20 months after the fire). This allowed us to capture changes in psychological symptoms as well as changes in social relationships between parents and caretakers. Among other measures, the interview instrument used standard scales to test for symptoms of Post-Traumatic Stress Disorder (WHO 1997) and Prolonged Grief Disorder (Prigerson et al. 2009). Following our analysis of network and well-being data, we conducted several semi-structured interviews with parents and caretakers. We reviewed government reports, the Mexico Supreme Court ruling, and other judicial reports, news items and academic reports on the fire, as cited in this chapter.

21.3   The Fire

At approximately 2:15 in the afternoon on June 5, 2009, sirens began to wail through the capital city of the state of Sonora, Mexico. Before long, word spread of a fire in a day care center in the southern part of Hermosillo. Ambulances, fire equipment, police vehicles, and parents converged on the ABC Day Care, where black smoke billowed from the building. Teachers, first responders, parents, and bystanders attempted to rescue children from the flames. Hector Ramirez drove his truck into the side of the building, opening large holes to aid in the effort (Ramirez became a hero in Hermosillo, and the local Chevrolet dealership replaced his truck with a new one). Parents ran from ambulance to ambulance looking for their children. The more fortunate found their children among the unhurt in what became known as the "green" house—a home a block from the fire where children released by the paramedics were taken to be claimed by family members.

Others began an agonizing search through the hospitals and clinics where the children were being treated. Emergency rooms were overwhelmed by the number of patients as doctors and nurses struggled to save as many as they could. One parent described walking into the emergency room: "I looked in and saw two doctors working on a child. They were both praying as they tried to save him. I did not know doctors prayed" (in Murphy 2009).

In an effort to organize the process, parents wore tags with the name of their child so staff could notify them easily if their child was identified. For many, it would be late on the morning of June 6 before they knew the fate of their children. In the end, 49 children died from their injuries and close to 100 had suffered minor burns, smoke inhalation, or severe burns over 85 % of their body. The most severely injured were taken for treatment to Shriner's Hospitals in Sacramento, California, and Cincinnati, Ohio.

Early reports suggested the fire began in a tire store next to the ABC Day Care Center, but attention soon focused on a government warehouse attached to the day care. Suspicion also arose as to the ownership of the center and its safety. If, as Seguro Social claimed, ABC had recently passed a safety inspection, some argued, how could such a tragedy have occurred? Why were the emergency exits locked? Why was a flammable false ceiling permitted in the building? More liberal members of the political elite in Hermosillo and nationally asked how Seguro Social—which had previously run these day care centers as a public service—could turn the care of children over to a capitalistic enterprise. As people sought answers and justice, focus shifted to the owners of the center and to the privatization of the public day care center system.

Nearly 5 years later, the impact of this fire is still evident throughout the community. There are three formal memorials to the children, one at the site of the fire and two in major public plazas. At each, 49 crosses include a child's name, often accompanied by a poster-sized photo of the child's face. In the plaza in front of the cathedral, 49 white crosses memorialize the "angelitos"—little angels in heaven. Many of the children were buried side by side in elaborate graves in the municipal cemetery. Even more striking are the billboards around the city with a deceased child's photo and a call for justice. Marches and demonstrations are commonplace.

The event has caused Mexico to reconsider its policy of franchising federally funded day care centers. On the day of our departure from a visit to Hermosillo in September 2010, a group of mothers holding placards of children's faces and the word "justice" blocked the entrance to the airport. Each year on the June 5th anniversary of the fire, several thousand community members march from the site to the downtown Plaza de Emiliana de Zubeldia. Seguro Social has stated that they have cancelled the contracts of 111 their 1,451 licensed day cares across Mexico (Latin America Herald Tribune 2011), and a comprehensive national law on child development was passed in mid-2011 because of the demands of, and issues highlighted by, parents and caretakers.

21.4   Structural Adjustment and the Privatization of Day Care in Mexico

In 1973, the law governing Seguro Social (Mexican Institute for Social Insurance) established day care up to age four as a right for all mothers working in the formal sector. Unlike many countries with similar social guarantees, Mexico undertook the route of direct provision through centers run by Seguro Social. By the mid-1990s, Seguro Social operated 497 day care centers through the country, caring for fewer than 60,000 children, about 5 % of those eligible (Knaul and Parker 1996; Staab and Gerhard 2010).

In 1997, as part of the reforms of the Zedillo administration (1994–2000), Seguro Social undertook a process of expanding its services through agreements with government-subsidized private day care providers (*guarderías subrogadas*) that would be funded and regulated by IMSS. By 2007, around 1,500 IMSS-regulated private day care centers served over 200,000 children in Mexica. This figure represents almost 20 % of the target population of children between age 43 days and 4 years whose mothers work in the formal sector (Staab and Gerhard 2010: 8). This rapid expansion took place without a concomitant rise in the ability of Seguro Social to carry out inspections, thus raising questions as to the standards set by Seguro Social and its ability to monitor and enforce regulations (Leal 2009). These issues were brought to full national attention by Hermosillo fire, 1 month ahead of gubernatorial elections in the state of Sonora.

21.5   Finding Meaning in the Call for Justice

The results from our two waves of network and wellbeing questionnaires and our subsequent qualitative ethnographic interviews indicate there is a need to understand the pathways these parents and caretakers of dead and injured children are taking to finding meaning and *justicia* after the event. The results suggest the primary paths parents used to find meaning after the event are: political activity seeking culpability; demanding compensation; interacting with other parents; dwelling on the event and generally languishing—in some cases allowing social relationships to deteriorate; and ignoring the event without engaging other parents and caretakers any more or less than before. Many attempted to reach out to others despite the depression and grief, not unlike Buffalo Creek, Love Canal, Exxon Valdez, 9/11, and the BP Gulf blow out (see for example, Erikson 1972; Schneider and McCumber 2004; Everest 1986; Brown and Mikkelsen 1990). Raphael (1986: 172) discusses similar states from a psychological perspective for victims of disasters.

In *Man's Search for Meaning*, Viktor Frankl (1992 [1946]) claimed that people can create meaning from trauma through work, love, and struggle. They can work to imagine a better future and struggle to build new meaning socially through story-telling, music, dance, religious ritual, funerary ritual, gathering of kin, cooking, serving others, and forgiveness (Touissant et al. 2010; Kalayjian et al. 2010). Indeed, grief involves attempting to discover new meaning and subsequent closure from suffering of a loss (Neimeyer 2015). The new meaning comes only after a long social process of acknowledgement, validation, reparation, facing negative perceptions, facing denial, gaining acceptance, and forgiveness (Kalayjian et al. 2010). Johnston (2015) notes, following Comas-Diaz (2012), that a next step in supporting mental health is to build on current recognition of individual, familial, and social and include societal aspects of wellbeing in the form of social justice.

There are relatively few examples in academic literature on groups forming after a disaster. In Argentina, mothers met regularly in the Plaza de Mayo seeking resolution for the disappearance of their loved ones at the hands of the dictatorships of the 1970s. They regularly held marches to denounce limited political freedoms, highlight their losses, and demand the punishment of those responsible for the disappearances (Kordon et al. 1988). The Bhopal chemical disaster also produced groups that mourned loved ones and sought accountability (Lapierre and Moro 2002; Fortun 2001; Mukherjee 2010). There is work on oil spills (e.g., Picou et al. 2004) that has generated insights into the negative aspects (i.e., secondary trauma) of getting involved with justice seeking. Indeed, Picou and colleagues point to the ways this justice seeking can create corrosive communities.

Danieli (2009) compared the search for reparative justice among Holocaust survivors' to many other cases of genocide and justice seeking by survivors. Danieli did not address the negative aspects of justice seeking, but noted its importance as a collective process in which there is sharing of grief, mourning, and. The larger community's consciousness is transformed; it will not forget the trauma.

Similar to other tragedies, the victims' individual responses in Hermosillo ranged from wanting to be left alone to go on with their lives, to making any variety of the following demands: retribution for responsible parties (e.g., lose license, lose job, fines, incarceration, public shame), medical support for living children, monetary compensation, political reform to eliminate corruption, regulatory reform, and safety improvements (see also Erikson 1972; Wagner 2008; Oliver-Smith 2002). For many, the fact that Seguro Social subsidized the day care center and was the governing authority over its safety meant the Mexican Government was responsible for taking care of the injured children and for indemnifying parents. In a process not unlike that described by Scheper-Hughes and Bourgois (2004) when discussing responses to political violence, some victims returned to a mindset that existed when Partido Revolucionario Institucional (PRI) was hegemonic, calling for the removal of those responsible from office. These calls were amplified as state elections would take place within a month of the fire. The main opposition party in Hermosillo, Partido Acción Nacional (PAN), seized on the issues to discredit PRI, which had held power in Sonora since 1929. The backlash from the fire effectively placed PAN in control of State Government.

21.6   Social Organization of Suffering and Political Action

In this study, we use social network analysis to capture the interdependence of survivors in their suffering. Two pieces of background information are important. First, parents had few if any substantive relationships with one another before the fire. They largely dropped children off and picked them up at this large day care center, chosen mainly because of its convenience to factories and other places of work. Second, child outcomes were virtually random. Whether a child lived or died in the fire was a consequence of chance, wholly undetermined by parental factors. In our interviews with 203 parents and caretakers, we asked them to name up to seven other people who had children in the day care at the time of the fire. We accepted answers like "Delfina's mom," since we were able to discern the identity of each individual was. Some interviewees could not name other parents at all. The network analyses yielded interesting findings relevant to understanding the emergence of community after mass trauma.

First, though most of the parents did not know each other before the fire, they could name other ABC parents in our interviews 8 months later. They were able to elaborate upon the kinds of relationships that had developed as a result of the fire. Mothers and fathers (mothers, particularly) were more active in relationships with others in the ABC community than were other caregivers (Norris 2012).

Next, almost a year after the event, two distinct groups of parents had emerged. These mapped closely to which parents had lost a child. Our survey and ethnographic research found that meaning in the form of seeking *justicia* varied between these groups. Parents with injured children were mostly concerned with ensuring long-term care and compensation for the injured children; parents who had lost children were more concerned with finding the relevant parties and holding them accountable. Some wanted compensation, while others emphasized awareness and prevention of another tragedy. A year later (20–23 months) after the fire, these two spheres of interaction had clearly split into four. Each of the original two groups split into a more active political subgroup and a less political subgroup.

Additionally, network participation was significantly and positively associated with distress. We measured this by finding the volume of social ties defined by how many people the interviewees could name, how often. The severity of Post-

Traumatic Stress Symptoms was a significant predictor of number of ties per individual in the overall sample, as was grief in a separate analysis of just the bereaved parents and caretakers (Norris 2012).

Finally, network participation was unrelated to perceptions of social support or social constraints. Many studies in trauma and social support suggest that social support from family and friends can help alleviate bereavement-related distress, but the research also shows that bereaved persons confront "social constraints" and "social ineptitudes" that can heighten or maintain their distress. Often unintentionally, those who would normally provide emotional support to the parent fail to do so in the case of a child's death—they are too uncomfortable. Further, the suffering of aunts, uncles, and grandparents is often underestimated or ignored by both formal and informal supports.

21.7 The Political Economy of Justice Seeking

Previous research on the design and building of public memorials indicates they are often the catalyst for fractures and divisions within grieving groups (Dwyer 2010; Wagner 2010; Sturken 2004). In the case of Hermosillo, the process was confounded by informal memorials that sprang up in front of the burned day care building, the cathedral, and the Plaza de Emiliana de Zubeldia in front of the University of Sonora. Each was the result of a constituency that found meaning in the event in a particular fashion and had its own concepts of *justicia* and commemoration. The "official" monument was built by the State Government in the City of Obregon, some 280 km (3.5 h) south of Hermosillo. Also, a memorial mural was painted his year in a community 80 km from Hermosillo. The mural depicted eight of the children being blessed by Jesus in heaven. Many wondered why *all* the children were not depicted.

Among the parents and caregivers, two major issues appear to define the groups that formed after the fire. The first is the question of medical support vs. indemnification. Parents of living injured children feared the short- and long-term impact of the fire on the health of their children; they wanted assurances that those responsible would pay for their care. In the short term, there was the question of immediate care for the critically injured. The Mexican government, through Seguro Social, ensured that severely injured children received the best care available to them either in Hermosillo, Mexico City, or the United States. Through UNICEF, Seguro Social also provided psychological counselling for parents (but not other caretakers) and children for the first year after the fire. In the long term, the greater concerns were over the impact of smoke and other injuries and the necessary care that might result. Seguro Social covers only workers employed in the formal sector of the Mexican economy, but a presidential degree provided all the children enrolled in the ABC day care with lifetime access to Seguro Social medical care, regardless of their employment status. In addition, children were granted care and medicines for injuries specific to the fire until age 18 *at a facility of their choice* (not just Seguro Social facilities). Parents who lost a child were indemnified $1,500,000 pesos (USD$150,000+), and women who either lost a child or had an injured child received lifetime disability coverage, paying the equivalent of their profession's minimum wage for life. Our interviews found that most parents were satisfied with those services and indemnifications.

The second issue defining groups that formed after the fire is the question of justice, which has become a primary concern—largely for parents who lost children in the fire. The meaning of *justice* varies considerably in our interviews, however, only some parents and caregivers focused on finding those responsible and bringing them before the legal system and the court of public opinion. While some parents advocate for jail time for those responsible (there is no death penalty in Mexico), most realize that is unlikely. The best they can hope for is the justice of public opinion directed at powerful and influential families they feel are responsible. As one parent expressed:

> We need to know who was responsible. Who paid off an inspector to ignore the problems in the day care? Who ordered the exit doors to be locked? It can't be the two or three minor people they have in jail. It had to be higher up. But, as the lawyer tells us they can't find a judge who will take on the case (parent, in Murphy 2011).

Mexico's justice system is Napoleonic: judges can take on cases and appoint investigators to dig into those like the ABC Day Care fire. This system works well in countries such as France, Spain, and Italy, where an independent judiciary has a tradition of bringing cases before the bench. In Mexico, with the opening of the formal political process and the nation's romance with multi-party democracy, Gutmann (2002) explains that the justice system does not yet seem to have the space, power, or technical capacity to exercise its rightful legal jurisdiction.

The Supreme Court investigated the incident at the ABC Day Care and found infractions had gone unheeded, inspectors had not enforced regulations, and there was a culture of collusion that included functionaries in state government. The Court found 19 local, state, and national functionaries responsible through negligence or unfulfilled duties.

Were the children's human rights violated? This question, addressed by the Supreme Court, confounded the meaning of justice. The court found in a split vote that human rights had not been violated because the fire was an accident; therefore, the Court had no jurisdiction over the case.

Subsequent to the Court's decision, in which a United States consulting firm suggested the fire was an accident started by a malfunctioning air conditioner, another U.S. expert found the fire to have been started by intentional burning of boxes of paper using an accelerant. This finding was confirmed again in mid-2013 through investigator interviews with warehouse workers (it is not uncommon to burn documents between political administrations, because a new administration might bring mid- and lower-level administrators from the previous administration before the Court in order to demonstrate its dedication to reform). In August 2013, a judge ordered the Attorney General to review all of the data in the case again. But the legal culture has not changed: it does not yet make sense to both elites and commoners nor can produce it results (cf. Jones and Murphy 2009). The people still search for varying but distinct forms of *justicia* and meaning, and the repeated litigation and justice-seeking may be viewed as a secondary trauma.

21.8 Conclusions

Everyday violence is usually "invisible or misrecognized" (see Scheper-Hughes 2004). Corrupt justice and political conditions around the world often result in violence and human rights violations, perpetuating the exclusion of the poor from justice (Haugen and Boutros 2014). When this is the, case even the non-poor find themselves excluded from justice and a meaningful resolution after an extreme event. The layers of diffused responsibility created by neo-liberal reforms, particularly in the face of lax or absent regulation, create the political and economic equivalents to the conditions that place the poor in harm's way when natural phenomenon such as hurricanes, floods, and earthquakes strike.

In Mexico, this complex context means tat those who lost loved ones in the ABC Day Care fire have difficulty identifying a focus for their rage and grief (Rosaldo 1989). Some direct their ire at owners, some at Seguro Social (and, by association, the state and federal governments), some at all three. It becomes difficult to assign the blame clearly enough so that any of these parties are held accountable. Many suffering caretakers and parents actually blame themselves for not noting the code violations or safety issues at the day care, for having had to use a day care at all, or for not picking up their child early that day. Their grief is compounded by the difficulty in finding meaning and *justicia*; for its flaws, the one-party system took care of problems politically, not legally. The new multi-party system is perhaps ill-prepared to mete out the justice many seek in this case.

As Grugel and Riggirozzi (2012: 15) point out, much of Latin America is entering a post-neoliberal period in which citizens are working to reclaim the state as a player in the protection of the welfare of its citizens. This is not a return to state capitalism or single-party rule as in the past, but a movement to develop a state that is "better able to defend the public interest" (Grugel and Riggirozzi 2012: 15). The difficulties in prosecuting this case occurred because political institutions such as the courts may not have developed sufficiently to provide the "horizontal forms of accountability, identity politics and voice within a democratic system" (Peruzzotti and Smulovitz 2006). A more established political context might have enabled groups such as these parents and caretakers to express their grief, achieve justicia, and find meaning in their suffering.

The reopening of the case by the Attorney General may indicate a turning point in the Mexican justice system. Yet, a drawn-out case keeps the victims in legal proximity to the perpetrators, something that often maintains rather than heals suffering, as we have seen in the cases protracted U.S. cases regarding the Exxon Valdez tanker spill, Hurricane Katrina's federal response, and the BP Gulf Oil Spill (Jones and Murphy 2009; Dyer 2009; Kalayjian et al. 2010). These cases demonstrate that even a well-developed legal structure in the context of entrenched political or economic interests is often unable to deliver "justice," let alone closure.

References

Brown, P., & Mikkelsen, J. (1990). *No safe place: Toxic waste, leukemia, and community action.* Berkeley: University of California Press.

Comas-Diaz, L. (2012). Psychotherapy as a healing practice, scientific endeavor, and social justice action. *Psychotherapy, 49*(4), 473–474.

Danieli, Y. (2009). Massive trauma and the healing role of reparative justice. *Journal of Traumatic Stress, 22,* 351–357.

Dwyer, L. (2010). Building a monument: Intimate politics of 'reconciliation' in Bali. In A. L. Hinton (Ed.), *Transitional justice: Global mechanisms and local realities after genocide and mass violence* (pp. 227–248). New Brunswick: Rutgers University Press.

Dyer, C. L. (2009). From the phoenix effect to punctuated entropy: The culture of response as a unifying paradigm of disaster mitigation and recovery. In E. C. Jones & D. M. Arthur (Eds.), *The political economy of hazards and disasters* (pp. 313–336). Lanhan: Alta Mira Press.

Erikson, K. T. (1972). *Everything in its path: Destruction of community in the Buffalo Creek flood.* New York: Simon and Schuster.

Everest, L. (1986). *Behind the poison cloud: Union Carbide's Bhopal massacre.* Chicago: Banner Press.

Fortun, K. (2001). *Advocacy after Bhopal: Environmentalism, disaster, new global orders.* Chicago: University of Chicago Press.

Frankl, V. E. (1992 [1952]). *Man's search for meaning.* Boston: Beacon Press.

Grugel, J., & Riggirozzi, P. (2012). Post-neoliberalism in Latin America: Rebuilding and reclaiming the state after crisis. *Development and Change, 43*(1), 1–21.

Gutmann, M. C. (2002). *The romance of democracy: Compliant defiance in contemporary Mexico.* Berkeley: University of California Press.

Haugen, G. A., & Boutros, V. (2014). *The locust effect: Why the end of poverty requires the end of violence.* New York: Oxford University Press.

Johnston, N. E. (2015). Healing suffering: The evolution of caring practices. In R. E. Anderson (Ed.), *World suffering and the quality of life.* New York: Springer.

Jones, E. C., & Murphy, A. D. (Eds.). (2009). *The political economy of hazards and disasters.* Walnut Creek: AltaMira Press.

Kalayjian, A., Moore, N., & Aberson, C. (2010). Exploring long-term impact of mass trauma on physical health, coping, and meaning: An examination of the Ottoman Turkish genocide of the Armenians. In A. Kalayjian & D. Eugene (Eds.), *Mass trauma & emotional healing around the world: Rituals and practices for resilience and meaning-making* (pp. 287–306). New York: ABC-CLIO.

Knaul, F., & Parker, S. (1996). Cuidado infantil y empleo femenino en Mexico: Evidencia descriptiva y consideraciones sobre las politicas. *Estudios Demograficos y Urbanos, 11*(3), 577–607.

Kordon, D., Edelman, L., Lagos, D., Nicoletti, E., & Bozzolo, R. (1988). *Psychological effects of political repression.* Buenos Aires: Sudamericana/Planeta.

Lapierre, D., & Moro, J. (2002). *Five past midnight in Bhopal: The epic story of the world's deadliest industrial disaster.* New York: Warner Books.

Latin American Herald Tribune. (2011). *On anniversary of deadly blaze, Mexico says daycares now safe.* Online [URL] http://laht.com/article.asp?CategoryId=14091&ArticleId=396418. June 6.

Leal, F. G. (2009). *El IMSS bajo el Foxismo.* Mexico City: UAM-Xochimilco.

Mukherjee, S. (2010). *Surviving Bhopal: Dancing bodies, written texts, and oral testimonials of women in the wake of an industrial disaster.* New York: Palgrave Macmillan.

Murphy, A. D. (2009, July). Field notes.

Murphy, A. D. (2011, June). Field notes.

Murphy, S., Braun, T., Tillery, L., Cain, K., Johnson, L. C., & Beaton, R. (1999). PTSD among bereaved parents following the violent deaths of their 12- to 28-year-old children: A longitudinal prospective analysis. *Journal of Traumatic Stress, 12,* 273–291.

Murphy, S. A., Johnson, L. C., & Lohan, J. (2002). The aftermath of the violent death of a child: An integration of the assessments of parents' mental distress and PTSD during the first 5 years of bereavement. *Journal of Loss and Trauma, 7,* 203–222.

Neimeyer, R. A. (2015). Meaning in bereavement. In R. E. Anderson (Ed.), *World suffering and the quality of life.* New York: Springer.

Norris, F. (2012). Four meanings of 'Community' in disaster. In C. S. Widom (Ed.), *Trauma, psychopathology, and violence: Causes, correlates, or consequences* (pp. 161–185). New York: Oxford University Press.

Oliver-Smith, A. (2002). Theorizing disasters: Nature, power, and culture. In S. M. Hoffman & A. Oliver-Smith (Eds.), *Catastrophe and culture: The anthropology of disaster* (pp. 23–47). Santa Fe: School of American Research.

Peruzzotti, E., & Smulovitz, C. (2006). http://www.upress.pitt.edu/htmlSourceFiles/pdfs/9780822958963exr.pdf

Picou, J. S., Marshall, B. K., & Gill, D. A. (2004). Disaster, litigation, and the corrosive community. *Social Forces, 82,* 1493–1522.

Prigerson, H. G., Horowitz, M. J., Jacobs, S. C., Parkes, C. M., Aslan, M., Goodkin, K., Raphael, B., Marwit, S. J., Wortman, C., Neimeyer, R. A., Bonanno, G., Block, S. D., Kissane, D., Boelen, P., Maercker, A., Litz, B. T., Johnson, J. G., First, M. B., & Maciejewski, P. K. (2009). Prolonged grief disorder: Psychometric validation of criteria proposed for DSM-V and ICD-11. *PLoS Medicine, 68,* e1000121. doi:10.1371/journal.pmed.1000121.

Raphael, B. (1986). *When disaster strikes: How individuals and communities cope with catastrophe.* New York: Basic Books.

Rosaldo, R. (1989). *Culture and truth.* Boston: Beacon.

Scheper-Hughes, N. (2004). Bodies, death and silence. In N. Scheper-Huges & P. Bourgois (Eds.), *Violence in war and peace: An anthology* (pp. 175–185). Malden: Blackwell.

Scheper-Hughes, N., & Bourgois, P. (2004). Introduction: Making sense of violence. In N. Scheper-Huges & P. Bourgois (Eds.), *Violence in war and peace: An anthology* (pp. 1–31). Malden: Blackwell.

Schneider, A., & McCumber, D. (2004). *An air that kills: How the asbestos poisoning of Libby, Montana, uncovered a national scandal.* New York: G.P. Putman's Sons.

Staab, S., & Gerhard, R. (2010). *Childcare service expansion in Chile and Mexico: For women or children or both?* (Paper No. 10, Programme on Gender and Development). Geneva: UNRISD.

Sturken, M. (2004). The aesthetics of absence: Rebuilding ground zero. *American Ethnologist, 31*(3), 311–325.

Toussaint, L. L., Peddle, N., Cheadle, A., Sellu, A., & Luskin, F. (2010). Striving for peace through forgiveness in Sierra Leone: Effectiveness of a psychoeducational forgiveness intervention. In A. Kalayjian & D. Eugene (Eds.), *Mass trauma and emotional healing around the world: Rituals and practices for resilience and meaning making. Volume 2, Human made disasters* (pp. 251–267). Santa Barbara: Praeger.

Wagner, S. (2008). *To know where he lies: DNA technology and the search for Srebrenica's missing.* Berkeley: University of California Press.

Wagner, S. (2010). Tabulating loss, entombing memory: The Srebrenica-Potočari memorial center. In E. Anderson, A. Maddrell, K. McLoughlin, & A. Vincent (Eds.), *Memory, mourning, landscape* (pp. 61–78). Amsterdam: Rodopi.

World Health Organization. (1997). *Comprehensive international diagnostic inventory, Version 2.1.* Geneva: World Health Organization.

Wortman, C., Battle, E., & Lemkau, J. (1997). Coming to terms with the sudden, traumatic death of a spouse or child. In R. David, A. Lurigio, & W. Skogan (Eds.), *Victims of crime* (2nd ed., pp. 108–133). Thousand Oaks: Sage.

Chapter 22
Community Quality-of-Life Indicators to Avoid Tragedies

Rhonda Phillips

22.1 Introduction

This chapter explores what can be learned from community indicators of quality of life (QOL) and other community-based approaches to community suffering and resilience. As Berkes (2006) explained, multiple levels of governance and external drivers of change need consideration to begin in order to address these types of questions. Engaging multiple stakeholders, including residents, in community-based planning and responses can lead to more effective construction and use of community quality-of-life indicators as gauges for change (particularly negative change such as that evidenced in tragedies). The resiliency literature provides insights connected to the use of community quality-of-life indicators, while work in disaster management and risk assessment illuminate indicators at the country level (such as the United Nations Development Program's Global Risk Vulnerability Index (United National Development Programme 2014)). Given the lack of local-level application, it is challenging to integrate indicators and related community-based approaches although local providers are the first responders to tragedy, and local governance needs to be an integral part of disaster management, risk assessment, and recovery. The ability of local organizations to respond will influence recovery time, quality, and directly influence residents' decisions after disaster. Thus, as Hahn et al. (2003: 7) point out, countries and communities need to "systemize and harmonize the presentation of risk information from the community level, [and] improve the capacity of decision-makers on local levels to measure key elements of disaster risk."

This piece looks at the connections among disaster management, risk assessment, and tragedy avoidance via use of viable and reliable community quality-of-

R. Phillips (✉)
Professor, Department of Agricultural Economics and Dean, Honors College,
Purdue University, West Lafayette, IN 47906-4238, USA
e-mail: rphillips@purdue.edu

© Springer Science+Business Media Dordrecht 2015
R.E. Anderson (ed.), *World Suffering and Quality of Life*,
Social Indicators Research Series 56, DOI 10.1007/978-94-017-9670-5_22

life indicators, and it includes both natural and anthropogenic (those created by humans) disasters. Drawing on studies about community quality-of-life indicators, I develop foundational concepts and present insights into how communities rebound after disaster and how others might learn how to avoid tragedy and alleviate suffering when it is unavoidable.

22.2   Context

There are several dimensions to address in the context of learning from community indicators of QOL and responses to suffering and resilience. First, I present some foundational concepts of suffering as related to communities. Second, I address the topic of community quality-of-life indicators in the context of the fundamental concepts. Third, I discuss disaster management and risk assessment. Finally, I explore the capacity for community quality-of-life indicators to help alleviate suffering.

22.2.1   *Community Suffering*

As Harvey discusses elsewhere in this volume, suffering can dominate a society. It can even become a distinguishing feature particularly in areas where residents are marginalized socially, economically, or politically (2014). Suffering can pervade the culture, becoming, as Harvey described, something the population "does". And no mistake, pain and suffering have always taken many forms in human life, whether in the micro aggressions of discrimination or in actual violence visited upon neighbors (Anderson 2014). Poverty is one major factor aligned with suffering, both in daily QOL and in its amplified form after disaster. Racism, too, impacts QOL; in some societies, it "extends to apartheid, genocide, or other institutionalized forms of oppression and elimination of one group by and for the privilege of another" (Karraker 2014). Surviving such atrocities as a collective is itself a story repeated throughout history: one need only look to the ancient plight of the Jewish people or to Trnka's 2008 account of political violence and community survival in Fiji.

Suffering is compounded by social inequities. In the U.S., many inequities are openly tolerated, and social, political, economic and environmental situations can lead to social injustices. For example, inequities can be experienced in areas of heavy industry (the lower Mississippi River Valley's "Cancer Corridor,") or housing and school quality inequities in economically comprised communities. Drevdahl (2013) writes:

> Only when one see one's relations with others from an ethical, moral, and human rights perspective does one begin to understand that the well-being of the one rests on the well-being of the collective "Other"; this obligates each person to ameliorate and, if possible, prevent the suffering of others. (53)

What many term "social suffering" thus demands a moral framework build around providing meaningful relief of others' suffering (Anderson 2014). As Anderson puts it:

> …Perhaps the greatest merit of the concept of social suffering is that it points out not only how horrifyingly inhuman many global acts continue to be, but also the role that institutional policies may play in producing greater suffering. (22)

Further, he explains that when another's suffering is relieved, their QOL is improved. Justifying QOL "as a concrete human need [with an] emphasis on *social* suffering as a qualitatively different type of suffering" (Anderson 2014: 22) leads to more inclusive and responsive perspectives. The relief of suffering, then, becomes a moral and societal imperative.

22.2.2 Community Quality-of-Life Indicators

Community quality-of-life indicators can be readily defined as points of information that combine to generate an overall picture of a local or regional system. They can yield valuable insight into whether a given community is improving, declining, or staying the same—or, most likely, some mix of all three (Besleme 1997; Maclaren 1996; Redefining Progress et al. 1997). The pertinent indicators are often selected by way of a community visioning process based in what residents value most in their area. A community relies heavily on social capital, cohesiveness, and the ability to work together to accomplish desired outcomes (Phillips and Pittman 2014), so a combination of indicators identified by residents can generate perhaps the most useful metrics to aid decision making (Chase et al. 2011; Hart 2003; Oleari 2000; Sirgy et al. 2013). Community quality-of-life indicators can gauge progress on many dimensions: economic, ecological, or social. Further, they "may or may not be part of a benchmarking process (i.e., a process that establishes numeric goals to measure progress), although some indicator projects are used for this purpose" (Phillips 2003: 5). They are vital in societies in which injustice, poverty, and inequities impede the community's quality of life for all its residents, in that community quality-of-life indicators can help call attention to issues that need addressing.

Policy makers have long used sets of information to aid in the decision-making process, just as community activists have used data to mobilize opinion leaders and influence change (Phillips 2003). Social indicators have been used at the community, regional, and country levels to track social trends, demographics, QOL, and more. Beginning in the World War II era, economic measures took precedence as the Gross National Product (GNP) and related measures became standards by which many countries looked at progress annually.

It was not until the late 1980s and into the 1990s that an interest in sustainability and sustainable development provided a new role for community quality-of-life indicators in policy and citizen engagement. Increasing public awareness of ecological issues and the need to balance with social and economic factors has prompted the popularity of community quality-of-life indicators as a way to gauge sustainability. Ideas such as the ecological footprint (a measure of the resources needed to support urban development) allow, for example, residents to see clearly how many resources are needed to support current lifestyles and development patterns. This may influence policy changes, or at least increase awareness of vulnerability and risk associated with limited resources. Vancouver, British Columbia is widely considered a sustainable and progressive city, yet its ecological footprint is 14 times the actual area of the city (Greater Vancouver Regional District 2001)—and even that is smaller than many other cities' footprints. In another example of integrating sustainability measures into decision-making at the community level is that of Seattle, Washington. When the city's annual salmon migration was threatened by pollution, citizens coalesced around environmental quality. Together, they created a community quality-of-life indicator system called Sustainable Seattle that has been emulated by communities across the U.S. and beyond (Phillips 2003; Besleme and Mullin 1997).

For years, Sustainable Seattle assessed the city's progress toward "long-term health and vitality." The model has been widely adopted because citizens could easily understand how its indicators affect their daily lives. Sustainable Seattle's model measures sustainability with 40 specific measures across the five categories listed below (SustainableSeattle.org).

Environment
    Wild Salmon
    Ecological Health
    Soil Erosion Neutral
    Air Quality Pedestrian- and Bicycle-Friendly Streets
    Open Space Near Villages
    Impervious Surfaces

Population and Resources
    Population
    Water Consumption
    Solid Waste Generated and Recycled
    Pollution Prevention
    Local Farm Production
    Vehicle Miles Travelled and Fuel Consumption
    Renewable and Nonrenewable
    Energy Use per Dollar of Income
    Employment Concentration
    Unemployment
    Distribution of Personal Income
    Health Care Expenditures

Economy
    Work Required for Basic Needs
    Housing Affordability
    Children Living in Poverty

Emergency Room for Non-Emergency Room Purposes
Community Reinvestment

Youth and Education
High School Graduation
Ethnic Diversity of Teachers
Arts Instruction
Volunteer Involvement in Schools
Juvenile Crime
Youth Involvement in Community Service
Equity in Justice
Adult Literacy

Health and Community
Low Birth Weight Infants
Asthma Hospitalization for Children
Voter Participation
Library and Community Center Use
Public Participation in the Arts
Gardening
Neighborliness
Perceived Quality of Life

The typology of indicators for most systems or projects can be considered instrumental, tactical, symbolic, political, or conceptual (Hezri and Dovers 2006). Common characteristics of the function of indicators fall into six key areas: finding, measuring, monitoring, setting, changing, and reflecting (Phillips et al. 2013). Table 22.1 provides additional information on the functions of indicators.

22.2.3   Disaster Management and Risk Assessment

The disaster management and risk assessment field has rapidly expanded over the last few decades. Increasingly large urban populations and rapid climate change intensifies the potential risk to larger numbers of people. In the past, a "command and control" type of planning and response was prevalent; now, there is more interest in community-oriented approaches (LaLone 2012). In a study of two cities experiencing floods in 2004, Kweit and Kweit (2004) found that the city pursuing citizen participation approaches experienced greater political stability and citizen satisfaction after the disaster. The city relying on organizational guidance experienced more changes in government structure, higher turnover of elected and appointed officials, and far less positive citizen evaluation. In other words, strong citizen participation—an underlying foundation of community development as well as an instrumental component of social capital and social community capacity building—makes a measurable difference in disaster impact and recovery efforts. It lowers the extent and duration of community suffering.

Table 22.1 Functions of indicators[a]

Key concept	Functions
Finding	Revealing core concerns
	Identifying information gaps
	Clarifying opportunities
	Information about past to present
Measuring	Tracking progress toward achieving result
	Evaluating performance
Monitoring	Monitoring collaboration between citizens, experts and decision-makers
	Producing a feedback system for decision maker
	Identifying emerging threats to community
	Early warning system
Setting	Setting community's priorities
	Predicting quantifiable thresholds
	Suggesting feasible goals
	Implementing choices underlain by clear goals
Changing	Shifting attention to particular area
	Keeping track the progress in new dimensions of human responsibility and concern
	The ability to changes in process and policy
Reflecting	Providing a broader perspective
	Sharing of decision-making power via better information, communication and dialogue
	Increasing public accountability

[a]Compiled from information by Gahin and Paterson (2001), Holden (2006), Land (1983), Maclaren (1996), Michalos (1997), Walker (2005), Phillips et al. (2013)

Similarly, Johnson et al. (2012) explored two communities in New Zealand after earthquakes and discovered that:

> …Effective survival and recovery from disasters depends not just on people's abilities to cope with the physical impacts of the event, but also on how the societal environment complements and supports the complex and protracted processes of community recovery. (252)

They propose that incorporating citizen and community participation reduces anxiety and trauma after disasters, and that collaboration across organizational resources is key to aiding recovery.

Others, too, have recognized the need to incorporate more community-oriented approaches into disaster management and risk assessment (Cutter et al. 2008). Paton and Johnson (2001) describe a model for promoting preparation by informing the community and integrating disaster management into the community development framework. The researchers recognize that community development is a foundation on which to build both social capital and resilience. It can also foster more effective disaster management, risk assessment, and recovery.

Within the geographic information system approaches, newer approaches include community factors alongside more traditional risk and prediction modeling. Miles and Chang (2011) describe such a system using spatial decision support for disaster mitigation and recovery planning. This is different from typical loss estimation models in that it incorporates measurements of community capital across multiple scales. Khazai et al. (2013) focuses on integrating indicators into a spatial framework to assess vulnerability and risk within industrial sectors. Included in their model are social indicators that assess risk based on multi-criteria decision theory. This approach is used to identify areas of vulnerability across regions.

22.3 Connections: Exploring the Use of Indicators for Tragedy Avoidance and Alleviating Suffering

One area where indicators connect to tragedy avoidance and the alleviation of suffering is that of social capital. Broadly defined as the networks and connections that make societies work effectively, social capital is an essential component of community capacity. Mattessich (2009) writes that community capacity:

> …includes the ability to: develop and sustain strong relationships; solve problems and make group decisions; and collaborate effectively to identify goals and get work done. Communities with high community social capacity can identify their needs; establish priorities and goals; develop plans, or which the members of that community consider themselves "owners"; allocate resources to carry out those plans; and carry out the joint work necessary to achieve goals. (50–51).

In other words, a community must have (or develop) some capacity to effectively plan for and respond to need. Tragedy is major and overwhelming, and those communities with social capacity are better able to prepare and recover. In this sense, social cohesion is a fundamental element in preventing or mitigating tragedy.

Others refer to social community capacity as resiliency—the ability to recover from difficulties. Social resilience, then, can be thought of as the ability of groups and communities to respond to or recover from crisis (Maguire and Hagan 2007). It is a multi-dimensional concept with various properties including resistance, creativity, and recovery (Maguire and Hagan 2007; Norris et al. 2008), and it is reflected in a set of adaptive capacities that Norris et al. (2008) identify as economic development, social capital, information and communication, and community competence. These four areas serve as a foundation for building a disaster management and recovery strategy. Further, they indicate that to strengthen resiliency, communities

> …must reduce risk and resource inequities; engage local people in mitigation; create organizational linkages; boost and protect social supports; and plan for not having a plan, which requires flexibility, decision-making skills, and trusted sources of information that function in the face of unknowns (127).

Maguire and Hagan (2007) find that social resilience does not necessarily emerge naturally in response to disaster; rather, it must be built and supported from within a community. Disaster management plans, in turn, build on that resiliency. Resilience can "help inoculate communities against potential threats and crisis… with perspectives, actions, and measures focusing on identifying, conserving and investing in the human, social, intellectual, and physical capital" (Zautra et al. 2009: 132).

22.3.1 Recovering in Communities

Notable examples of community capacity and resilience include those communities within New Orleans that recovered rapidly as neighbors helped neighbors, or recovery in Bangladesh and the Philippines where local and international organizations worked together to provide relief. The literature is plentiful with studies from sociological, economic, and anthropological perspectives on community recovery. For example, Chang (2010) provides a detailed framework for assessing patterns of disaster recovery through statistical indicators. Using the case of Kobe City, struck by Japan's 1995 earthquake, Chang's study applies indicators to gauge recovery rather than to preventing unavoidable tragedy.

A more recent book, *Building Resilience: Social Capital in Post-Disaster Recovery* by Aldrich (2012), brings the elements of social capital and resilience into the analysis of post-tragedy recovery. The author hones in on four well-known disasters: a devastating 1923 earthquake in Tokyo; the 1995 earthquake in Kobe; the Indian Ocean Tsunami's landfall in Tamil Nadu in 2004; and Hurricane Katrina, which devastated New Orleans and much of the United States' Gulf Coast in 2005. Aldrich finds that communities with stronger social networks and social capital (what I have called social community capacity) are more capable of recovery—these resources able to provide information and allow for faster responses. These strong communities also prevented the outmigration of residents, thus keeping resources in the community after disaster. The presence of robust social capital and social networks implies that resilience is further strengthened after it is tested in disaster (Bretherton and Ride 2011).

22.3.2 Potential Models

Clearly, traditional disaster response plans must integrate more community-based planning and participation. While there are an increasing number of such community-based disaster plans and approaches (Islam et al. 2013; Zhang et al. 2013), full integration is not yet apparent. The positive benefits of this cohesion need to be more widely recognized (Jordan and Javernick-Will 2013), and community development foundations and indicators should strive to measure and build social capital and social community capacity.

Wells et al. (2013) agree that community resilience is a priority for preparedness, but laments that few models exist. A pilot study was undertaken by the team of researchers in Los Angeles to devise a community-partnered, participatory approach to help support resident workgroups in developing community-based plans. These plans included a toolkit for individual preparedness as well as community responses. The process included three stages: vision (planning), valley (implementation), and victory (products, dissemination). Each stage included organizing, action, and feedback in partnership with the Los Angeles County Community Disaster Resilience Initiative. The approach prioritized building community capacity prior to and in the absence of any impending disasters. Chandra et al. (2013) describe the project as being aimed at merging disaster preparedness and community health promotion to build stronger partnerships (they found, in a baseline survey conducted before the Disaster Resilience Initiative, low community resilience and little preparation by health departments and community-based organizations for disaster management). While L.A. County's approach does not specifically integrate community quality-of-life indicators, it provides a participatory model for addressing disaster planning and recovery from tragedy via building community resilience.

Another model for encouraging community-based resiliency, is place-based and relies heavily on the concept of resilience, has been proposed by Cutter et al. (2008). Providing a "conceptualization for understanding and measuring community-level resilience to natural hazards," it "presents resilience as a dynamic process dependent on antecedent conditions, the disaster's severity, time between hazard events, and influences from exogenous factors" (604). The Cutter model is operationalized by ecological, social, economic, and institutional, indicators, as well as community competence, infrastructure categories, and resilience metrics. Specific indicators include: wetlands acreage and loss; social networks and social embeddedness; values-cohesion; participation in hazard reduction programs; emergency response plans; interoperable communications; local understanding of risk; counseling services health and wellness (low rates of mental illness, stress-related outcomes); and QOL measures (high satisfaction). It is a good start toward a disaster response model that integrates a wide variety of community quality-of-life indicators to serve as a reflection of community need and, over time, of the success of suffering alleviation efforts.

22.4 Summary

Disaster recovery and risk assessment is a vast and growing domain. It is urgent to prevent, plan for, and regain after disaster strikes, so as to mitigate social suffering. Some response models have begun to integrate community quality-of-life indicators as a means to gauge and monitor tragedy avoidance and alleviate suffering through effective recovery. The types and approaches vary from descriptive and predictive modeling based on quantitative data and spatially focused GIS-based systems to inclusive, citizen-led initiatives to protect valued assets and identify potential risks. Whichever approach is taken, incorporating community quality-of-life indicators can help all stakeholders prepare and prioritize citizens' specific needs. Social community capacity is a key concept within this context—by building capacities in advance, communities are better able to avoid, prevent, or respond and recover. This social community capacity leads to greater resilience, or the ability of a community to "bounce back," which, in turn, can help regain vital functions and retain residents and resources in the area.

Community quality-of-life indicators, given that they are meant to represent the spectrum of the community's values and desires, as well as the resources citizens want to protect, can serve as a bridge between community-based planning and traditional disaster and risk assessment approaches. They also represent a way to illustrate social community capacity as reflected in the often community-based, participatory process of identification and implementation. Indicators can also be used to identify inequities and issues to address social suffering, or suffering of the community collective, that may occur independently or in tandem with a natural or anthropogenic disaster.

References

Aldrich, D. P. (2012). *Building resilience: Social capital in post-disaster recovery*. Chicago: University of Chicago Press.

Anderson, R. E. (2014). *Human suffering and quality of life*. Dordrecht: Springer.

Berkes, F. (2006). From community-based resource management to complex systems: The scale issue and marine commons. *Ecology and Society, 11*(1), 45.

Besleme, K. K. (1997). Community indicators and healthy communities. *National Civic Review, 86*(1), 43–52.

Besleme, K., & Mullin, M. (1997). Community indicators and healthy communities. *National Civic Review, 86*(1), 43–52.

Bretherton, D., & Ride, A. (2011). *Community resilience in natural disasters*. New York: Palgrave Macmillan.

Chandra, A., Williams, M., Plough, A., Stayton, A., Wells, K. B., Horta, M., & Tang, J. (2013). Getting actionable about community resilience: The Los Angeles county community disaster resilience project. *American Journal of Public Health, 103*(7), 1181–1189. doi:10.2105/AJPH.2013.301270.

Chang, S. E. (2010). Urban disaster recovery: A measurement framework and its application to the 1995 Kobe earthquake. *Disasters, 34*(2), 303–327. doi:10.1111/j.1467-7717.2009.01130.

Chase, L., Amsden, B., & Phillips, R. (2011). Stakeholder engagement in tourism planning and development. In M. Uysal, R. Perdue, & M. J. Sirgy (Eds.), *Handbook of tourism and quality-of-life research: Enhancing the lives of tourists and residents of host communities*. Dordrecht: Springer.

Cutter, S. L., Barnes, L., Berry, M., Burton, C., Evans, E., Tate, E., & Webb, J. (2008). A place-based model for understanding community resilience to natural disasters. *Global Environmental Change, 18*(4), 598–606. doi:10.1016/j.gloenvcha.2008.07.013.

Drevdahl, D. J. (2013). Injustice, suffering, difference: How can community health nursing address the suffering of others? *Journal of Community Health Nursing, 30*, 49–58.

Gahin, R. R., & Paterson, C. (2001). Community indicators: Past, present, and future. *National Civic Review, 90*(4), 347–361.

Hahn, H., De Leon, J., Villagran, C., & Hidajat, R. (2003). *Comprehensive risk management by communities and local governments*. Washington, DC: Inter-American Development Bank, Regional Policy Dialogue, Preliminary Draft.

Hart, M. (2003). What is an indicator of sustainability?. Available at www.sustainablemeasures. com/Indicators/WhatIs.html. Accessed 26 August.

Harvey, D. (2014). The geography and culture of suffering. In R. Anderson (Ed.), *World suffering and quality of life*. Dordrecht: Springer.

Hezri, A. A., & Dovers, S. R. (2006). Sustainability indicators, policy and governance: Issues for ecological economics. *Ecological Economics, 60*(1), 86–99. doi:10.1016/j. ecolecon.2005.11.019.

Holden, M. (2006). Revisiting the local impact of community indicators projects: Sustainable Seattle as prophet in its own land. *Applied Research in Quality of Life, 1*(3–4), 253–277. doi:10.1007/s11482-007-9020-8.

Islam, M. N., Malak, M. A., & Islam, M. N. (2013). Community-based disaster risk and vulnerability models of a coastal municipality in Bangladesh. *Natural Hazards, 69*(3), 2083–2103. doi:10.1007/s11069-013-0796-6.

Johnston, D., Becker, J., & Paton, D. (2012). Multi-agency community engagement during disaster recovery. *Disaster Prevention and Management, 21*(2), 252–268. doi:10.1108/09653561211220034.

Jordan, E., & Javernick-Will, A. (2013). Indicators of community recovery: Content analysis and delphi approach. *Natural Hazards Review, 14*(1), 21–28.

Karraker, M. W. (2014). Community action to alleviate suffering from racism: the role of religion and caring capital in small city, USA. In R. Anderson (Ed.), *World suffering and quality of life*. Dordrecht: Springer.

Khazai, B., Merz, M., Schulz, C., & Borst, D. (2013). An integrated indicator framework for spatial assessment of industrial and social vulnerability to indirect disaster losses. *Natural Hazards, 67*(2), 145–167. doi:10.1007/s11069-013-0551-z.

Kweit, M., & Kweit, R. (2004). Citizen participation and citizen evaluation in disaster recovery. *TheAmericanReviewofPublicAdministration,34*(4),354–373.doi:10.1177/0275074004268573.

LaLone, M. B. (2012). Neighbors helping neighbors: An examination of the social capital mobilization process for community resilience to environmental disasters. *Journal of Applied Social Science, 6*(2), 29–237. doi:10.1177/1936724412458483.

Land, K. C. (1983). Social indicators. *Annual Review of Sociology, 9*, 1–26.

Maclaren, V. (1996). Urban sustainability reporting. *Journal of the American Planning Association, 62*(2), 184–202.

Maguire, B., & Hagan, P. (2007). Disasters and communities: Understanding social resilience. *Australian Journal of Emergency Management, 22*(2), 16–20.

Mattisich, P. (2009). Social capital and community building. In R. Phillips & R. Pittman (Eds.), *Introduction to community development*. London: Routledge.

Michalos, A. (1997). Combining social, economic, and environmental indicators to measure sustainable human well-being. *Social Indicators Research, 40*(1), 221–258.

Miles, S. B., & Chang, S. E. (2011). ResilUS: A community based disaster resilience model. *Cartography and Geographic Information Science, 38*(1), 36.

Norris, F. H., Stevens, S. P., Pfefferbaum, B., Wyche, K. F., & Pfefferbaum, R. L. (2008). Community resilience as a metaphor, theory, set of capacities, and strategy for disaster readiness. *American Journal of Community Psychology, 41*(1), 127–150. doi:10.1007/ s10464-007-9156-6.

Oleari, K. (2000). Making your Job easier: Using whole-system approaches to involve the community in sustainable planning and development. *Public Management, 82*(12), 12–16.

Paton, D., & Johnston, D. (2001). Disasters and communities: Vulnerability, resilience and preparedness. *Disaster Prevention and Management, 10*(4), 270–277. doi:10.1108/ EUM0000000005930.

Phillips, R. (2003). *A Planner's guide to community indicators* (Planners Advisory Service (PAS) Report, No. 517). Chicago: American Planning Association.

Phillips, R., Sung, H., & Whitsett, A. (2013). State-level applications: Developing a policy support and public awareness indicator project. In J. Sirgy, R. Phillips, & D. Rahtz (Eds.), *Community quality-of-life indicators: Best cases VI* (pp. 99–118). Dordrecht: Springer.

Phillips, R., & Pittman, R. (Eds.). (2014). *Introduction to community development* (2nd ed.). London: Routledge/Taylor & Francis Group.

Redefining Progress, Tyler Norris Associates, & Sustainable Seattle. (1997). *The community indicators handbook*. San Francisco: Redefining Progress.

Sirgy, J., Phillips, R., & Rahtz, D. (Eds.). (2013). *Community quality-of-life indicators: Best cases VI*. Dordrecht: Springer.

Trnka, S. (2008). *State of suffering, political violence and community survival in Fiji*. Ithaca: Cornell University Press.

United Nations Development Programme. (2014). Accessed July 1 at www.undp.org.

Walker, D. M. (2005). Key national indicator systems: An opportunity to assess national progress, improve performance and strengthen accountability. *Journal of Government Financial Management, 54*(2), 10–14.

Wells, K., Fogleman, S., Plough, A., Tang, J., Lizaola, E., & Jones, F. (2013). Community resilience and public health practice: Applying community engagement to disaster planning: Developing the vision and design for the Los Angeles county community disaster resilience initiative. *American Journal of Public Health, 103*(7), 1172.

Zautra, A., Hall, J., & Murray, K. (2009). Community development and community resilience: An integrative approach. *Community Development, 39*(3), 130–147.

Zhang, X., Yi, L., & Zhao, D. (2013). Community-based disaster management: A review of progress in china. *Natural Hazards, 65*(3), 2215–2239. doi:10.1007/s11069-012-0471-3.

Chapter 23
Community Action to Alleviate Suffering from Racism: The Role of Religion and Caring Capital in Small City USA

Meg Wilkes Karraker

23.1 Introduction

Endowed with arresting natural beauty, classic eighteenth century architecture, and a genuinely friendly populace, Bluffton is a lovely place to spend a quiet weekend along the Mississippi River. But Bluffton has had some ugly recent history as well. This chapter tells the story of Bluffton's encounter with diversity and how that city "had the guts to do something about racism."

Like so many other Midwestern cities (as aptly described in Wuthnow's [2011] *Remaking of the Heartland*), Bluffton has a long history as a predominantly, almost exclusively white city. In 1980, Bluffton had a total population around 60,000 but less than 400 people of color. In the last years of the twentieth century, more black families arrived, attracted by employers and the efforts of a task force charged with bringing more diversity to the city. Nonetheless, a visible minority of Bluffton's citizens expressed violent disapproval of diversity efforts, throwing bricks through the windows of black homes. The city counted more than six cross-burnings in less than 6 months. At a time when membership in the Ku Klux Klan had dwindled (again, this was only about 30 years ago), a KKK rally in Bluffton drew over 100 participants.

Nonetheless, by the early twenty-first century, Bluffton had become home to small but visible numbers of immigrants from over 50 countries. During the same years, Bluffton faced population and economic decline, due in no small part to substantial employment lay-offs when the city's largest employer left town. Immigrants and especially people of color living in Bluffton came to be viewed by some whites with suspicion, as competition for the diminishing supply of blue-collar jobs and even as a source of the kind of urban violence shown on television (though not yet seen in Bluffton). The city found itself struggling with race, ethnicity, and immigration, but

M.W. Karraker (✉)
Department of Sociology, Faculty of Sociology, Family Studies & Women's Studies,
University of St. Thomas, Mail #4048, 2115 Summit Ave, St. Paul, MN 55105, USA
e-mail: mwkarraker@stthomas.edu

© Springer Science+Business Media Dordrecht 2015   305
R.E. Anderson (ed.), *World Suffering and Quality of Life*,
Social Indicators Research Series 56, DOI 10.1007/978-94-017-9670-5_23

also its self-image as place with a respectable quality of life peopled with citizens who cared for one another.

In late 2008, I embarked on a 3-year, mixed-methods community study of Bluffton. I collected my data during 2009–2012. During that time I conducted face-to-face interviews with 28 civic and religious leaders, including Catholic sisters. I also studied city and congregational histories, newspaper stories, and other publically accessible accounts. During the period of my research I was a regular on-line reader of Bluffton's daily newspaper, as well as the weekly newspaper of her Catholic archdiocese. I was also a frequent visitor to Bluffton's official Web site, as well as the Web sites of Bluffton's civic partners. Finally, I spent time in Bluffton's public and private places: dining in her cafes and restaurants; strolling her city streets and along her riverbank; visiting her churches, libraries, and museums; walking the campuses of her colleges and universities. During each research visit, I shared meals with sisters and stayed overnight in one or another of the motherhouses (formerly called convents) of Bluffton's congregations.

In this study I sought to understand how civic and religious values and networks come together around diversity and inclusion for the common good—in other words, the social and caring capital, at Bluffton's civic heart. I came away with a sense of how a small city like Bluffton could relieve suffering and insure the quality of life across her civic landscape, even in the face of racism by some members of her community against others.

23.2   Racism, Suffering, and Quality of Life

Writing about social problems and quality of life, Lauer and Lauer (2013) teach that racism affects quality of life in at least four areas: the rights of citizenship (including equality before the law), the right to equal employment opportunities (including the acquisition of income and wealth), the right to life and happiness (including not only life chances, but also freedom from fear), and the right to dignity as a human being (including the myth of inferiority). In some societies, racism extends to apartheid, genocide, or other institutionalized forms of oppression and elimination of one group by and for the privilege of another. Scholars of suffering have labeled this "social suffering" (Klienman et al. 1997; Wilkerson 2005). Also discussed under the rubric of social suffering are distresses from any stigmas assigned to social characteristics such as disability, gender, poverty, low social status (Anderson 2014: 8–24).

My research attempts to assess the daily experiences of racism suffered by excluded groups in contemporary America. Two stories from Bluffton help reveal the micro-level costs to quality of life borne by individuals and families, friends, and other groups as a result of racism. Almost 10 years after Bluffton's hate crimes, the son of one of the black families targeted by cross-burning spoke of the physical danger and fear his family experienced. Now living in another city in the Midwest, he described additional suffering he experienced at the personal level. The cross-burnings were horrendous, but the subsequent media and community attention directed toward his family left him feeling stigmatized and excluded, with a strong sense of resentment toward white people in Bluffton.

A second story reveals the work yet to be done to close the Bluffton's racial gap in the quality of life. At a recent annual breakfast in honor of Rev. Dr. Martin Luther King, Jr., two men described their friendship, which had begun at their workplace. The white man spoke of being witness to the indignities and discrimination suffered by his black friend. He noted that even their shopping experiences are different: his black friend is often required to show two forms of identification when using a credit card, and, when using cash, the white man receives his change in his hand, but the black man's change is left on the counter. He recounts the extra scrutiny accorded his black friend, as when a store intercom alerts a manager to "assist a customer in aisle three," when the only customer in that aisle needs no assistance, only surveillance.

Forty decades of sociological and psychological research confirm that stressors in the form of chronic strains, negative events, and trauma have substantial negative physical and mental health consequences (Thoits 2010). Racial-ethnic, along with gender, marital status, social class and other inequities, tax quality of life in particular ways, as minority-group members suffer from discrimination and stressors that are compounded across the life course and over generations, widening gaps between the health, well-being, and quality of life between under-privileged and privileged groups (Thoits 2010).

Using indicators such as the Index of Race-Related Stress and the World Health Organization's inventory, research teams led by Shawn Utsey have demonstrated that racial and ethnic group membership is associated with race-related stress and quality of life among black Americans (Utsey et al. 2002a, b; Utsey and Constantine 2008; Utsey and Payne 2000). Some research indicates that those effects can be moderated by cognitive ability and social support (Utsey et al. 2006). These mediators include mastery and self-esteem (Thoits 2010), as well as cultural, sociofamiliar, and psychological resources (Utsey et al. 2008). In sum, people of color experience more acute stressors and chronic strains, but they also experience chronic stressors and strains particular to their racial or ethnic group (Pearlin 1989; Thoits 1991). As a result, people of color suffer in terms of mental and physical health, socioeconomic status, and life satisfaction (Coke and Twaite 1995).

The stories of the man whose family suffered from the cross-burnings and the two friends building inter-racial friendship reveal how Bluffton's citizens have confronted the suffering of racism at personal and interpersonal levels. Indisputably, the far greater everyday suffering in both cases is experienced by the black person. These accounts reveal what we might call secondary or vicarious compromises to community, which correlate to a middle-range unit of Anderson's (2014) individual-to-global conceptualization of suffering. Although Wilkinson (2005: 16) includes "social isolation and personal estrangement" as an element of suffering, opportunities to build friendships or other intimate connections is a poorly attended part of this scholarship. While white persons are certainly far more privileged (and even able to overlook racism), my respondents' accounts attest to co-suffering and the interpersonal costs of suffering.

Racism and exclusion compromises and engenders suffering at the individual and interpersonal level, but also across broad demographic categories. For example, being a person of color dramatically increases one's chance of being poor. In Bluffton, Hispanics are more than twice as likely and blacks more than six times as likely as whites to be poor. Furthermore, disparities around poverty and citizenship are even more marked in Bluffton than in the rest of the state and in the greater United States. In 2010, 62 % of blacks in Bluffton were poor, compared to 43 % in the state and 27 % in the United States. Likewise, Bluffton has an lower percentage of foreign-born residents who are naturalized citizens than in either the state or the nation. Whereas only 31 % of Bluffton's foreign-born citizens are naturalized citizens, the percentages in the state and in the nation are 37 and 44 %, respectively (United States Census Bureau 2010).

It is probably fair to say that the racial discrimination that emerged in the last decades of the twentieth century caught Bluffton a bit off-guard. Until then, Bluffton's population had been so overwhelmingly white that community leaders, including Catholic Sisters, could easily overlook differential treatment accorded to Bluffton's few black or other racial or ethnic minorities. However, as the storm of racism approached, the city's civic leaders realized, to remain competitive and shrug off negative perceptions of their city as racist, they must work to create a more inclusive, welcoming culture.

Bluffton began to institutionalize values and norms through offices and organizations to vigorously address not only economic but also civil rights agendas. Building on the efforts of the original task force charged with bringing more racial and ethnic diversity to the city, leaders set a goal of bringing 100 families of color to Bluffton within 5 years. They mounted a community education campaign around multicultural competency, with broad support across the community, from city employees to Girl Scouts, the city's daily newspaper, and 300 businesses.

At the forefront of those earliest efforts were the city's religious leaders. Seeing the need to bring members of the community together face-to-face, Bluffton's Catholic Sisters did what they do so well: extended hospitality. They opened one of their motherhouses to the community and organized the first breakfast to honor the Rev. Dr. Martin Luther King, Jr.'s birth. Now entering its third decade, the annual breakfast is a community-wide, inter-faith celebration, sustained by the Bluffton Community Foundation with sponsorships that stretch across the community to include parochial and public schools, major employers, Bluffton's Civil Rights Commission, and the NAACP. Now part of the national Circles® initiative, the Bluffton initiative sponsors essay, poster, and multimedia contexts in celebration of the vision of Dr. King and extends awards to community leaders who have worked to eliminate discrimination, build resources, and strengthen community.

In recent years, Bluffton and its civic leaders have been recipients of awards like the National League of Cities' National Black Caucus of Local Elected Officials (NCB-LEO) City Cultural Diversity Award for achieving excellence in diversity.

But what of the suffering generated by racism and exclusion at the broader community level? In the late 1900s, Bluffton was starting to see that it was viewed in the news media and elsewhere as unwelcoming, intolerant, and, in light of the cross-burnings, the embodiment of long-held racism. Such an image could not but help to contribute to the population loss already plaguing Bluffton: companies would be unlikely to consider moving their headquarters to Bluffton, and adult children were unlikely to choose to live there if they had other options.

Bluffton is by no means unique in confronting the suffering caused by racism. Often, once-homogenous communities find themselves in the midst of what Bloom (2000) calls "culture clashes." Such clashes seem paradoxical, given the assets that these newcomers bring to their communities–often struggling with declining populations that have left small towns and farming communities with too few workers and too few consumers. For example, federal immigration policies strike, ironically, at the very employers who have the greatest demand for a cheap labor force (even if it means "no questions asked" about documentation of citizenship). On May 12, 2008, U.S. Immigration, Customs, and Enforcement (ICE) conducted a raid on Agriprocessors, a Kosher meatpacking plant in the small, northeastern Iowa town of Postville. With just 2,000 citizens, Postville had been struggling to stay afloat until Agriprocessors arrived, bringing with it a flood of immigrant workers and their families, who arrived with their new language, customs, religious practices, and other traditions (Strandberg 2008). Immigrants, documented or otherwise, were a welcome part of Postville's future prosperity, but the ICE raid threatened it again.

Back in Bluffton, the city had created a civil rights office, and its head national told reporters who descended on the town after the cross-burnings, "The difference between Bluffton and big cities like Chicago was that Bluffton had the guts to do something about racism." Why *was* Bluffton able to move from a desire to act for the common good to the ability and action to improve their community? This is one of the core processes of community development: "the ability of communities to act collectively and enhancing the ability to do so" (Phillips and Pittman 2009: 3). These factors can qualify some of the concerns that may arise during community development, concerns around relationships, structure, power, shared meaning, communication for change, motivations for decision making, and integration of disparate concerns (Hustedde 2009).

23.3   Religious Culture[1] and Caring Capital

My research indicates that Bluffton had mobilized across civil society, building social capital inspired by caring capital rooted in Bluffton's faith community and, in particular, her Catholic Sisters. Essential to Bluffton's story is what I have called "the sixty-five percent solution" (Karraker 2013: 55). From the time of its founding, Bluffton had been not only predominantly white, but also predominantly Catholic. In 2000, two thirds (65 %) of the city's residents claimed the Catholic faith

---

[1] Another aspect of religion and suffering, the Christian teaching of faith as a "cultural resource to live through and beyond" hardship, stress, and trauma, is well-addressed by Wilkinson (2005: 33).

(Association of Religion Data Archives 2012). While the region and the country were experiencing precipitous declines in religious identification of any sort (referred to as "nones"), Bluffton's Catholic population changed little in the last half of the twentieth century.[2]

Anyone who follows the social teachings of the Catholic Church and especially the outcome of the Second Vatican Council (known as Vatican II), the engagement of Catholics in diversity efforts in cities like Bluffton comes as no surprise. As one Sister told me, injustice like racism is a "summons to act on behalf of others" and to "answer the call of God." Such a call is embodied in the long-held traditions of all three Abrahamic faiths (Judaism, Christianity, and Islam); their teachings instruct all to care for "the stranger" and the immigrant. In the New Testament's Book of Matthew (25: 35), Jesus praises his disciplines: "for I was hungry, and you gave me food, I was thirsty and you gave me something to drink, I was a stranger and you welcomed me." Likewise, *imago dei*, the principle that every person is created in the image of God, inspires Christians to engage in social action (Jones 2008). For Christians, welcoming the stranger is welcoming Christ (Knoll 2009; United States Conference of Catholic Bishops 2000).

Likewise, Vatican II instructed Catholic adherents, including Sisters, to live within the social world and engage in apostolic ministries that would bring both lay and vowed religious in direct contact with "the least of these"—that is, the most oppressed in society (Benestad 2010). As a result, Catholic women religious and their congregations have become a progressive, visible, and welcoming element of civil society. Catholic Sisters, along with other vowed religious and lay women and men, have answered calls from their Church to provide hospitality and care and to treat everyone as welcome guests. They have often placed themselves on the front lines of social conflicts involving disenfranchised members of society, including civil rights.

American Sisters have a distinguished history of investing their economic and human capital in their community. In Bluffton, Sisters whose congregations had originated in Germany, Ireland, and cities in the Eastern United States founded and funded, managed and staffed many educational, health care, and social service insti-tutions. This included two of Bluffton's original three hospitals, her six parochial schools, and a women's college. The congregations worked on their own and col-laborated with civic agencies to shelter and advocate on behalf of women and chil-dren suffering from violence or homelessness. Led by a charismatic Sister, one congregation established a center where newcomers to Bluffton could achieve English language, citizenship, and other skills and where college students and other volunteers could participate in helping these new citizens. Sisters even served in appointed and elected positions in Bluffton's government.

The Catholic Sisters were universally held in the highest esteem. A former member of Bluffton's human rights commission told me, "Bluffton *loves* her Sisters!" After all, these are the women who have taught Bluffton's children and educated her

---

[2] The percentage of Catholics in Bluffton dipped to 58 in 1990, but by the time of my study, it had risen to slightly surpass 1980 levels (Association of Religious Data Archives 2012).

adults. (One informant volunteered, "Sisters... *are* education in Bluffton!") They had cared for those who were hurting or in need, while conducting much of the day-to-day work of the Archdiocese that served Bluffton's majority-Catholic population. These women were on the front-lines, responding to the most critical needs of Bluffton's most vulnerable, including women, children, and, as the need arose, immigrants.

Across Bluffton's civil sector, the eight government, philanthropy, social service, journalism, and business leaders with whom I conducted interviews were very strong in the approbations they extended to Catholic Sisters. On a Likert-type scale, where seven equals "strongly agree," these leaders responded 5.3, 5.3, and 4.8 to three indicators[3] of Sisters' reputation in the community. This esteem held for not only Catholic, but also for Protestant and Jewish leaders. Perhaps not surprising, given their greater familiarity and often collaboration with Sisters' ministries, the mean responses by the five faith leaders to the three indicators of Sisters' reputation in the community were even higher: 6.8, 6.8, and 6.3.

Every one of these leaders volunteered considerable elaboration on the important work of Sisters in Bluffton:

"Sisters see the big picture."
"Sisters have been in the trenches."
"Nuns, who have traveled the world, return with worldly experience, which they bring back to the community conversation."

These leaders often commented specifically on Sisters' contributions to the quality of life in those terms:

"Sisters are always ready, willing, and most of all able to work to improve the quality of life."

23.4 Community Strategies to Relieve Suffering and Enhance Quality of Life

My research found that Sisters generated a highly valued system of social networks, social capital, and caring capital through their abilities and assets, as well as their lived faith in service to alleviating suffering:

"Sisters have the gift to 'tell the story' [of human suffering] in a compelling way."
"They [Sisters] have the ability to leverage other resources to make positive change in Bluffton."
"Sisters take on social concerns around Gospel teachings for the 'least of these' when no one else will do so."

From published histories, news accounts, and informal conversations with residents of Bluffton, I gathered data that revealed that Catholic Sisters and their

---

[3] 1: Catholic Sisters have a reputation for doing good work in our community. 2: Our community is a better place because of the work of Catholic Sisters. 3: If I knew an immigrant who needed assistance, I would refer that person to a program run by Catholic Sisters.

congregations had been central nodes in Bluffton's coming to terms with diversity. I had found the same in my home towns of Saint Paul and Minneapolis, Minnesota. There, for example, the Sisters of St. Joseph of Carondelet have long served the Twin Cities through ministries including Sarah's… An Oasis for Women, which serves women seeking refuge from across the world. I had found the same in Rome, where, for example, *Suor Buon Pastore* (Sisters of the Good Shepherd) were involved in not only serving the victims of sex trafficking, but also in providing critical global leadership around such issues through the collaborations at the highest levels of the Church (Karraker 2010, 2011a, b).

Where Bluffton's Sisters were critical nodes in the social and caring capital of this small city, they answered the Knight Foundation's question as to what

> …makes people embrace a community and, in turn, want to work there and help it prosper? …[T]he drivers that create emotional bonds between people and their community are consistent in virtually every city and can be reduced to just a few categories …Interestingly, the usual suspects – jobs, the economy and safety – are not among the top drivers. Rather, people consistently give higher ratings for elements that relate directly to their daily: an area's physical beauty, opportunities for socializing and a community's openness to all people. (Knight Foundation 2011)

Quality of life, as defined by the Knight Foundation's *Soul of the Community* research project (Stehling 2012) relies heavily on aesthetics, social offerings, and (key to Bluffton) openness or the view of a city as welcoming for racial and ethnic minorities and immigrants, older people, child-free adults, and gay men and lesbians.

The Resiliency Capacity Index (RCI) offers a multi-variate assessment of the quality of life across 361 American cities (Institute of Government Studies 2011). Perhaps not surprising for a city of her size, Bluffton ranks in the bottom third on economic diversification. However, on the other 11 indicators, Bluffton's rankings are most impressive. Bluffton scores high on two economic indicators (affordability and business environment), three socio-demographic indicators (educational attainment, without disability, and health-insured), and three community connectivity indicators (civic infrastructure, metropolitan stability, and homeownership). But it is Bluffton's rank in the top 50 of all cities on three indicators pertinent to quality of life–income equality, out of poverty, and voter participation–that bode particularly well for the city's quality of life (Karraker 2013).

23.5 Conclusion: Lessons Learned from One Small City

Albeit still predominantly white and Catholic, in other ways, Bluffton is like the places where an increasing proportion of Americans live. In 2012 16 % of Americans lived in an incorporated place with a population of 50,000–99,999 (US Census Bureau 2012). Still, the politics, economics, and cultures of smaller communities are different from the larger cities, which have been the subject of much community research regarding diversity and racism. Smaller communities are generally much more homogenous than metropolitan areas (Lingeman 1980; Pedersen 1992) and, even in the face of dramatically declining populations, groups based in national, ethnic, religious, and other traditions may hold tight to cultural segregation (Bloom 2000). We would expect higher suffering from racism for those people of color in these smaller communities unless their citizens make a concerted effort at inclusion.

As the case of Postville testifies, small communities also confront the mixed challenges of economic resource competition and shifting population demographics. Bluffton's experiences with diversity are shared by other communities. America is far from a "post-racial" society, and minorities and other "strangers" continue to suffer the effects of prejudice in communities from Bluffton (where there was another cross-burning in 2012) to Sanford, Florida (where unarmed teen Trayvon Martin was shot in the same year (NY Times 2013)).

Bluffton *is* unique in its religious affiliation—not only the proportion of her citizens who claim religious affiliation, but those who are specifically self-avowed Catholics. Still, change is clearly on the horizon even here. Although weekly Mass participation remains higher in this Archdiocese than in the state and in many places across the United States, the percentage of Catholics in Bluffton dropped 14 % between 2000 and 2010, leading to the archdiocese's decision to close two parishes. Conversely, the percentage of those claiming no religious identification has grown from 12 % in 1960 to 21 % in 1980 and 32 % in 2010 (Association of Religion Data Arches 2012).

Since we have established the centrality of the Catholic Sisters to Bluffton's successful community-building efforts, it is also important to note the dramatic demographic decline among Sisters in Bluffton and throughout the United States. The drop gives pause as to the future of faith-driven efforts to relieve suffering and improve the quality of life in the face of racism and other challenges in inclusion. As the proportion of the population who are committed to a faith tradition declines, what will happen to local cultures once explicitly connected to that faith tradition? Will the values and norms remain, though religious affiliation drops?

In the face of such changes in the foundations of caring capital, it is difficult to measure the caring capital communities like Bluffton have successfully banked against future suffering. Perhaps the best indicator that a community like Bluffton has moved forward to alleviate suffering in the face of racism is the extent to which the city has institutionalized caring capital investments. In 2012, a cross was, once-again, burned in the front yard of a mixed-race family. The ashes could hardly have been cold before the mayor issued a powerful statement condemning the action and committing the full force of Bluffton's law enforcement behind solving the case.

Beyond such symbolic gestures (however forceful), Bluffton has embraced intercultural competency among government officials, city staff, agencies, and partnerships that stretch across the city. As I was completing my research, Bluffton was recognized for community engagement programs around the needs of a multicultural population, and a recent self-study identified efforts to make Bluffton a more inclusive place that benefits from and welcomes the contributions of *all* her citizens. While recognizing the work yet to be done, the study charged the entire community with getting involved.

The city's website features a quote from William James: "Act as if what you do makes a difference. It does." Indeed, something around institutional, interpersonal, and individual compassion *happens* in Bluffton. I was frequently told by civic and religious leaders, "We know and care about each other and about this city." Such a commitment to the common good has clearly been nurtured by Catholic religious identification and, especially, articulation of a caring capital by Bluffton's Sisters.

Faith-based organizations are known to effectively build bridging capital across racial, ethnic, and even religious backgrounds (Kaiser 2010). Further:

> Civil society …benefits from caring or charitable acts, because caring often fosters recipro-
> cal relationships, which may reinforce social capital of the bonding variety, which in turn
> builds social solidarity. (Anderson 2012: 480)

I also agree with Alexander (2006: 9), "Civil society is a project. It cannot be fully achieved." The building of a strong, connected, and inclusive community is work without an end.

In the conclusion to *Diversity and the Common Good* (Karraker 2013: 114), I asked: "Can Bluffton be a beacon for other communities that hope to make a good society during trying times?" Over two centuries ago, Alexis de Tocqueville (1835/2002) observed the powerful connection between Americans' commitment to religious organizations and civic engagement, and in a large body of work, Robert Wuthnow (1991, 1996, 1998, 1999, 2006) has linked acts of compassion and caring capital to religion and, thereby, religion to civil society, especially as communities face increasing challenges from diversity (Wuthnow 2007). Even as affiliation drops, the basic exhortation to "love one's neighbor" remains. Religious organizations are, in the United States, also community organizations that enable citizens to study social issues and engage in opportunities to serve the community, providing a place to acquire some of the "transferable skills" of civil society. Churches, religious bodies, and faith-based organizations (Adkins et al. 2010; Saguaro Seminar on Civic Engagement in America 2013) serve as foundations for the social and caring capital they build as citizens work with others to address suffering and social problems.

References

Adkins, J., Occhipinti, L., & Hefferan, T. (Eds.). (2010). *Not by faith alone: Social services, social justice, and faith-based organizations in the United States*. Lanham: Lexington Books.
Alexander, J. C. (2006). *The civil sphere*. New York: Oxford University Press.
Anderson, R. E. (2012). Caring capital websites. *Information, Communication, and Society, 15*, 479–501.
Anderson, R. E. (2014). *Human suffering and the quality of life*. New York: Springer.
Association of Religious Data Archives. (2012). U.S. congregational membership reports. Retrieved October 27, 2013, from http://thearda.com/rcms2010/r/c/19/rcms2010
Benestad, J. B. (2010). *Church, state, and society: An introduction to Catholic social doctrine*. Washington, DC: Catholic University of America.
Bloom, S. G. (2000). *Postville: A clash of cultures in heartland America*. Orlando: Harcourt.

Coke, M. M., & Twaite, J. A. (1995). *The black elderly: Satisfaction and quality of later life*. New York: Haworth Press.

de Tocqueville, A. (1835/2002). *Democracy in America* (H. C. Mansfield & D. Winthrop, Trans.). Chicago: University of Chicago Press.

Hustedde, R. J. (2009). Seven theories for seven community developers. In R. Phillips & R. H. Pittman (Eds.), *An introduction to community development* (pp. 20–37). London/New York: Routledge.

Institute of Governmental Studies. (2011). *Building resilient regions*. Retrieved from http://brr. berkeley.edu/

Jones, R. P. (2008). *Progressive & religious*. Lanham: Rowman & Littlefield.

Kaiser, A. (2010). *Bridging social capital formation in a faith-based organization*. Doctoral dissertation. Retrieved from http://digitalcommons.wayne.edu/oa_dissertations/93/

Karraker, M. W. (2010). *Charism, networks, and charisma: Catholic women's congregations' ministries to migrant women and children*. Paper presented at the triennial conference of history of women religious, Scranton.

Karraker, M. W. (2011a). *Charisms, contacts, and communities: Catholic Sisters in religious and civic networks around immigration*. Paper presented at the annual meetings of the Society for the Social Scientific Study of Religion and the Religious Research Association, Milwaukee.

Karraker, M. W. (2011b). Religious, civic, and interpersonal capital: Catholic Sisters in one community's response to migrant families. *Forum on Public Policy, 2011*(2). Retrieved from http://forumonpublicpolicy.com/vol2011.no2/globalconflict2011vol2.html

Karraker, M. W. (2013). *Diversity and the common good: Civil society, religion, and Catholic Sisters in a small city*. Lanham: Lexington.

Kleinman, A., Das, V., & Lock, M. (Eds.). (1997). *Social suffering*. Berkeley: University of California Press.

Knoll, B. R. (2009). "And who is my neighbor?" Religion and immigration policy attitudes. *Journal for the Scientific Study of Religion, 48*, 313–331.

Lauer, R. H., & Lauer, J. C. (2013). *Social problems and the quality of life* (13th ed.). New York: McGraw Hill.

Lingeman, R. (1980). *Small town America: A narrative history, 1620-the present*. New York: G. P. Putnam and Sons.

New York Times. (2013). *Trayvon Martin case* (George Zimmerman). Retrieved from (http://topics.nytimes.com/top/reference/timestopics/people/m/trayvon_martin/

Pearlin, L. I. (1989). The sociological study of stress. *Journal of Health and Social Behavior, 30*, 241–256.

Pedersen, J. M. (1992). *Between memory and reality: Family and community in rural Wisconsin, 1870–1970*. Madison: University of Wisconsin Press.

Phillips, R., & Pittman, R. H. (2009). A framework for community and economic development. In R. Phillips & R. H. Pittman (Eds.), *An introduction to community development* (pp. 3–19). London/New York: Routledge.

Saguaro Seminar on Civic Engagement in America. (2013). *Better together: Religion and social capital*. Retrieved from http://www.bettertogether.org/pdfs/Religion.pdf

Stehling, S. (2012). *Community philanthropy: Improving*. Minnesota Council on Foundations. Retrieved from http://www.mcf.org/news/giving-forum/community-philanthropy

Strandberg, S. (2008, November 18). *Decorah helps Guatemalan detainees*. Decorah Newspapers. Retrieved from http://www.decorahnewspapers.com/main.asp?Search=1&ArticleID=18709&SectionID=2&SubSectionID=13&S=1

The Knight Foundation. (2011). *Issues produce strong connection*. Retrieved from http://www.knight-foundation.org/press-room/press-mention/quality-life-issues-produce-strong-connection-stud/

Thoits, P. A. (1991). On merging identity theory and stress research. *Social Psychology Quarterly, 43*, 101–112.

Thoits, P. A. (2010). Stress and health: Major findings and policy implications. *Journal of Health and Social Behavior, 51*, 541–553.

United States Census Bureau. (2010). *American factfinder.* Retrieved from http://factfinder2.census.gov/faces/nav/jsf/pages/index.xhtml

United States Census Bureau. (2012). *Growth in urban population outpaces rest of nation.* Retrieved from http://www.census.gov/newsroom/releases/archives/2010_census/cb12-50.html

Utsey, S. O., & Constantine, M. G. (2008). Mediating and moderating effects of racism-related stress on the relation between poverty-related risk factors and subjective well-being in a community sample of African Americans. *Journal of Loss and Trauma, 13,* 186–204.

Utsey, S. O., & Payne, Y. A. (2000). Differential psychological and emotional impacts of race-related stress. *Journal of African American Men, 5,* 56–72.

Utsey, S. O., Chae, M. H., Brown, C. F., & Kelly, D. (2002a). Effect of ethnic group membership on ethnic identity, race-related stress, and quality of life. *Cultural Diversity and Ethnic Minority Psychology, 8,* 366–377.

Utsey, S. O., Payne, Y. A., Jackson, E. S., & Jones, A. M. (2002b). Race-related stress, quality of life indicators, and life satisfaction among elderly African Americans. *Cultural Diversity and Ethnic Minority Psychology, 8,* 224–233.

Utsey, S. O., Lanier, Y., Williams, O., III, Bolden, M., & Lee, A. (2006). Moderator effects of cognitive ability and social support on the relation between race-related stress and quality of life in a community sample of Black Americans. *Cultural Diversity and Ethnic Minority Psychology, 12,* 334–346.

Utsey, S. O., Giesbrecht, N., Hook, J., & Stanard, P. N. (2008). Cultural, sociofamiliar, and psychological resources that inhibit psychological distress in African Americans exposed to stressful life events and race-related stress. *Journal of Counseling Psychology, 55,* 49–62.

United States Conference of Catholic Bishops. (2000). *Welcoming the stranger among us: Unity in diversity.* Retrieved April 4, 2012, http:usccb.org/issues-and-action/cultural-diversity/pastoral-care-ofmigrants-refugees-and-travelers/resources/welcoming-the-stranger-among-us-unity-indiversity.cfm#summary

Wilkinson, I. (2005). *Suffering: A sociological introduction.* Cambridge: Polity.

Wuthnow, R. (1991). *Acts of compassion: Caring for others and helping ourselves.* Princeton: Princeton University Press.

Wuthnow, R. (1996). *Christianity and civil society: The contemporary debate.* Valley Forge: Trinity Press International.

Wuthnow, R. (1998). *Loose connections: Joining together in America's fragmented communities.* Cambridge: Harvard University Press.

Wuthnow, R. (1999). Mobilizing civic engagement: The changing impact of religious involvement. In T. Skocpol & M. P. Foirina (Eds.), *Civic engagement in American democracy* (pp. 331–363). Washington, DC: The Brookings Institute.

Wuthnow, R. (2006). *Saving America? Faith-based services and the future of civil society.* Princeton: Princeton University Press.

Wuthnow, R. (2007). *America and the challenges of diversity.* Princeton: Princeton University Press.

Wuthnow, R. (2011). *Remaking the heartland: Middle America since the 1950s.* Princeton: Princeton University Press.

Chapter 24
Suffering in Online Interactions

Katrin Döveling and Katrin Wasgien

24.1 Introduction

In today's "global village" (McLuhan 1962: 31), online communication fosters a conglomerate of information, opinions, and attitudes. It enhances overall interaction, especially in the communication of personal suffering. Rapidly growing online exchange of emotional messages challenges our understanding of users' motives as well as the diverse forms and communicative functions of interpersonal online communication within suffering processes. Founded in an extensive literature overview, one notes that the domain of online-suffering still leaves many questions unanswered. Not only "digital natives" (Prensky 2001: 2) make use of the Internet to share their emotions (Döveling and Wasgien 2014; Rimé et al. 1991), all age groups share in the virtual interactional processes equally. This study provides new, empirically grounded insights in shared suffering in online communities and the role of emotional exchange in suffering processes. These findings pertain to both shared offline and online suffering, equally investigating potential differences and similarities between adults and children.

This chapter focuses on a specific form of online suffering, as previous findings revealed that the social web allows mourners to find emotional support within an emotional community (Döveling 2012). The study was designed to address several research questions. Motives and potential gratifications for shared emotions were assessed, along with patterns and mechanisms of the emotional communication. Emotion management processes triggered by online social sharing of emotions were disclosed.

K. Döveling (✉) • K. Wasgien
Institute of Communication and Media Studies, Department of Empiric Research
in Communication and Media, University of Leipzig, Dresden, Germany
e-mail: katrin.doeveling@uni-leipzig.de; kwasgien@gmail.com

© Springer Science+Business Media Dordrecht 2015
R.E. Anderson (ed.), *World Suffering and Quality of Life*,
Social Indicators Research Series 56, DOI 10.1007/978-94-017-9670-5_24

24.2   Suffering and Grief: An Interdisciplinary Perspective

Suffering has been a topic in a wide range of scholarly disciplines (Kleinman et al. 1997; Nagappan 2005; Ferrel 2005; Francis 2006). From a psychological point of view, it "encompasses mild unpleasantness to excruciating torture and intense agony" (Anderson 2011: 2). Cassell (1991) states that when exploring suffering, mind and body should not be separated, because "suffering occurs when an impending destruction of the person is perceived" (p. 32). If body and mind are both taken into account, one would think that *suffering* and *pain* should be used in a similar way, but the two terms can be defined differently—*pain* being a physical discomfort, a neurological sign, while *suffering* can be understood as the *interpretation* of that neurological sign (Anderson 2011: 2; Cassell 1991).

In the case of the loss of a loved one, the bereaved does not only suffer physically, but due to the loss of an immediate tie to a social bond a bereaved person also experiences an extremely excruciating form of mental suffering: *grief* (Charmaz and Milligan 2006; also see Neimeyer 1998, 2015).

While *grief* and *sadness* are often used as interchangeable terms, we find it important to define the variations and clear characteristics of both. Izard writes that "Sadness is the predominant emotion in grief" (1991: 203), indicating that sadness is a basic human emotion. Grief, however, is a highly aversive emotional condition "that generates various molecular components, including a range of specific emotions" (Bonanno et al. 2008: 798) and appears to be a more complex construct (cf. Döveling 2014). Most dominantly, but not exclusively, sadness is included in this set of emotions (Bonnano et al. 2008). While sadness as a basic human emotion lasts only a few seconds, minutes, or hours (Ekman 1984), grief and the construct surrounding it can last for months or years (Bonnano 2004). In addition, "[s]uffering is pervasive, if not always shared." (Anderson 2014: 10).

Grief as a specific form of suffering is also regarded as a basic and evolutionary founded human emotion (Ekman and Friesen 1971). Grief characterizes the process in which dismay, abjection, and suffering are present during the emotionally challenging situation caused by the loss of a significant other (Bonanno et al. 2008) and the cognitive understanding of the experience (Izard 1991). The focus of such pain is tied to someone or something that is missing and will not return in the future, an irrevocable loss (Parkes 1993).

Suffering, grief, sadness, and the correlated *mourning* (Izard 1991) are socially rooted, interrelated processes associated with the occurrence of other emotions (cf. also Jakoby 2012b). Their sharing needs to be regarded as a transformational process that equally incorporates the bonding emotions of *empathy* and *compassion*. Morse notes:

> …enduring and suffering are fundamental and normal responses to catastrophic loss, yet strangely these two basic states have not been extensively explored using qualitative methods. Both states occur commonly as a human response to illness, injury, and bereavement (2000: 1).

The confrontation with the suffering, from a perspective of process-orientation in the positive sense and outcome, is also known as *coping* (Aldwin 2007) with the incorporated goal of reaching a "new reference" to oneself (Kast 1982: 5).[1] Likewise, Neimeyer concludes that a central feature of grieving is *the attempt to reaffirm or reconstruct a world of meaning that has been challenged by loss"* (Neimeyer in this volume and cf. Neimeyer 1998).

A central characteristic of coping is *social support*, given and received as an *emotional resource* (Pierce et al. 1996). A dual process of *loss-oriented* and *restoration-oriented* coping displays a natural strategy of managing an emotionally challenging situation (Stroebe and Schut 1999: 213). Suffering and grieving, then, are directly interrelated processes that rarely occur in an isolated situation, but are rather *social phenomena*, correspondingly influenced by social structure and group norms (Jakoby 2012a; Rimé et al. 1991). Accordingly, "social sharing of emotions" (Rimé et al. 1991) represents a fundamental strategy of coping. Therefore, in a social setting, suffering might lead to a deeper reflection of the precipitating event. The need for shared collective experiences with other humans is vital in understanding such coping processes. *Interpersonal communication* of one's grief can:

– help to realize and find a meaning for the loss (Luminet et al. 2000),
– cause reciprocal understanding (Rimé 2009), and
– lead to the much needed social support and empathy from the social environment (Rimé et al. 1991).

When scrutinizing emotions in the online exchange of grief, the emotional expression of empathy becomes evident. Online users are able to react to one another with emotional support because of *empathic mechanisms*, that is, one must be able to notice and feel one's own emotions in order to relate with someone else's (Hoffman 2008). Collins characterizes those mechanisms as "emotional energy" (Collins 1984, 1990: 33). Interacting harmoniously and supporting the other has direct positive effects on any form of social solidarity, online or otherwise. Collins highlights that, in the course of interaction, group-specific symbols that represent the affiliation have the potential to engender "interaction ritual chains" (Collins 1987: 198). Due to growing trust and confidence, social interaction about a sensitive emotional topic primarily happens face-to-face, but if the emotional process is restrained by "disenfranchised emotions" (Doka 2008) or if, on account of social norms, emotion management is imposed by the societal surrounding (Hochschild 1983; Döveling 2005; Southam-Gerow 2013), then social sharing of grief may be extended to a group of anonymous individuals, such as that found in *online support communities* (Turner et al. 2001; Radcliffe et al. 2010).

---

[1] So called *phase* or *stage models*, as most notably, Kübler-Ross' (1969) well known stage model, implying a logical development in grief work, have been intensively criticized as they do not take the complexity and distinctness in grieving processes into account. Grief is thus a complex emotional process (cf. Stroebe and Schut 1999; cf. also Neimeyer in this volume). As Klass et al. (1996) note, grieving can also entail a continuous bond with the deceased.

In the virtual community of Social Network Sites, mourners generate resources, share experiences, and provide social support. Bambina (2007) differentiates two communicative role patterns: "[G]ivers, who supply each other and the takers with support and takers, who do not provide anyone with support" (Bambina 2007: 115). Based on this concept, we take into account that the exchange of emotions structures social situations in the "real" and virtual worlds (Döveling 2005, based on Collins' concept of emotions, cf. Collins 1987). Emotions are socially exchanged resources. Within this "social sharing of emotions" (Rimé et al. 1991), emotion regulation and management might take place (Rimé 2007; Döveling 2014). We understand these processes as dynamic interpersonal and intrapersonal processes that include conscious or unconscious strategies that modify the emotional burden of suffering. As equally highlighted by Gross and Thompson (2007) these regulation processes of emotions also include the selection of specific situations, as in our case is the choice to turn to the social web (for further analysis of 'emotion regulation' see Döveling 2014).

Furthermore, emotions tend to follow an *associative logic* (Kappas and Müller 2006) and in day to day interactions are primarily dominated by *mimic*, *gesture*, and *intonation* (Geise 2011). Purely text-based online communication might hinder or impede this associative logic. This is where emotional symbols come into play. So-called emoticons help in online emotional communication, as they are simplified visual signals of emotions (cf. Derks et al. 2008, Misoch 2006). The use of a multiplicity of emoticons and other symbolic communications in text-based support opens a broader array of possibilities for emotional expression online (Misoch 2006).

24.3   Study Design and Research Method

After having laid out the theoretical basis and the complexity of emotional interactions for the study, the focus turns to the analysis of motives, processes and potential outcomes in the online "social sharing of emotions" (Rimé et al. 1991). The qualitative content analysis (cf. Strauss and Corbin 1998; Mayring 2000) was conducted from 11/2012 to 4/2013 of 179 postings across three different platforms (N=56 in "TrauerVerlustForum", N=59 in "YoungWings" and N=67 in "MeineTrauer"[2]).

By choosing a random sample, we avoided the bias resulting from selecting a sample on the basis of convenience. In a first step, the central characteristics of postings were explored. These characteristics led to categories which were revised, condensed to main categories, and operationalized according to theory and material.

---

[2] Trauerverlustforum [sadnesslossplatform] will be abbreviated TVF; Youngwings will be abbreviated YW; MeineTrauer [MySadness] will be abbreviated MT. The research project was led and supervised by Katrin Döveling and conduced in a team at the TU Dresden: Supervisor: Katrin Döveling, Research Team: Katrin Wasgien, Kevin Klamert, Charlotta Knigge, Lisa Krämer, Carolin Pohl, Anne Schier.

The categories were underlined with prototypical text passages from the postings and their coding reliability was tested and confirmed. Coding rules for the distinctive categories were formulated. The material was then analyzed according to the categories. Based on this, hypotheses were generated, each of which will be given and illustrated in the following section.[3] A model that portrayed the central mechanisms in a conceptual form was built. The qualitative content analysis was found well-suited in understanding the complex, inherent mechanisms in this sensitive topic (For the subsequent quantitative analysis, see Döveling 2014).

24.4 Results

Through *qualitative content analysis* the motives and mechanisms of shared online grief were identified. We noted communicative processes disclosing patterns of emotional interaction, which will be laid out and illustrated in the following sections.

24.4.1 Missed Support

One common feature within online communication was the verbalization of missed support in the offline world. Bereavement platforms were substantially used as an extension of one's own personal social environment, particularly when the bereaved does not feel the needed emotional support offline, from family or other loved ones.

> H. in MT: *"I cannot share my feelings with anyone. That's why I ended up in this community and try to write down, what tortures me."*
> L. in YW: *"Hello, I would like to tell you my story, because I have no one to really talk to."*

Various postings reveal similar statements which led to the first hypothesis:

If the bereaved feels left alone or not understood in his or her suffering in the offline world, he or she will turn to online platforms.

24.4.2 Feeling of Cohesiveness

A common communicative aspect in all bereavement platforms is the open disclosure of formerly 'intimate' emotions. The bereaved verbalize a strong sense of togetherness and shared understanding. This intimate interaction of personal

---

[3] For the follow up quantitative analysis see Döveling, K. (2014). Emotion regulation in bereavement: searching for and finding emotional support in social network sites, *New Review of Hypermedia and Multimedia*, DOI: 10.1080/13614568.2014.983558

feelings corresponds to findings in the offline communication of bereavement. The platform is considered a refuge, as mourners find a common ground that binds them and leads to mutual emotional support. As Stylianos and Vachon (1993) highlight in their analysis of 'offline' social support, finding meaning of death, encountering one's own perspectives and communicating about one's struggles are vital elements in understanding support in bereavement. This is equally true in online bereavement.

> A. in MT: *"We are here for you. We feel the same."*
> J. in MT: *"You see—you are not alone."*
> S. in MT: *"You have found your way to us—that's a good start… Here you will find many Moms and Dads that are in the same situation like you!"*

This led to the second hypotheses:

The stronger the feeling of community is topic for the bereaved, the more online socio-emotional support is expressed.

24.4.3   Interaction Patterns in Online Communication

Users of online platforms apply different mechanisms within their emotion regulation and can integrate themselves into the community to different degrees or intensities. Users who have evolved and feel stronger in their suffering may be more supportive to others than users who have just recently faced their source of grief. Thus, *different interaction patterns* were found. Users who *supported* other users were defined as care-giving, while users who seek and potentially *received* emotional support were defined as care-seeking. The following excerpt illustrates the reciprocity within this relationship:

> R., care-giving in TVF: *"I just want to hug you and let you know that I send supporting thoughts. Please endure what maybe cannot be understood. You are not alone, wherever you are! Letting out your thoughts and emotions may be the only thing that I can suggest to you."*
>
> S., care-seeking in TVF: *"Thank you! I don't know what to do. We were already separated since January. Do you think I should visit his parents? Or maybe call? I am just helpless right now."*

The social web creates an *emotional proximity*, enabling the open communication of grief, empathy and gratitude.

The findings reveal that reciprocal communication patterns regulate the development of interaction ritual chains (Collins 1987: 198). With increasing confidence in the other members of the community, online communication on a delicate and complex emotional topic is enabled, empowering emotion regulation and interactive emotion management in the reciprocity of care-giving and care-seeking.

> L. in YW: *"I just can't do it anymore… Last week I found my boyfriend dead in his apartment. He had just killed himself. […] My entire plan of life just burst away! At night when I really want to sleep the pictures come, the accusations and the deep grief I feel for losing him…"*

Answer from J. in YW: *"I can't put into words what I would like to say to you right now. I sometimes feel like language wasn't built for emotions that strong. [...] Right now you need to be good to yourself and try not to let the dark thoughts take over! Even if that is really, really hard!"*

As the above quote illustrates, a care-seeking message is followed by a care-giving message, enabling regulative emotion processes. Likewise, the findings show that a care-seeking person who is more stable in his emotional management may proceed to care-giving.

J. in YW: *"As I wrote that, all the pictures in my head came up again and I had to fight tears. But still I think it was good to finally get it out of my head and write it all down."*

J. in YW (Further on in the conversation): *"I am very sorry about what happened to your father and that you couldn't talk after your fight—it must be so hard for you, I can only imagine! At least I was able to talk to him one last time and prepare for it... I am so sorry for you!"*

This led to the third hypothesis:

When a support seeker has moved on in his emotion regulation within his coping process, his or her messages will become care-giving.

24.4.4 Emotional Visuals

In addition to text-based communication, online-shared emotions are commonly supported by visuals online. *Emoticons* as well as *ritualistic symbols* (such as candles) function as reinforcement of text messages. The social web enables corresponding emotional communication in suffering and coping processes that are comparable to communication patterns in real life.

During online interaction, visual communication displays a relevant means of communicating emotions and framing messages. As the online social net platform does not allow direct signals in face to face exchange, nonverbal communication patterns are transmitted through the use of visual elements, so called emoticons and ritual elements such as virtual candles, into the communication patterns. Visual communication stimuli were used in 34.4 % of all messages (For more quantitative results, see Döveling 2014).

24.4.5 Communicative Topic Development

Children and young adults are particularly adaptive. They develop inherent communicative exchange patterns within online communication. Emotional proximity, intensity, familiarity, and mutual trust are gained, leading to communicative patterns comparable to those in offline interactions. This finding corresponds to the concept of self-disclosure as found in offline surroundings. Within the development

of an interpersonal relationship, the communication evolves to a more open, intimate and personal nature (cf. Derlega et al. 1993). While adult users predominantly
address topics of death, grieving, and dying, adolescent and young mourners open
up to discuss topics of everyday life that do not deal with their bereavement.

> M. in YW: *"no, I don't speak any further languages. I am more of a mathematical talent.
> Have you been born in Hungary?"*

Based on those findings, the fourth hypothesis is:

> The longer a conversation is held within one thread of the youth platform, the less
> the conversion will deal with the suffering.

24.5   Process Model of Online Coping

The communication in the online environment is not solely related to death, dying,
and grief, but equally as a means of mutual sharing and understanding personal loss.
We interpret this finding as a sign of *returning to life* or finding relief from suffering.
The social network site enables emotion regulation away from grief and toward
emotions of friendship and cohesiveness. This directly influences the bereaved in a
positive way.

The findings reveal that in *virtual interaction chains*, empathic emotions become
a vital resource. Based on empathic reactions and taking into account the anonymity
of the social network site, *emotional gratifications* become evident (see Fig. 24.1).
Through the communicative function of an *emotional agenda* (Döveling 2005),
interactive chains are unveiled that—through encoding and decoding—lead to a

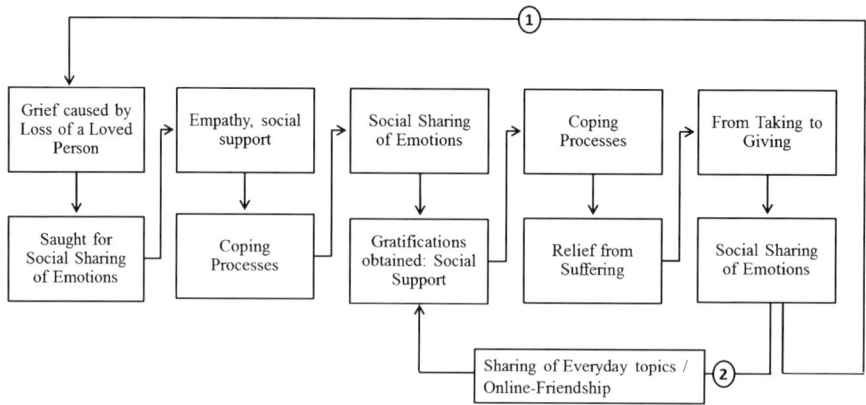

1. Commucative Development in Online Bereavement Platforms
2. Development of Online Friendships through Sharing of Emotions

Fig. 24.1 Process model of online coping

reciprocal understanding of online gratification in the sense of obtaining social support engendering coping in grieving processes.

Social Internet usage thus plays an essential role in coping with bereavement, particularly when there is a void in supportive offline interactions. The social net platform allows mourners to act and interact freely, finding mutual reciprocal exchange of support. The *process model of online coping* exemplifies how virtual sharing of emotions within a community can lead to emotion regulation in bereavement and felt relief from suffering. We continually found communication structures as laid out in the model above in online grief communities.

24.6 Discussion and Implications: Online Emotion Regulation in the Process of Suffering

Throughout this study, insights into the motives, forms, and mechanisms involved in online suffering have been identified. The bereaved turn to social network platforms, as these enable a common ground of understanding and much needed social support, especially in the absence of other, more visceral support. Formerly privately shared emotions are often expressed within online communities.

A relevant aspect of online suffering is the *meeting of likeminded*. Online platforms provide a social space in which bereaved individuals who have lived through the same or similar emotional distress may bond and participate in a process of mutual understanding. The magnitude of messages acknowledging missed support in the offline-environment highlights the relevance of feeling membership within an online community. Young users especially do not solely search for someone to talk to about death and dying, but forge relationships of mutual support, and cultivate friendships that allow conversations to extend beyond suffering and into the more mundane topics of life that signal a reduction of suffering or especially grief.

According to findings on (offline) bereavement (Klass and Walter 2001), grieving caused by the loss of a loved one needs to be considered a reoccurring emotional process. A person may feel better one day and worse the next. Yet, when the mourner feels better, has found or rediscovered meaning (cf. Neimeyer in this volume) in the sense that he is in the recovery process as Strobe and Schutt (1999) highlight for offline communication, he can provide the assistance a care seeker needs. Due to mutual understanding, these role patterns enable online emotion regulation of grief (cf. Döveling 2014).

Within the online-bereavement community, users who have proceeded in their regulation of grief provide help, hope, and socio-emotional and informational support as well as affirmation to other users who are at the beginning of their emotional regulation process. Communication patterns underline those *interactional patterns* and engender *emotion management and regulation* within the community (cf. Döveling 2014).

Alongside emotions shared with friends and family, online-shared emotions help manage emotional distress and provide support. The analysis demonstrates that online-shared emotions should not be overlooked within the scientific community. The Internet is highly relevant to suffering processes and its study contributes to a deeper understanding of virtual communication .

Online platforms can be considered places where one can find likeminded from all over the world to connect with, share emotions, and give and receive social support.

Online suffering is a new field of communication research, and this study outlines basic mechanisms and structures via a qualitative analysis of relevant platforms in Germany(cf. Döveling 2014, for quantitative analysis).

Further insight will be obtained by applying other research methods such as quantitative content analysis (cf. Döveling 2014) and interviewing the suffering. Relevant future research might widen the cultural perspective to analyze emotional communication patterns in other countries. Is the described phenomenon only valid for Germany or is it—as is strongly suggested by the theoretical background—also relevant in other countries and cultures? Another next step will be to focus on more detailed research questions, taking into account factors such as cultural impact, age and gender differences, the influence of religion, and the diversity of emotion regulation patterns and approaches.

This quote by Kübler-Ross, a pioneer in the field of grief and suffering, captures the essence of our respect for those expressing their bereavement emotions online:

> The most beautiful people we have known are those who have known defeat, known suffering, known struggle, known loss, and have found their way out of the depths. These persons have an appreciation, a sensitivity, and an understanding of life that fills them with compassion, gentleness, and a deep loving concern. Beautiful people do not just happen (Kübler-Ross 1975: 96).

References

Aldwin, C. M. (2007). *Stress, coping, and development. An integrative perspective*. New York: The Guilford Press.

Anderson, R. E. (2011). *World suffering—Conceptualization, measurement, and findings.* Paper presented at the 2011 meeting of the American Association for Public Opinion Research (AAPOR) in Phoenix. Retrieved from http://www.compassionatesocieties.org/attachments/article/684/Suffering-paper-for-aapor2011-18may11.pdf. Accessed 17 Apr 2013.

Anderson, R. E. (2014). *Human suffering and quality of life conceptualizing stories and statistics*. New York: Springer.

Bambina, A. (2007). *Online social support. The interplay of social networks and computer-mediated communication*. Youngstown: Cambria Press.

Bonanno, G. A. (2004). Loss, trauma, and human resilience: Have we underestimated the human capacity to thrive after extremely aversive events? *American Psychologist, 59*(1), 20–28.

Bonanno, G. A., Goorin, L., & Coifman, K. G. (2008). Sadness and grief. In M. Lewis, J. M. Haviland-Jones, & L. Feldman Barrett (Eds.), *Handbook of emotions* (3rd ed., pp. 797–810). New York: Guilford Press.

Cassell, E. J. (1991). *The nature of suffering and the goals of medicine*. Oxford/New York: Oxford University Press.

Charmaz, K., & Milligan, M. J. (2006). Grief. In J. E. Stets & J. H. Turner (Eds.), *Handbook of the sociology of emotions* (pp. 516–543). New York: Springer.

Collins, R. (1984). The role of emotion in social structure. In K. R. Scherer & P. Ekman (Eds.), *Approaches to emotion* (pp. 385–396). Hillsdale/London: L. Erlbaum Associates.

Collins, R. (1987). Interaction ritual chains, power and property: The micro–macro connection as an empirically based theoretical problem. In J. C. Alexander, B. Giesen, R. Münch, & N. J. Smelser (Eds.), *The micro–macro-link* (pp. 193–206). Berkeley/Los Angeles/London: University of California Press.

Collins, R. (1990). Stratification, emotional energy, and the transient emotions. In T. D. Kemper (Ed.), *Research agendas in the sociology of emotions* (pp. 27–57). Albany: State University of New York Press.

Derks, D., Fischer, A. H., & Bos, A. E. R. (2008). The role of emotion in computer-mediated communication: A review. *Computers in Human Behavior, 24*(3), 766–785.

Derlega, V., Metts, S., Petronio, S., & Margulis, S. T. (1993). *Self-disclosure*. Thousand Oaks/London: Sage.

Doka, K. J. (2008). Disenfranchised grief in historical and cultural perspective. In M. S. Stroebe, R. O. Hansson, H. Schut, & W. Stroebe (Eds.), *Handbook of bereavement research and practice* (pp. 223–240). Washington, DC: American Psychological Association.

Döveling, K. (2005). *Emotionen—Medien—Gemeinschaft: eine kommunikationssoziologische Analyse* [Emotions—Media—Community: A media-sociological perspective]. Wiesbaden: VS Verlag für Sozialwissenschaften.

Döveling, K. (2012). Emotionsmanagement im Netz: Bewältigung von Krankheit, Sterben und Tod in Sozialen Netzwerken. Emotional Sharing = Coping [Emotion management in the internet: Coping with illness, dying and death in social networks. Emotional sharing = Coping]. *Zeitschrift für Palliativmedizin, 13*(05). Retrieved from https://www.thieme-connect.com/ejournals/abstract/10.1055/s-0032-1322890. Accessed 17 Feb 2013.

Döveling, K. (2014). Emotion regulation in bereavement: searching for and finding emotional support in social network sites. *New Review of Hypermedia and Multimedia*, published online 6 December 2014. doi:10.1080/13614568.2014.983558

Döveling, K, & Wasgien, K. (2014). Emotionsmanagement im Netz. Kindertrauer online. Ein aktueller Forschungsbeitrag [Emotion management in the Web. Children's sadness online. Current Research]. In Franziska Röseberg und Monika Müller (Eds.), *Handbuch Kindertrauer* (pp. 421–434). Göttingen: Vandenhoeck & Ruprecht.

Ekman, P. (1984). Expression and the nature of emotion. In K. Scherer & P. Ekman (Eds.), *Approaches to emotion* (pp. 319–343). Hillsdale: Erlbaum.

Ekman, P., & Friesen, W. V. (1971). Constants across cultures in the face and emotion. *Journal of Personality and Social Psychology, 17*(2), 124–129.

Ferrel, B. (2005). Ethical perspectives on pain and suffering. *Pain Management Nursing, 6*(3), 83–90.

Francis, L. E. (2006). Emotions and health. In J. E. Stets & J. H. Turner (Eds.), *Handbook of the sociology of emotions* (pp. 591–610). New York: Springer.

Geise, S. (2011). *Vision that matters*. Wiesbaden: VS Verlag für Sozialwissenschaften.

Gross, J. J., & Thompson, R. A. (2007). Emotion regulation. Conceptual foundations. In J. J. Gross (Ed.), *Handbook of emotion regulation* (pp. 3–26). New York: Guilford Press.

Hochschild, A. R. (1983). *The managed heart. Commercialization of human feeling*. Berkeley: University of California Press.

Hoffman, M. (2008). Empathy and prosocial behavior. In M. Lewis, J. M. Haviland-Jones, & L. Feldman Barrett (Eds.), *Handbook of emotions* (3rd ed., pp. 440–455). New York: Guilford Press.

Izard, C. E. (1991). *The psychology of emotions*. New York: Plenum Press.

Jakoby, N. (2012a). Trauer als Forschungsgegenstand der Emotionssoziologie [Grief as scholarly topic in emotion-sociology]. In A. Schnabel & R. Schützeichel (Eds.), *Emotionen, Sozialstruktur und Moderne* (pp. 407–424). Wiesbaden: VS Verlag für Sozialwissenschaften.

Jakoby, N. (2012b). Grief as a social emotion: Theoretical perspectives. *Death Studies, 36,* 679–711.

Kappas, A., & Müller, M. G. (2006). Bild und Emotion—ein neues Forschungsfeld [Picture and emotions—a new field of study]. *Publizistik, 51*(1), 3–23.

Kast, V. (1982). *Trauern: Phasen und Chancen des psychischen Prozesses* [Grieving: Phases and chances of the psychological process]. Freiburg: Kreuz Verlag.

Klass, D., & Walter, T. (2001). Processes of grieving: How bonds are continued. In M. S. Stroebe, R. O. Hansson, W. Stroebe, & H. Schut (Eds.), *Handbook of bereavement research: Consequences, coping and care* (pp. 431–448). Washington, DC: American Psychological Association.

Klass, D., Silverman, P. R., & Nickman, S. L. (Eds.). (1996). *Continuing bonds. New understandings of grief.* Washington, DC/Bristol/London: Taylor & Francis.

Kleinman, A., Das, V., & Lock, M. (Eds.). (1997). *Social suffering.* Berkeley/Los Angeles: University of California Press.

Kübler-Ross, E. (1969). *On death and dying.* New York: Scribner.

Kübler-Ross, E. (1975). *Death: The final stage of growth.* New York: Simon & Schuster.

Luminet, O., Bouts, P., Delie, F., Manstead, S. R., & Rimé, B. (2000). Social sharing of emotion following exposure to a negatively valenced situation. *Cognition and Emotion, 14*(5), 661–688.

Mayring, P. (2000). *Qualitative Inhaltsanalyse. Grundlagen und Techniken* [Qualitative content analysis: Basics and techniques] (7th ed.). Weinheim: Beltz.

McLuhan, M. (1962). *The Gutenberg galaxy. The making of typographic man.* Toronto/Buffalo/London: University of Toronto Press.

Misoch, S. (2006). *Online-Kommunikation* [Online-communication]. Konstanz: UVK.

Morse, J. M. (2000). Responding to the cues of suffering. *Health Care for Women International, 21*(1), 1–9.

Nagappan, R. (2005). *Speaking havoc: Social suffering & South Asian narratives.* Seattle: University of Washington Press.

Neimeyer, R. A. (1998). *Lessons of loss: A guide to coping.* New York: McGraw Hill.

Neimeyer, R. (2015). Meaning in bereavement. In R. Anderson (Ed.), *World suffering and quality in life.* New York: Springer.

Parkes, C. M. (1993). Bereavement as a psychosocial transition: Processes of adaptation to change. In M. S. Stroebe, W. Stroebe, & R. O. Hansson (Eds.), *Handbook of bereavement* (pp. 91–101). Cambridge: Cambridge University Press.

Pierce, G. R., Sarason, I. G., & Sarason, B. R. (1996). Coping and social support. In M. Zeidner & N. S. Endler (Eds.), *Handbook of coping. Theory, research, applications* (pp. 434–451). New York: Wiley.

Prensky, M. (2001). Digital natives, digital immigrants. *On the Horizon, 9*(5), 2–6.

Radcliffe, A. M., Lumley, M. A., Kendall, J., Stevenson, J. K., & Beltran, J. (2010). Written emotional disclosure. Testing whether social disclosure matters. *Journal of Social and Clinical Psychology, 26*(3), 362–384.

Rimé, B. (2007). Interpersonal emotion regulation. In J. J. Gross (Ed.), *Handbook of emotion regulation* (pp. 466–485). New York: Guilford Press.

Rimé, B. (2009). Emotion elicits the social sharing of emotion. Theory and empirical review. *Emotion Review, 1*(1), 60–85.

Rimé, B., Mesquita, B., Boca, S., & Philipot, P. (1991). Beyond the emotional event. Six studies on the social sharing of emotion. *Cognition and Emotion, 5*(5/6), 435–465.

Southam-Gerow, M. A. (2013). *Emotion regulation in children and adolescents. A practitioner's guide.* New York: Guilford Press.

Strauss, A. L., & Corbin, J. M. (1998). *Basics of qualitative research: Techniques and procedures for developing grounded theory* (2nd ed.). Thousand Oaks/London/New Delhi: Sage.

Stroebe, M. S., & Schut, H. (1999). The dual process model of coping with bereavement: Rationale and description. *Death Studies, 23,* 197–224.

Stylianos, S. K., & Vachon, M. L. S. (1993). The role of social support in bereavement. In M. S. Stroebe, W. Stroebe, & R. O. Hansson (Eds.), *Handbook of bereavement: Theory, research, and intervention* (8th ed., pp. 397–410). Cambridge: Cambridge University Press.

Turner, J. W., Grube, J. A., & Meyers, J. (2001). Developing an optimal match within online communities: An exploration of CMC support communities and traditional support. *Journal of Communication, 51*(2), 231–251.

Chapter 25
Cosmopolitan Perspectives on Suffering

Laura Robinson

25.1 Introduction

Drawing on empirical data from Brazilian, French, and American digital discourse spaces, the analysis in this chapter illuminates the use of universalistic and transnational identity frames to identify with those suffering in the wake of 9/11/01. More specifically, this chapter asks three questions. First, what was the range of cosmopolitan stances used to classify others' suffering as worthy of compassion? Second, what forms of identity work facilitated empathy with those suffering? Third, what cultural frames influenced how individuals framed similarities or erased boundaries between themselves and those suffering?

To answer these questions, this chapter analyzes the construction of cosmopolitan identity categories used to make sense of victims' identities on 9/11/01. To make these connections, the analysis explores how individuals performed identity work that created expansive identity categories as a means of expressing solidarity. The analysis of cosmopolitan identity work presented here points to the potential of inclusionary identity work in which the suffering of others is shared. As the Brazilian case tells us, when such thinking predominates, "humanity" becomes the primary identity category of importance.

In so doing, this chapter contributes to the literature on cosmopolitanism. Often cosmopolitan thinking refers to "moral cosmopolitanism" defined as the "moral ideal of a universal human community" (Kleingeld and Brown 2011). However, cosmopolitan identities exist along a continuum and allow individuals to identify with a range of supranational communities. At their most narrow, cosmopolitan

L. Robinson (✉)
Santa Clara University, Santa Clara, USA
e-mail: laura@laurarobinson.org

© Springer Science+Business Media Dordrecht 2015
R.E. Anderson (ed.), *World Suffering and Quality of Life*,
Social Indicators Research Series 56, DOI 10.1007/978-94-017-9670-5_25

identities produce empathy when observers make connections between themselves and those suffering. Further along the continuum, cosmopolitan identities may be transnational and build upon similarities linking citizens of different nation states. In their broadest incarnation, cosmopolitan identities can be completely universalistic and have the power to compete with national identities in importance (Jameson 1982). When individuals espousing a cosmopolitan stance regard themselves as world citizens, the suffering of all of humanity becomes equally salient and worthy of solidarity. Thus we see that contrary to much social science literature assuming the nation state as the dominant identity category (Beck 2000), cosmopolitan identities may also yield considerable salience.

25.2   Data and Methods

Scholarship continues to show the importance of the Internet as a venue to collect data on narratives of suffering (Anderson 2014). This chapter follows this tradition by drawing on data from three discourse communities hosted by flagship newspapers in Brazil, France, and the U.S.: *O Estado de São Paolo, Le Monde*, and *The New York Times*. Part of a larger project (Robinson 2005, 2008, 2009), the sampling frame is the universe of contributions posted to the three sites during the week following the attacks. From September 11 to September 17, 2001 individuals wrote 2,905 posts to *The New York Times'* "A Nation Challenged," 2,264 posts to *Le Monde's* "The September 11th attacks in the United States," and 1,119 posts to *O Estado's* "The First War of the Century."

Data in this chapter come from posts expressing solidarity with the victims, their families, and/or concern with collective suffering. Therefore, the data include only posts specifically addressing these themes analyzed through iterated coding and recoding. I began open coding to demarcate analytic categories. Subsequently, I wrote initial memos concentrating on core themes identified in open coding before proceeding to focused coding to refine the analytic categories. Rounds of focused coding and integrative memos grounded the analysis in the data.

25.3   Universalistic Cosmopolitanism

Brazilian cosmopolitans identify with those suffering as members of the human family independent of any other identity category. The Brazilian case offers an exemplar of cosmopolitanism at its most universalizing. For Brazilian cosmopolitans, the suffering of all members of humanity is equally relevant:

> It is when the other is suffering, when the consequences are such that all must help each other and ask for help… The worst is when one does not want to see one's sick and sad brother and one does not pray together to ask for peace for mankind and good will to men.

Further, these cosmopolitans frame the extension of empathy as a moral imperative. As one Brazilian cosmopolitan argues: "Anyone with a conscience should mourn the death of thousands of civilians and ask God to comfort the families of the unfortunates." By using this inclusionary strategy, cosmopolitanism extends empathy to the suffering other and marginalizes other identity categories: "We have no right to sacrifice any human life for political motives or other ideologies. Terrorism is a great error. I mourn and pray for the dead in this sad act that they may have peace."

By including all members of humanity as "brothers," they explicitly denationalize victims and dismiss any other identity category as irrelevant. This Brazilian cosmopolitan writes: "The best thing we can do is for all countries to show their solidarity with our American brothers. In these moments, differences do not exist!" Another adds: "The value of life is the same in all places: priceless." A third contributes: "It is a pity that so many innocents died in this terrible story. Humanity must evolve a great deal here on earth." Brazilian cosmopolitans employ the category of humanity to unite themselves with those suffering: "Humanity watched… those innocent human beings of innumerable nations that were assassinated in this horrible and unforgettable day." Further, they extend empathy to those left behind: "What I am terribly sad for are the loved ones of those who have died." Another adds: "I feel terribly for these people's deaths and would like to tell their families that only God can measure the depth and intensity of their pain, indignation, and sadness." Whether in reference to the victims themselves or their loved ones, cosmopolitan Brazilians emphasize humanity as the only salient aspect of the victims' identities:

> Imagine the families' desperation looking for their relatives. They are lives and lives that were lost. How many fathers, family men, di--people who never think of political oppression. We should cry for this tragedy just as we should cry for people who die of violence in Brazil… We are all human… right?

Another exhorts: "My condolences to the Brazilian and American families, but principally to humanity, a small part of which died yesterday." In making these claims, Brazilian cosmopolitans erase boundaries between themselves, the victims, their families, and the rest of humanity.

Further, Brazilian cosmopolitans make larger commentaries on what it means to be human—at its best and worst. One describes: "Horror… horror… horror… I feel shame to be a human being." Another comments: "Human beings are the greatest guilty party in all of this that has happened, for through global greed humanity respects no one." Yet a third contributes: "I believe that what I am thinking is not terribly different than what the rest of the world is imagining. We are ashamed to be part of the same race as those responsible for this!" This cosmopolitan asserts: "How is it possible that the human race has decided to bring itself so low? We are all guilty in this tragedy. We all carry within us the feelings of hatred and intolerance." These Brazilian cosmopolitans frame humanity as the ultimate symbolic perpetrator of 9/11/01. They believe that because humanity is capable of great evil, as members of humanity, every human shares in the guilt. As this cosmopolitan asserts: "What has happened is the fruit of greed, religion, politics, economics, in short what we call being human." Thus, Brazilian cosmopolitans argue that 9/11/01 provides an opportunity to reconsider what it should mean to be human: "Nothing justifies these acts. Perhaps humanity will think more about things that have been so forgotten like love, the environment, prosperity and equality between mankind. I hope that we can learn this lesson," and "I hope that those responsible will be punished and made examples of and the world will come back to be more HUMAN"

Brazilian cosmopolitans contribute the strongest expression of cosmopolitanism as an ideology that symbolically divides humanity against those that would destroy it. For them, every human faces the fundamental choice between the good and evil both present in humankind:

> Terrible? Brutal? We humans need to stop and reflect about all that happened, is happening, and will happen, about evil created by human beings, we need to understand and stop and think of ourselves and use our free will, each of us to change the World. If the World continues selfishly, evilly, and continues to shut its eyes to poverty, pain, etc. the end will be next, much worse than we think! But there is time; we can all change. My thoughts go to the victims.

Others also divide the world into the "human" and "inhuman." One relates: "…all of humanity suffers the consequences of the inhuman acts committed today." The use of the word "inhuman" is significant and taken up by others: "An attack of these proportions demonstrates to the world the extreme treachery of these groups of terrorists… the death of thousands of people, innocent victims of this brutal attack is an inhuman act." For Brazilian cosmopolitans, all members of humanity must make their choice and choose a side:

> For me it was obvious that there are two worlds that are absolutely different: the first is made up of people who are born and work for their neighbor, for society. People like us, who despite whatever difficulty, day-to-day struggle for what is best. The second type of being, which we cannot call human, only is born to grow up to sow hatred, destruction, unjustified death, in truth the horsemen of the Apocalypse who decide who will live and who will die. We must not allow ourselves to be influenced by this feeling of hatred and in turn create more destruction.

Brazilian cosmopolitans frame this choice as the ultimate identity marker and the choice that must be made by all members of humanity in response to every kind of human suffering.

25.4 Transnational Cosmopolitanism

Turning to the French forum, identity work may resemble discourse in the Brazilian forum at first glance, but closer inspection reveals important differences. Like their Brazilian counterparts, French cosmopolitans link 9/11/01 victims with the victims of other tragedies, such as terrorist bombing in Paris:

> I feel so close to those who have died. I work in a tower at La Défense, and the images of those towers collapsing haunt me. Those who worked there worked many kinds of jobs, secretaries, accountants, janitors, etc. like those whose paths I cross every day at my work. They were not soldiers. They must have been of all races and religions.… Human history is no more than a vast repetition; the same horrors repeat themselves…

Also parallel to Brazilian cosmopolitans, French cosmopolitans frame those suffering as worthy of solidarity:

> The authors did not choose their target to destroy an American landmark; they wanted and determined to destroy the greatest number of human lives, regardless whether they were Christian, Muslim, or Jewish. They were all present in and around the WTC towers. They spared no one.

At first French discourse may seem similar to the universalistic cosmopolitanism expressed by Brazilians. However, whereas Brazilian cosmopolitans employ the concept of "humanity," even the most expansive French cosmopolitans rarely refer to "humanity" when expressing empathy.

Rather, French cosmopolitans emphasize their nationality when asserting the transnational bond: "I understand your heartache and I share it, yet understand that I myself am French… accept from me and from many others the assurance that, despite a few insignificant quibbles, we are at your side." Another writes: "I am not American, I am French… you can count on your longtime friends… This pattern is also clear regarding the three minutes of silence observed in the European Union to honor the victims on the Friday following 9/11/01. French cosmopolitans describe the three minutes of silence as an expression of Franco-American unity:

> The French news showed how the 3 minutes of silence were observed throughout the country. It was gut wrenching. It made me proud to be French… Make no mistake, some of us French people are ready to die for America like your grandfathers died for us.

Another echoes: "Today, the French observed 3 minutes of silence in memory of the victims of the attacks and I assure you that I could read real emotion on the faces of those people around me." Other French cosmopolitans also highlight French nationality in their expressions of transnational solidarity: "The real France stood still for three minutes today to honor your deaths… The real France was deeply shocked by the attacks… We really felt attacked. The real France is with you."

In lieu of "humanity," the French adopt a more transnational cosmopolitanism based on shared democratic values. French cosmopolitans' solidarity with those suffering is expressed as a function of the democratic heritage they share with the U.S. as citizens of the French Republic: "I entirely approve of the affirmation of support given to the United States by the President of the Republic and the Prime Minister; in the case of grave crisis like this one, democracies must forget their differences and close their ranks against their adversaries." Here it is important to note the use of the word adversaries used to define those who commit acts of terror, particularly terrorist acts framed as targeting democratic ideals or the democratic state: "Democratic values allow us to resolve our weaknesses, our contradictions, and our cowardice. Today I have chosen my camp and I support the American people. – An ordinary citizen." French emphasis on democracy indicates that this form of cosmopolitanism is rooted in shared transnational values, as well as a shared sense of vulnerability to terrorism: "I believe that many people on this forum showed their solidarity with Americans because they are conscious that in attacking the Americans, it is the way of life and the values that we, the French, share that is attacked." French expressions of transnational solidarity rely on erasing boundary differences between France and the U.S. as "democracies," rather than between all members of "humanity." In the eyes of French cosmopolitans, the French system is the actualization of Western goals and values that serve as a model for other nations such as the United States. Therefore, the French cosmopolitans that express solidarity with the victims do so based on their shared commitment to democracy, as this cosmopolitan writes: "This CRIME must simply be condemned. Compassion and indignation. DEMOCRACY."

25.5 Nationalism, Transnationalism, and Cosmopolitanism

In the American forum we see the full spectrum of identity frames that range from universalizing cosmopolitanism, to more circumscribed transnational cosmopolitanism, to nationalism. Regarding nationalism, not surprisingly, in immediate response to 9/11/01 many Americans call for national unity. While a number of Americans reference larger collectivities, they do so in tandem with expressions of national identity. While they may refer to collectivities beyond American borders, they simultaneously define the object of empathy as closer to home: "…I think it is imperative that we stand by our American brothers and sisters in this time of crisis, remaining firmly committed to the democratic ideals that unite us across religious and ethnic boundaries." For these Americans, national unity is paramount even when used in parallel with transnational identity frames:

> As I write, I am sitting in my office, in New York, watching as the sun prepares to set over the Hudson River. It is clear and beautiful out. Democracies are funny thing--anti-western despots can never understand them… they mistake our openness for weakness; our dynamic capitalism for self-centeredness. How do we answer them? E pluribus Unum. Out of many, one. America, and especially New York, will come out of this stronger than before.

In the days following the attacks, Americans are compelled by the forces of cultural trauma to situate themselves first and foremost as Americans who are also members of larger collectivities. When such Americans reference supranational identity frames, they typically couple them with references to national identity.

These Americans are joined on the forum by hundreds of citizens of other nations also expressing their solidarity. When the forum opens on the morning of September 12th, a flood of international empathy flows into the forum. As one explains, "Registering with this *New York Times* Message Board was the only way I could think of to communicate with some of the citizens of New York from a small town in the north of England." These international cosmopolitans present themselves as symbolically united with the victims in New York, Washington D.C., Pennsylvania, and the larger U.S. They come to the forum "…to let the inhabitants of New York and America know that they are not alone." The phrase "you are not alone" appears repeatedly: "I merely wanted to say to all who read this that you are not alone… and once again I say you are not alone."

Yet there are important differences in the international cosmopolitans participating in the American forum. Similar to the discourse in the French forum, European and "Anglosphere" (Vucetic 2011) cosmopolitans are more likely to rely on transnational cosmopolitan identity frames based on membership in "democracies" or the "free" world. One declares: "This attack was not just on America, it was an attack on all the good and just people of the free world." Such references to the "free world" resemble transnational discourse in the French forum much more closely than the universalistic cosmopolitanism dominant in the Brazilian forum. As this Australian cosmopolitan writes:

> What I saw shook me to the core. I can't begin to express the horror/shock/pain I felt. I've never been to the U.S. but somehow I've always felt that the U.S. represented the free world, & therefore my world. Since then I've sat glued to my television every moment I can, mourning with the families who've lost loved ones, praying with those still searching, rejoicing with each rescue of a victim & wishing for justice for those who organized this terrible thing. It's frightening to have this happen to America, the country that represents strength, freedom & democracy. Seeing New York & Washington violated in such a way made me realize how unsafe we all are against such attacks.

Another Spanish cosmopolitan declares: "Time for a Coalition of Democracies against Terrorism… We have a common enemy and let us work." On behalf of her family, a German cosmopolitan adds:

> Me and my family would like to assure you (and the American people) that we are very shocked about what happened not only to NY and Washington but also to the whole civilized world… We hope very much that the democratic countries will manage one day to stop terrorism.

While these transnational self-identifications are expansive, they frame solidarity in terms of the "democratic" or "free" world, thus mirroring the transnational cosmopolitanism on the French forum.

In parallel, expressions of universalizing cosmopolitanism are more likely to be contributed by citizens of democratic nations such as India. Contributions by these international cosmopolitans are parallel to the Brazilian use of "humanity" as the master identity frame. One writes: "We condemn the gravest act of barbarism against humanity where innocent people-men, women and children were so brutally massacred. May God receive them in heaven with open arms!" Another Indian cosmopolitan visits the American forum to express kinship with the victims and to condemn the attacks on "humanity":

> I offer my heartfelt condolences to the families of the innocent victims who tragically lost their lives in the worst ever attack on humanity, democracy and freedom… These acts are not against a nation but against humanity as a whole.

Significantly, coming from the world's largest democracy, this Indian cosmopolitan places "humanity" ahead of either democracy or freedom because the terrorist attacks violate "humanity as a whole." Finally, this Argentine cosmopolitan also employs universalistic discourse similar to that on the Brazilian forum: "From Argentina, what I can say is that here [the attacks] are seen as an act of cruelty… what they did was against humankind… The ones behind this to me can't be considered human anymore…" Like Brazilian commentary dividing the world into the "human" and the "inhuman," these Argentine and Indian cosmopolitans make connections between the acts of 9/11/01 and what it should mean to be a member of humanity.

25.6 Conclusions

Across the cases, cosmopolitans do identity work to symbolically unite victims of 9/11/01 with larger collectivities. This being said, there are important differences between the identity frames at play. Brazilian cosmopolitans offer a completely inclusionary form of cosmopolitanism. In the Brazilian case, "humanity" grounds cosmopolitan identity frames that include all individuals united in the "day-to-day struggle for what is best" as members of the human family. By using "humanity" as the single most important identity category, they render the suffering of any human being as equally worthy of empathy and underscore the conviction that all members of humanity share in each other's pain. Even more expansive, Brazilians make connections between those suffering on 9/11/01 and larger commentaries on what it should mean to be human. These findings resonate with previous research indicating the relevance of universalizing belief systems in contemporary Brazil (Pew-Templeton 2013). Brazilian references to "free will" and the "Horsemen of the Apocalypse" are part of larger spiritual belief systems for over 85 % of the population (65 % self-identify as Catholic and 22 % as Protestant) (Pew-Templeton 2013). For these Brazilians, Catholicism and Protestantism are salient cognitive authorities (Burdick 1996).

In the French forum, the forms of cosmopolitan discourse articulated are related to very different cultural factors. French cosmopolitans adopt a more circumscribed version of transnational cosmopolitanism that nonetheless builds unity with those suffering. French cosmopolitans draw on national identity and link it to transnational kinship based on the long-shared history between the French Republic and the U.S. This emphasis on French national identity and the French Republic stems from the idea of "l'exception française" or "l'exception culturelle." Both concepts refer to the idea of French exceptionalism in the realm of culture both at home and abroad: "The idea that France is somehow unique is deeply embedded in the nation's self-image… It reflects the conviction that France has an exemplary, universal role as a civilizing force…" (Jenkins 2000:112). Further, many of the French contributing to this forum would have lived through two series of terrorist bombings in France in the mid-1980s and 1990s. For these reasons, French cosmopolitans frame their solidarity in terms of democratic values they share with other democratic nations across time and space — values threatened by the specter of terrorism in both France and the United States.

Turning to the American forum, we see nationalism, transnational cosmopolitanism, and universalistic cosmopolitanism side by side. What is most interesting about the American forum is the mingling of multiple identity frames by international participants. Here we see important parallels between the French and Brazilians. Significantly, European and "Anglosphere" (Vucetic 2011) contributors are more likely to reference "democracy" as a shared transnational identity frame. While these self-identifications are expansive, they are similar to the French case. By contrast, nationals of democracies like India and Argentina are more similar to Brazilians in their use of the expansive identify frame of "humanity."

In making these connections, the chapter makes several contributions. First, it reveals the assumptions about the social world used to bolster the use of cosmopolitan identity frames. Second, the findings show how cosmopolitan perspectives allow us to frame the "other" as similar to ourselves. Third, the analysis points to new connections between cultural context and forms of cosmopolitanism. Finally, while 9/11/01 is a specific case, it demonstrates the range of discursive grammars or templates available to construct cosmopolitan identities as a means to express solidarity with victims of any disaster including those created by acts of political violence. By drawing on empirical evidence to distinguish between more and less universalizing forms of cosmopolitanism, this chapter indicates how cosmopolitan identity work in its many forms may offer important insight into world citizens' ability to help mitigate the suffering of unknown and distant others.

References

Anderson, R. (2014). *Human suffering and the quality of life: Conceptualizing stories and statistics*. New York: Springer Books.

Beck, U. (2000). The cosmopolitan perspective: Sociology of the second age of modernity. *British Journal of Sociology, 51*(1), 79–105.

Burdick, J. (1996). *Looking for god in Brazil*. Berkeley: University of California Press.

Jameson, F. (1982). *The political unconscious: Narrative as a socially symbolic act*. Ithaca: Cornell University Press.

Jenkins, B. (2000). French political culture: Homogenous or fragmented? In W. Kidd & S. Reynolds (Eds.), *Contemporary French cultural studies* (pp. 111–126). New York: Oxford University Press.

Kleingeld, P., & Brown, E. (2011). Cosmopolitanism. In E. N. Zalta (Ed.), *The Stanford encyclopedia of philosophy*. http://plato.stanford.edu/archives/spr2011/entries/cosmopolitanism/. Accessed 3 June 2013.

Pew-Templeton Global Religious Futures Project. (2013, July 18). *Brazil's changing religious landscape*. http://www.pewforum.org/2013/07/18/brazils-changing-religious-landscape/. Accessed 19 July 2013.

Robinson, L. (2005). Debating the events of September 11th: Discursive and interactional dynamics in three online fora. *The Journal of Computer-Mediated Communication, 10*(4).

Robinson, L. (2008). The moral accounting of terrorism: Competing interpretations of September 11, 2001. *Qualitative Sociology, 31*(3), 271–285.

Robinson, L. (2009). Cultural tropes and discourse: Brazilians, French, and Americans Debate September 11, 2001. *The International Journal of Communication, 3*.

Vucetic, S. (2011). *The Anglosphere: A genealogy of a racialized identity in international relations*. Stanford: Stanford University Press.

Chapter 26
Iconography of Suffering in Social Media: Images of Sitting Girls

Anna Johansson and Hans T. Sternudd

26.1 Introduction

Mental suffering, for example depression, stress, and anxiety, is said to have increased among young people in Western societies and is particularly common among young women (Rutter and Smith 1995; Collishaw et al 2004; Torsheim et al. 2006). Furthermore, ways of expressing suffering are often intimately tied to social categories such as gender or age. As digital media are today integral to the lives of young people, it is important to understand how experiences of suffering are mediated in online contexts.

Many argue that digital culture entails increasing emphasis on visual communication, and our previous studies on self-injury and teen mental distress in online settings have shown how young people's communication about these issues is sometimes framed by certain aesthetic forms (Sternudd 2012). In YouTube videos on self-injury, for example, distinctive combinations of textual, visual, and sonic elements are drawn on to convey gendered feelings of unhappiness, pain, and misery (cf. Johansson 2013), and similar designs can also be seen when mental suffering is dealt with in other social media contexts. While highly stylized depictions of suffering are rarely new or unique to contemporary culture, they may be produced, shared, and used in specific ways through digital media – something that, in turn, may affect how people conceptualize and cope with troublesome feelings.

Anna Johansson's contribution to this paper is part of her work in the Media Places research programme, funded by the Knut and Alice Wallenberg Foundation.

A. Johansson (✉)
HUMlab, Umeå University, Umeå SE-901 87, Sweden
e-mail: anna.johansson@humlab.umu.se

H.T. Sternudd
Department of Music and Art, Faculty of Art History and Visual Culture,
Linnaeus University, Växjö, Sweden
e-mail: hans.sternudd@lnu.se

© Springer Science+Business Media Dordrecht 2015
R.E. Anderson (ed.), *World Suffering and Quality of Life*,
Social Indicators Research Series 56, DOI 10.1007/978-94-017-9670-5_26

This paper draws on one particular visual trope as the starting point for a discussion of the iconography of suffering in social media: the sitting girl.[1] This character first caught our attention in the YouTube videos mentioned above. These videos were mainly montages composed of a number of sequenced still photographs and dialogue intertitles. The sitting girl, often on the floor or on the ground but also on a swing, on a pier, and on a railway track, struck us as emblematic, and similar or identical images appear in many videos. In this paper, we aim to investigate the meaning and significance of this as a trope of suffering. By taking the sitting girl as a case in point, the paper also sets out to discuss the ways in which digital technologies may inform the aesthetics of suffering in ways that both reinforce and challenge hegemonic ideas about gender and mental health.

26.2   Perspectives on Suffering

The concept of suffering can be used to describe a wide range of sensory and emotional responses varying in intensity and resulting from different causes. Ron Anderson (2014: 10) defines suffering as "distress resulting from threat or damage to one's body or self-identity," identifying three distinct categories: physical, mental, and social suffering. Whereas the first two are relatively straightforward, social suffering, as described by Kleinman et al. (1997: ix), "results from what political, economic, and institutional power does to people and, reciprocally, from how these forms of power themselves influence responses to social problems." The threefold typology is useful in that it allows for distinctions between different forms and causes of suffering, although it has to be acknowledged that it builds on a mind/body dualism and that the categories often merge or overlap; moreover, every instance of suffering is both individually experienced and culturally and socially shaped. In accounts of self-injury, for example, the three categories are sometimes inseparable: the sensation of pain is intertwined with mental or emotional difficulties and distress following from structural inequalities related to, for example, gender or class. Online social networks also tend to merge individual and collectively shared dimensions of suffering.

Notwithstanding this intertwinement, the main focus of this paper is on the iconography of *mental* suffering. A general definition includes depression, anxiety, grief, and existential suffering (Anderson 2014: 44), hardships that are typically assigned to the domains of psychiatry, psychology, or biomedicine. In other words, mental suffering is often framed in terms of illness or disorder, and the problem is

---

[1] The noun "girl" has been used throughout because, while the age of the person is not known, the attributes and contexts of the images generally articulate young femininity. Girlhood, then, should be understood as a social construction rather than being indicative of an exact chronological age (cf. Aapola et al. 2005). We acknowledge that by using the term, we may reproduce precisely the stereotypes that we wish to problematize; however, our hope is that the chapter sheds light on how intersections of gender and age are co-constructed with mental suffering in some online contexts.

located within the individual. This view has been criticized for ignoring how social factors such as poverty or discrimination may cause mental suffering and how definitions of illness are always culturally shaped (Busfield 2000; Ussher 2011). Feminist scholars in particular have emphasized that conceptions of mental illness and mental suffering are intimately tied to notions of femininity, following from a dualist model of gender in which women are associated with attributes such as weakness, fragility, and emotionality (Showalter 1985; Tatman 2012). In contemporary Western culture, mental suffering (not necessarily defined in terms of illness) is also claimed to be more widespread among women than men (Anderson 2014: 55–56).

Our interest in this paper lies with processes of meaning production, where we understand mediated content to be a means of making sense of suffering that simultaneously builds on and (re)produces existing discourses. Anderson (2014: 16–23) outlines eight major conceptual frames for understanding suffering – including the views of it as, for example, a punishment, a reward, and a natural destiny – that structure the experiences of the individual sufferer. Our main point here is that suffering needs to be communicated in order to be acknowledged. Thus, the one who suffers must present as such through linguistic, embodied, and visual performances (Grace 1997; cf. Tatman 2012: 43) and, in order to be recognizable, these need to be modeled on culturally intelligible scripts. Such scripts usually vary according to gender, class, and age, which means that ways of "doing" mental suffering intersect with other identity performances (Johannisson 2006). While the trope of the sitting girl in many ways builds on a long tradition of suffering aesthetics and mental illness iconography (e.g., Huberman 2004), we set out to understand how connectivity and circulation through digital media may shape the ways in which mental suffering is enacted and rendered meaningful today.

26.3 Methods and Materials

As a major video-sharing site, YouTube allows users to upload and share video clips that may be searched for, commented on, and "liked" or "disliked" by other people. The site has sometimes been described as a prominent example of participatory culture (Burgess and Green 2009), although it is driven not only by users but also by commercial interests (Snickars and Vonderau 2009). A YouTube search for "self-injury" returns tens of thousands of results, ranging from informational materials to video blogs to the kind of montages discussed here. A large proportion of the videos appear to be posted by people with personal experience of self-harm, predominantly cutting, and the purpose when indicated is often to raise awareness of self-injury.

Reviewing the first 20 videos returned from a search for "self-harm," we identified 51 unique images of sitting persons in video montages (three of which appeared more than once).[2] The majority were persons identified as females (n = 46, 81 %)

---

[2] The search was performed in August 2012.

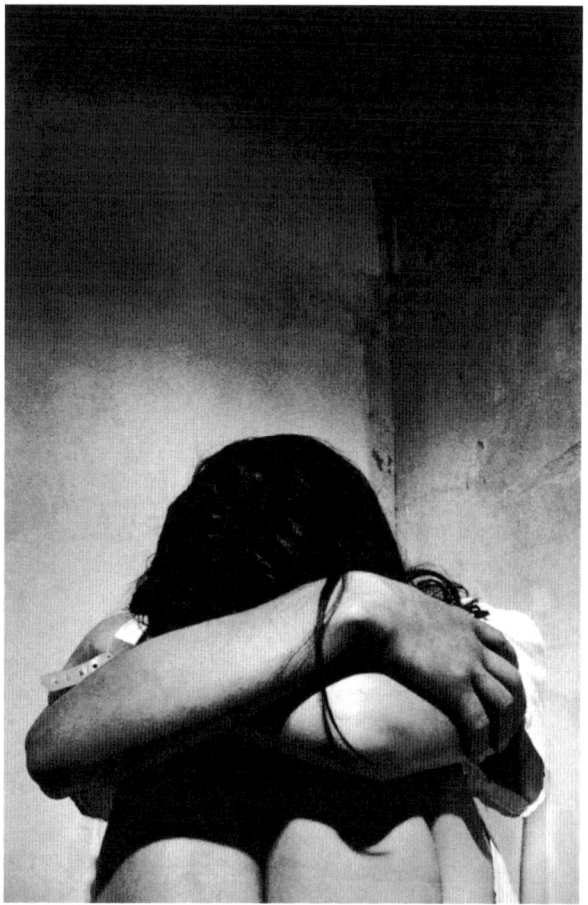

and the posture was predominantly sitting with knees bent up (n = 24, 67 %). Other findings were that the gaze of the person was in most cases hidden (n = 38, 78 %), as the head was bent down between the knees in a hunched-over position (see Fig. 26.1) or turned away from the viewer.

In this article we present an analysis of two such images of sitting girls. The selection is partly governed by copyright regulations, as these are the images for which the copyright holders could be found. However, the two images are representative of the larger sample in their depiction of seemingly young individuals sitting down, hunched over, with their eyes hidden or turned away from the viewer. First, we analyze the respective images, and in the next step we extend the analysis to their context: the narratives of the video montages and the YouTube interface. The analysis is guided by an iconographical and discourse analytical approach, in which we pay specific attention to how elements – that is, formal (e.g., Adams 1996) and representational content as well as media-specific features – are articulated together (Laclau and Mouffe 1985: 105) in constructions of suffering. Examining the online iconography of mental suffering involves analyzing the manner in which this theme is expressed visually (i.e., the interpretation follows the outlines in Panofsky's iconographical analysis (1982: 41)).[3] Meaning is seen as established through inter-textual relations with and references to other texts and images, which means that images of the hunched-over sitting girl found outside the context of YouTube are also of great interest.

Inspired by multi-sited ethnography and George Marcus's (1995) concept of "following the thing," we therefore deployed image search tools Google Search by Image and TinEye Reverse Image Search through which users can search for images by uploading files or pasting images into the search field. Such a "reverse image search" retrieves information about other contexts in which the image has been used and thus makes it possible to track an image's online existence, although the two tools are slightly different. TinEye cannot recognize content and returns results only for exact and altered copies of the image (TinEye 2014). Google, on the other hand, shows results in three categories: a "best guess" search term suggesting a way of conceptualizing the image together with a few top results; "visually similar images" that resemble the searched one; and links to "pages that include matching images" with more or less exact matches (Google 2014). Our main focus here was on the last category.

By tracking a selection of 10 images as digital-material "things," we found that the sitting girls were used in many contexts relating to mental health outside of YouTube. It should be noted that the results are shaped by search algorithms, of which we know very little (cf. Beer 2009), and with the use of other tools our results may have been different. However, our findings in this last step are intended to be neither exhaustive nor representative of online suffering; instead, we understand them to be one example of how iconographies of suffering surface online. Tracking the various contexts in which the hunched-over sitting girl occurred hence furthered our understanding of suffering and gender, while also extending the last step of the analysis to the larger context of social media and the way they construct particular aesthetics of suffering.

26.4   The Sitting Girl as a Visual Trope of Suffering

This section introduces the hunched-over sitting girl as a trope of mental suffering by presenting an analysis of two photos from the YouTube montage videos.

The first image (Fig. 26.1) is a black and white photograph that shows a person sitting down, her arms holding her bent legs close to her body. A more careful inspection reveals a patient bracelet on the person's arm. The position of the girl at the bottom of the image, with a black shadow hanging over the figure, may signify suppression and/or depression, which is accentuated by the dark character of the photo. Furthermore, the location in a corner is important, as it could signify a person

---

[3] Iconography is used here in a "loose sense" (Rose 2012: 205) that corresponds more to a con-structivist discourse perspective than the essentialist tendencies in Panofsky's classic iconographic method. For an introduction to this method see, for example, Panofsky (1982: 26–54).

Fig. 26.2 Screen shot from
Self injury – pictures
(GRAPHIC)

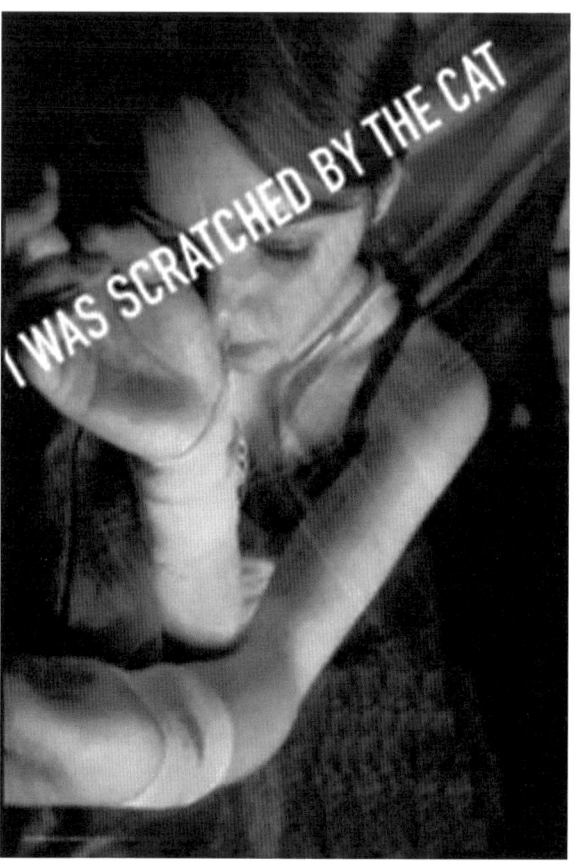

redeeming her actions (being in the naughty corner) or someone who seeks
protection from the walls.

Figure 26.2 is originally a color photograph showing a person with their eyes
shut and their wrists covered in blood stained bandages. A diagonal text overlay
reads, "I was scratched by the cat." The photo has several features in common with
Fig. 26.1: they both show a person alone in a dark place, partly hiding her body and
her face with her arms. In both examples, the room also lacks perceived depth, a
visual quality that, according to Mulvey (1989: 14–26), reduces the possibility of
interpreting the person as active. Both images show the person close to the picture
plane – in Fig. 26.2, for example, the arms seem to approach the viewer as they
nearly reach out of the picture's frame. None of the photos shows what the person
is sitting on. Figure 26.2 has a vaguer composition than Fig. 26.1; it is slightly
unbalanced due to the posture of the body and the lack of an element balancing the
composition in the lower right corner. Another aspect contributing to the ambiguity
of Fig. 26.2 is that the person is actually lying down, which is revealed when the
image is turned 90 degrees counter-clockwise. This is particularly interesting,

considering the fact that the image is used in a way that puts the lying person in a sitting position.

The bodies are largely hidden from view, and yet the images invoke a reading of the characters as girls or young women, evidenced also from the use and interpretation of them in other contexts (see Sternudd and Johansson forthcoming). We argue that this is due not only to the presence of gendered features such as the long hair in Fig. 26.1 or the red lips, mascara, and shoulder straps in Fig. 26.2, but that the "girling" of the characters is also an effect of the images' simultaneous articulation of mental suffering. Suffering and young femininity/infantility are mutually constitutive here, in the sense that both inform the interpretation of the other. There is nothing inherent in someone sitting down that warrants an understanding of them as either a sufferer or a young woman; a sitting person can be seen as a discursive element open to many different interpretations. However, when this particular figure is articulated with other elements, such as the YouTube context, the tonality of the images, the hunched-over position, and the objects referring to medical treatment – the patient bracelet and bandages – this effects a temporary fixation of meaning that transforms the sitting person into a suffering girl.

A particularly important element here is the head or eyes turned away from the viewer. This is, we argue, a fairly familiar way of depicting sadness that invokes a reading of the person as protecting herself from the gaze of others in an act of shame or rejection of the world. Articulated with the sitting position, this lends itself well to representing suffering. In a previous publication (Sternudd and Johansson forthcoming), we draw on research by Goffman (1979), Shields (1989), and Atkinson (2003) in suggesting that the practice of sitting on the floor or on the ground may evoke associations of subordination and helplessness. The position indicates power imbalance, and could therefore be read as an expression of inferiority and infantility: "The sitting body is a docile body and the sitting character, it could be argued, is thus constituted as a docile (feminine) subject." The sitting girl, then, "could be read as performing mental suffering through gendered subordination" (Sternudd and Johansson forthcoming). Whereas sitting may also represent the opposite of docility – sitting on the street or on the pavement has often been associated with protest and opposition – the fact that the girl in our sample images sits all by herself, "without peers or fellow protesters, could perhaps be seen as reducing her subversive agency. At the same time, her loneliness emphasizes the sense of alienation in the image, and thus constructs not only a position of vulnerability" (ibid.) but also a position that, in turning away, seems to actively reject being part of the world.

Our point here is that the articulation of formal qualities, the subordinated or docile position, and the alienated or vulnerable character corresponds not only to hegemonic understandings of suffering but also to constructions of contemporary young femininity. Through the turned away head, the character seems to turn her attention inwards, thereby reproducing a normative performance of suffering girlhood that precludes any externalizing practices, such as aggressive outbursts or collective action. This hunched-over sitting girl, then, emerges as an iconographic sign in a discourse that articulates girlhood with suffering as an individualized problem.

26.5   YouTube Video Montages of Suffering

Let us now proceed by turning to the contexts where we found the sitting girls: the YouTube video montages. We define montages here as videos composed of sequenced still images and text slides. Self-injury video montages are best described as a genre of their own, with specific stylistic conventions and similar contents, that usually narrate a story about a self-harmer or provide facts and information on the issue of self-injury. In many ways, these videos build on the principles of remix: the creation of something new out of existing content produced by others (Lessig 2008; cf. Navas 2010), a feature characteristic of contemporary digital media (Manovich 2005). Figure 26.2 is an example of such a remix in which a text block and logotypes have been removed from the original (see Fig. 26.3), a poster of the World Health Organization (WHO 2014).[4]

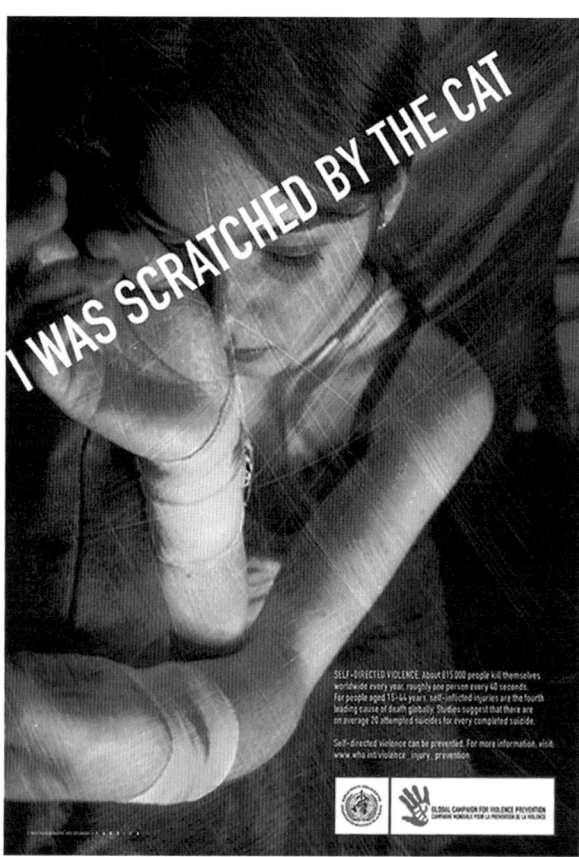

Fig. 26.3 *"I was scratched by the cat"* © World Health Organization, 2003, printed with permission from World Health Organization

---

[4]The removed text: "About 815,000 people kill themselves worldwide every year, roughly one person every 40 s. For people aged 15–44 years, self-inflicted injuries are the fourth leading cause of death globally. Studies suggest that there are on average 20 attempted suicides for every completed suicide."

The video montages are themselves examples of another type of remix, in which modified images from various sources are assembled and mixed with intertitles. Furthermore, the YouTube interface may itself be seen as a remix in that it links videos to each other, either through active choice by the user to post a video response to an existing video, or through the algorithm that offers a selection of suggested – usually topically related – videos to the viewer.

The video in which Fig. 26.1 appears (jellyfish 2008) contains 46 slides with 11 of these being intertitles. Figure 26.2, on the other hand, appears in a video that includes 32 slides, out of which 8 are intertitles (oxKaylaa2xo 2010). In both videos, the majority of intertitles are written in a matter-of-fact style, often reproducing medical or psychological discourses – such as in "self harm (SH) or self injury is deliberate injury inflicted by a person upon their own body without suicidal intent" (jellyfish 2008). Both videos also entwine these informative intertitles with photos of self-injury in various stages of progress. These graphic photos are one main category of images in the montages; the other category includes the generic photos or staged artworks represented by Figs. 26.1 and 26.2. This second category seems to be used as a marker of emotional response – for instance, empathy – and such images serve to illustrate – and thereby make sense of – the emotional qualities involved in the act of self-injury. Our interpretation that these images are used to produce pathos is supported by the surrounding intertitles. In the intertitle that follows Fig. 26.2, for example, user oxKaylaa2xo gets personal and reaches out to fellow self-injurers by stating, "You can and will stop, it just take time. […] I have faith and hope in you." Furthermore, Fig. 26.1 follows an intertitle with the text: "when people self/harm they often/feel isolated/trapped && alone."

Several video montages explicitly narrate the lives of young women through the use of gendered names and pronouns in intertitles. Self-injury, especially in the form of cutting, is considered more prevalent among women and can be described as an embodied performance of gender as well as of mental suffering (Johansson 2013). However, the videos not only tend to reproduce this understanding of self-injury, but the imagery, narratives, video titles, comments, and usernames speak of a more general conceptual link between (young) femininity and mental suffering, where girls are depicted as sad, depressed, stressed, and abused.

The strong emphasis on loneliness, alienation, and possibly shame noted in the individual images is also prominent in video montages. Here, mental suffering is conceptualized as a hidden secret, and the need to keep up a façade is construed as central to the management of suffering – seen not least in the apologetic text overlay of Fig. 26.2, "I was scratched by the cat." This individualization may seem paradoxical given the social character of YouTube: the videos are created for the purpose of reaching out to other people, and the intention to seek support, or raise awareness about mental suffering, is often explicitly stated. Whereas suffering is described as something dealt with in private, the video sharing is thus simultaneously a public performance of suffering – but the line between personal and nonpersonal is often carefully straddled. The videos seem to tell us about personal experiences, but this is usually done from a third person point of view, as in the example above describing how "they [self-harmers] often feel isolated, trapped and alone."

Furthermore, producers of video montages are generally anonymous (as compared to, for instance, producers of video blogs), and the images used rarely show identifiable individuals. Studying the use of photographs in digital storytelling,[5] Vivienne and Burgess (2013: 291) claim that generic stock images are often chosen due to "limited time or in some cases [producers'] lack of confidence in their own creative capacities." Stock images also work as substitutes for personal photos, as they provide a greater degree of anonymity (ibid.). This may be part of the explanation for the prevalence of generic sitting girls in the video montages. Also, too realistic or graphic depictions of self-injury tend to be heavily criticized and even removed from YouTube (Johansson 2013), which might be one further reason why self-injury is often depicted using images of a less provocative character.

26.6 Tracking the Online Aesthetics of Mental Suffering

Perhaps the trope of the hunched-over sitting girl is not new in itself (see e.g. Johannesson 2003). But digital media may change the way it is used and circulated, not least because digital technologies offer means for sufferers to engage in public meaning-making and processes of identity construction. By tracking 10 of our 51 photos through image searches, we were able to discern how these were made use of outside of YouTube. Search results almost exclusively pointed to contexts in which these images were drawn on to illustrate texts about mental suffering, ranging from informational websites on mental disorders to blog posts about unrequited love. Several of the images could be traced back to stock-photo collections and artists' websites: they had been taken up – with or without legal permission – and modified, then articulated in a new context and thereby passed on for others to use.

It has been claimed that digital photography changes the way we engage with everyday images, not least because personal photography has become an important means for identity construction in social media (van Dijck 2008; Murray 2008). However, our study shows that this is true not only for personal photos but also for already existing images that can be found online and then recombined for the purpose of self-presentation. Through the image search, Fig. 26.1, for example, was tracked back to Getty Images Inc.'s large stock-photo bank. Stock images are produced for commercial purposes and thus need to be decontextualized and generic enough for use in a variety of contexts (Machin 2004). At the same time, they must still "encourage a specifically appropriate and relevant interpretation" (Frosh 2001: 638). This preferred interpretation is indicated in the agencies' classifications of images. In the Getty Image bank, Fig. 26.1 is tagged with the following search terms:

---

[5] Digital storytelling refers here to the creation of short autobiographical multimedia narratives in video form, in which personal photos or art are combined with narration and music. This is usually conducted during workshops, and the videos may be shared online (Vivienne and Burgess 2013: 283). The format of such digital stories is similar to the video montage narratives in our study.

People, Depression, Social Issues, Healthcare And Medicine, Vertical, Three Quarter Length, Indoors, Black And White, Grainy, Patient, Sitting, One Person, Head In Hands, Hiding, Adult, One Woman Only, Photography, Unrecognizable Person, Mental Illness, Adults Only (Getty Images 2013).

While some of these terms are mainly factual and descriptive, others are more abstract notions meant to be invoked by the image: depression, social issues, healthcare and medicine, and mental illness – all confirming that this is intended to be a visualization of mental suffering, or perhaps even a script for how suffering should be properly performed.[6] Frosh (2003: 105) describes the stock image as "the visual correlate to cultural stereotypes," and while this photo easily builds on and thereby reproduces the articulation of mental illness and femininity, it also seems to underscore the importance of keeping one's suffering to oneself.

The generic, or stereotypical, character may be what makes images of hunched-over sitting young women useful in various mental health contexts. Broadly speaking, we found that our 10 sample images were used as parts of a wide range of different aesthetic styles. Two of them were especially striking as they to some extent represented different approaches to suffering. On the one hand, Christian help sites and sites run by support organizations and healthcare institutions often used imagery and design that were light, clean, and easy to navigate, including color photos of families and nature, a particular aesthetic that is reminiscent of the web design Thompson (2012) identifies in her study of a mental health community. Looking at the long-term development of a specific site, Thompson (2012: 396) describes a "trend towards greater use of visual imagery and new media to convey ideological messages about wellness and disorder" where stock photos and other visual elements are used to market wellness as "an ideal to pursue." The support-oriented websites we found similarly inscribed suffering in a medical–psychological discourse, in which health and well-being are construed as ideals and suffering is, accordingly, seen as manageable through therapy and medication (cf. Anderson 2014: 21–22).

This can be contrasted with another aesthetic style, which was also more similar to the aesthetics of the YouTube montages. These sites were generally darker and collage-like, and included monochrome photographs with occasional details in red or pink and text overlays showing quotes about self-hatred and despair: often a messy multitude of reposted images and texts that appeared as "personal media assemblages" (Good 2012). This was predominantly seen on blogs and image-sharing sites – that is, in contexts with a high degree of interactivity and user-generated content, such as Tumblr, Pinterest, and Weheartit (as opposed to the previous aesthetic that was more often seen on static web pages). Several of our images also appeared in online image banks providing graphic design elements for social network sites (e.g. the Punjabi site www.Desicomments.com).

Both of these contexts largely emphasize visual display and formal elements in their framing of suffering. Obviously, the two contexts overlap insofar as the same

---

[6] Interestingly, however, the image is tagged here as depicting an adult woman. Whereas this may suggest a preferred interpretation, our study also demonstrates that the image can be reappropriated as a signifier of young femininity when articulated with particular elements and in other contexts.

or very similar images appear in both contexts – which is why we found them at all – but they are partly distinct in the way they make use of these images. Our suggestion would be that the former represents an institutional, or even normative, approach to suffering, while the latter is more of a vernacular style showing how young people, often presenting as women, make sense of their emotional and mental hardships. As Robert Howard (2008) points out, vernacular and institutional discourses are hybridized through digital media, something seen, for example, in how "facts" are used in the montage videos, in how personal blogs draw on medical–psychological discourse, and in how care institutions use similar photos to those used by video makers.

At the same time, the two contexts described here are clearly distinguishable. While the normative or institutional approach explicitly promotes positive thinking, well-being, and ways to cope with suffering, the alternative or vernacular approach more often includes dwelling on experiences of mental and existential suffering in poems or blog posts, or through graphics. This is not to say that the latter involves an outspoken glorification of suffering, but it is clear that the vernacular aesthetic to some extent is linked to the embracing of a suffering identity. In this respect, we think of it as an alternative conceptualization of suffering that in some ways challenges the institutional focus on light, cleanness, and healing. Formally, the vernacular aesthetic is also reminiscent of subcultural styles such as Goth, Punk, or Emo, which adds to the sense of "alternativeness." Many of the sites bear resemblance to the DIY aesthetics of cut-and-paste collage, but instead of scissors and glue it is the materiality of social media platforms and online archives of photos and graphic design elements that are the building blocks enabling the creation and circulation of these particular performances of mental suffering.

26.7 Concluding Remarks

Gender and mental health discourses, digital photography, social media technologies, and remix culture all in different ways contribute to the pervasiveness of the hunched-over sitting girl as a trope of suffering. This paper has attempted to discuss some of these processes. It is clear that the character of the sitting girl appeals to many people, evidenced not least by its presence in commercial stock image collections. Part of the attraction may lie in how the suffering person is simultaneously conceptualized here as vulnerable or docile and as actively refusing to engage with the world around her, thus making the image open to various readings and identifications. This, we argue, is also what makes the trope suitable for use in institutional as well as vernacular contexts. Generally, the images reproduce a well-known and much-criticized discourse on girls as delicate and in need of help, but they can also be used to invoke a sense of rebellion or opposition. Articulated with a medical–psychological discourse and the imperative to seek help, the understanding of the suffering person as frail and dependent is foregrounded. In such contexts, the sitting girl images also often stand out as different from the rest of the design; the sites on which they appear are dominated by colorful imagery of smiling people embodying the ideal of "health" or "wellness." In the context of the vernacular or DIY-like aesthetic and approach, however, focus is instead directed to the trope as representing a deliberate rejection of conventional ideals. Mental suffering is traditionally associated with deviancy and stigma, but this particular aesthetic of suffering – made possible through participatory as well as commercial elements of digital media – seems to reclaim this "otherness," framing it as a valued part of a sufferer's identity. Suffering, here, may be construed as either good or bad, or both, at the same time.

What bearing could the findings of this study have as regards quality of life (QOL)? Following Anderson's (2014) argument that the reduction of suffering is an important factor for improving the QOL, and considering that we see the trope of the hunched-over sitting girl as highly normative, our analysis may indicate that the use of the image in some contexts could increase suffering. This gendered performance includes elements that, according to Anderson, are associated with *mental suffering*, such as shame and loneliness, and with *social suffering*, such as social exclusion, incapacitation and disability (2014: 11). If the sitting girl is seen as normative in terms of how suffering is to be conceptualized, and if these "multiple types of suffering occur together", this may multiply their individual effect rather than adding them to one another (ibid., 63).

At the same time, the aestheticization of suffering through tropes such as the sitting girl may also help to alleviate suffering, as it provides an opportunity for active participation in meaning-making around one's personal issues. Furthermore, through the use of this trope in social media, instances of individualized mental suffering are brought out into the public sphere where they form the basis for collective recognition, community building, and social support – factors that may relieve suffering and increase quality of life.

References

Aapola, S., Gonick, M., & Harris, A. (2005). *Young femininity: Girlhood, power and social change*. New York: Palgrave Macmillan.

Adams, L. S. (1996). *The methodologies of art: An introduction*. New York: Westview Press.

Anderson, R. (2014). *Human suffering and quality of life: Conceptualizing stories and statistics*. New York: Springer.

Atkinson, R. (2003). Domestication by cappuccino or a revenge on urban space? Control and empowerment in the management of public spaces. *Urban Studies, 40*, 1829–1843.

Beer, D. (2009). Power through the algorithm? Participatory web cultures and the technological unconscious. *New Media and Society, 11*(6), 985–1002.

Burgess, J. E., & Green, J. (2009). *YouTube: Online video and participatory culture*. Cambridge: Polity.

Busfield, J. (2000). Introduction: Rethinking the sociology of mental health. *Sociology of Health & Illness, 22*(5), 543–558.

Collishaw, S., Maughan, B., Goodman, R., et al. (2004). Time trends in adolescent mental health. *Journal of Child Psychology and Psychiatry, 45*(8), 1350–1362.

Frosh, P. (2001). Inside the image factory: Stock photography and cultural production. *Media, Culture and Society, 23*(5), 625–646.

Frosh, P. (2003). *Image factory: Consumer culture, photography and the visual content industry*. Oxford: Berg Publishers.

Getty Images. (2013). http://www.gettyimages.se/detail/foto/woman-sitting-resting-her-head-on-her-knees-bildbank/AB08685#. Accessed 13 Dec 2013.

Goffman, E. (1979). *Gender advertisements*. London: Macmillan.

Good, K. D. (2012). From scrapbook to Facebook: A history of personal media assemblage and archives. *New Media and Society, 15*(4), 557–573.

Google. (2014). *Reverse image search*. https://support.google.com/websearch/answer/1325808?p=searchbyimagepage&hl=en. Accessed 11 Dec 2014.

Grace, V. (1997). Reading the silent body: Women, doctors and pelvic pain. In M. de Ras & V. Grace (Eds.), *Bodily boundaries, sexualised genders & medical discourses* (pp. 85–98). Palmerston North: Dunmore Press.

Howard, R. G. (2008). The vernacular web of participatory media. *Critical Studies in Media Communication, 25*(5), 490–513.

Huberman, G. D. (2004). *Invention of hysteria: Charcot and the photographic iconography of the Salpêtrière*. Cambridge, MA: MIT Press.

jellyfish. (2008). *self harm/injury **TRIGGERING***. YouTube. http://www.youtube.com/watch?v=rLiEyC4Mf0E. Accessed 1 Feb 2013.

Johannesson, L. (2003). Sittandets semiotik och den kvinnliga modernismen. In Y. Eriksson & A. Göthlund (Eds.), *Från modernism till samtidskonst: svenska kvinnliga konstnärer* (pp. 22–47). Lund: Signum.

Johannisson, K. (2006). Sjukdomsestetik och kultur: Exemplen hysteri, anorexi och apati. In J. Beskow & L. Berglund (Eds.), *Att se det osedda: Vänbok till Ann-Sofie Ohlander* (pp. 29–55). Stockholm: Hjalmarson & Högberg Bokförlag.

Johansson, A. (2013). Hybrid embodiment: Doing respectable bodies on YouTube. In S. Lindgren (Ed.), *Hybrid media culture: Sensing place in a world of flows* (pp. 16–32). London: Routledge.

Kleinman, A., Das, V., & Lock, M. (Eds.). (1997). *Social suffering*. Berkeley: University of California Press.

Laclau, E., & Mouffe, C. (1985). *Hegemony and socialist strategy*. London: Verso.

Lessig, L. (2008). *Remix: Making art and commerce thrive in the hybrid economy*. New York: Penguin Press.

Machin, D. (2004). Building the world's visual language: The increasing global importance of image banks in corporate media. *Visual Communication, 3*(3), 316–336.

Manovich, L. (2005). *Remixability and modularity*. http://www.manovich.net/articles.php. Accessed 15 Mar 2014.

Marcus, G. (1995). Ethnography in/of the world system: The emergence of multi-sited ethnography. *Annual Review of Anthropology, 24*, 95–117.

Mulvey, L. (1989). *Visual and other pleasures*. Bloomington/Indianapolis: Indiana University Press.

Murray, S. (2008). Digital images, photo-sharing, and our shifting notions of everyday aesthetics. *Journal of Visual Culture, 7*(2), 147–163.

Navas, E. (2010). Regressive and reflexive mashups in sampling culture. In S. Sonvilla-Weiss (Ed.), *Mashup cultures* (pp. 157–177). Vienna/New York: Springer.

oxKaylaa2xo (2010). *Self injury – Pictures (GRAPHIC)*. YouTube. http://www.youtube.com/watch?v=_o2wowMysc4. Accessed 27 Nov 2012.

Panofsky, E. (1982 [1955]). *Meaning in the visual arts*. Chicago: The University of Chicago Press.

Rose, G. (2012). *Visual methodologies: An introduction to researching with visual materials* (3rd ed.). London: Sage.

Rutter, M., & Smith, D. J. (Eds.). (1995). *Psychosocial disorders in young people: Time trends and their causes*. Chichester: Wiley for Academia Europaea.

Shields, R. (1989). Social spatialisation and the built environment: The West Edmonton mall. *Environment and Planning D, 7*, 147–164.

Showalter, E. (1985). *The female malady: Women, madness and English culture 1830–1980*. New York: Pantheon Books.

Snickars, P., & Vonderau, P. (Eds.). (2009). *The YouTube reader*. Stockholm: National Library of Sweden.

Sternudd, H. T. (2012). Photographs of self-injury: Production and reception in a group of self-injurers. *Journal of Youth Studies, 15*, 421–436.

Sternudd, H. T., & Johansson, A. (forthcoming). *The girl in the corner: Aesthetics of suffering in a digitalized space*. Oxford: Inter-Disciplinary Press.

Tatman, L. (2012). The other thing about suffering. In J. Malpas & N. Lickiss (Eds.), *Perspectives on human suffering* (pp. 43–48). New York: Springer.

Thompson, R. (2012). Looking healthy: Visualizing mental health and illness online. *Visual Communication, 11*(4), 395–420.

TinEye. (2014). *Frequently asked questions*. http://www.tineye.com/faq. Accessed 15 Mar 2014.

Torsheim, T., Ravens-Sieberer, U., Hetland, J., et al. (2006). Cross-national variation of gender differences in adolescent subjective health in Europe and North America. *Social Science & Medicine, 62*(4), 815–827.

Ussher, J. M. (2011). *The madness of women: Myth and experience*. London: Routledge.

van Dijck, J. (2008). Digital photography: Communication, identity, memory. *Visual Communication, 7*(1), 57–76.

Vivienne, S., & Burgess, J. (2013). The remediation of the personal photograph and the politics of self-representation in digital storytelling. *Journal of Material Culture, 18*(3), 279–298.

WHO. (2014). *Violence and injury prevention, "Explaining away violence" poster series*. World Health Organization (WHO). http://www.who.int/violence_injury_prevention/publications/violence/explaining/en. Accessed 25 Mar 2014.

Part V
Research and Policy Challenges for the Future

Chapter 27
The Neurosociology of Social Rejection and Suffering

David D. Franks

27.1 What Is Neurosociology?

Neurosurgeon Bogen et al. (1972) first used the term "neurosociology" to refer to neuroscience studies that focused on the social aspects of the brain. Shortly after that, neuroscientist Brothers (1977) was the first to succinctly describe our social natures and to directly show how neuroscience could fit in with sociological social psychology. (See Brothers 1977: xii.) Within sociology proper, Jonathan Turner (2000) echoes this opinion. Neurosociology has put an end to the old belief that there is no such thing as human nature. Human nature is social. Leading social neuroscientists Cacioppo and Patrick (2008) voiced the same conclusion in their book: *Loneliness: Human Nature and the Need for Social Connection.* In 2013, *The Handbook of Neurosociology* suggested that neurosociology had come of age as a field of inquiry (Franks and Turner 2013). One could legitimately ask why we need neurosociology when there is already a well-developed field of social neuroscience that has been developed by cognitive psychologists. Much of the need for two fields has to do with keeping their distinctive boundaries clear. This does not mean that one field needs to reign above the other. As I have argued before (Franks 2010) the two can be quite useful to each other. The important difference has to do with keeping true to our units of analysis. Sociology is interactional and the focus is on at least two people and how they influence each other. This is not the case in psychology that has to do with the singular person and personality. The two fields can actually compliment each other but it is nonetheless important to keep the boundaries between them distinct.

Using a shared symbolic language, actors in social interaction can view themselves as they think others do and use this to guide their own conduct. This is a

D.D. Franks (✉)
Department of Sociology, Emeritus Professor of Sociology, Virginia Commonwealth University, 821 West Franklin Street, Richmond, VA 23284, USA
e-mail: daviddfranks@comcast.net

© Springer Science+Business Media Dordrecht 2015
R.E. Anderson (ed.), *World Suffering and Quality of Life*,
Social Indicators Research Series 56, DOI 10.1007/978-94-017-9670-5_27

distinctive sociological perspective pioneered by Mead (1934) who had a distinctive social theory of the *act*, which directly contrasts with deterministic learning theory. He saw us as being pulled along by our own anticipations of completing the act. Here the person becomes thoroughly social because the other person's anticipated response is incorporated into one's own developing lines of action. In cognitive psychology's learning theory we are pushed passively into behavior because of stimuli outside of the person. It is not a matter of one or the other since role taking develops after conditioning and does not preclude the latter.

Psychology's version of role taking is referred to as "theory of mind". This is not a general theory of mentality; it is the actor's own belief about what is going on in the mind of the other. In this perspective, actors operate on their own as do the other actors. There is not any necessary focus on an incorporation of the other's responses into one's own.

While neurosociology is necessary to keep these units of analysis separate, the two fields can also compliment each other.

27.2 Rene Spitz and the Pain of Infant Social Isolation

In the mid-1900s, Rene Spitz published his findings of infants who had been raised in two very different kinds of environment (Spitz 1966). The first one contained a normal social environment where expectant mothers took care of other mother's babies. The other another put such a high priority on medical sanitation that infants were deprived of any meaningful contact with adults and each other. While the babies fared well in the first environment, the results in the medically sanitized hospital were ironically tragic with literally all the babies psychologically and intellectually impaired for life. One reason for this was that as long as they were isolated from the emotional attentions from others they could not grow emotionally themselves. Intellectual capacity cannot arise without a firm emotional base.

Even more disastrous was their psychological condition. All were severely depressed and would cry when anything new, including Dr. Spitz himself, came into the room. The situation was so bad that despite the rigid sanitation, normal childhood diseases ended in unusually high rates of death.

27.3 One Brain Structure for Both Physical and Social Pain: Implications

Leslie Brothers (1977) gave neurosociology strong support by her arguments about our thoroughly social nature. Lieberman and Eisenberger (2006) have called our attention to the fact that linguistically and thus metaphorically, we assume that both social and physical pain are anatomical processes as when we say, "he broke my heart" or "go ahead, eat your heart out". According to Lieberman (2013) researchers found that people in fifteen other countries, including non-European ones, use words for physical pain to describe social pain. It is not surprising therefore that Lieberman and Eisenberger (2006) propose that social and physical pain are also literally lodged in the brain to the extent that a common brain structure enables both. This structure is the cingulate cortex. The upper front of this structure enables physical pain and the back enables social pain from social rejection or social isolation. Social pain is, indeed, actually physical insofar as it is enabled from a physical part of the cingulate cortex and the two can be differentiated only cognitively by their separate causes. One can locate physical pain specifically in their anatomy, but this is harder to literally do with social pain. Most "heart-broken" persons would no doubt agree.

Lieberman and Eisenberger (2008) follow this by an important statement: "… other brain parts than the one making physical and social pain possible may also be involved in these feelings". This is a common occurrence in the brain where interconnections are the norm. In this case these parts are the somatosensory cortex, insular and the right ventral prefrontal cortex.

27.4 Our Social Natures as Functional in Evolution

Panksepp (1998) has observed that drugs intended to cure physical pain also worked to ease the pain of social isolation. This lead Nelson and Panksepp (1998) to suggest that in evolutionary terms "the social attachment system may have piggybacked onto, or developed out of, the physical pain system which has older phylogenetic roots than the social pain system" (Lieberman and Eisenberger 2006: 169).

Popular images of early man depict him heroically fighting mastodons with long spears, but such was not the case. Homo sapiens at that time were lowly scavengers and this too had its dangers since all kinds of animals were determined to get their share. One of Homo sapiens' advantages was the ability to get others of his kind to cooperate in warding off the other competing parties. Our early social natures were most likely utilized here including the ability to read the emotions portrayed in the faces of others. See Turner (2000).

An advantage of the human social group in contrast to other species also competing for food was that hominids could engage in the reciprocity and normative structures that enabled them to share what they scavenged, even before spoken language was available. While other mammals and birds shared food only with their young, hominids shared among all members of their group.

Macdonald and Leary (2005) and Leary (2007) suggest that the brain's shared enablers of physical and social pain were an evolutionary development to aid social animals in responding to threats of exclusion. All mammals have cingulated cortexes. Mammals that herd are particularly sensitive to isolation because the herd protects them, which is critical for their survival. For example, among wild horses young colts frequently nip grown horses and like most youngsters, act in inappropriate ways. This causes the lead female horse to expel them from the herd. She lets him back only if he hangs his head and whimpers at which time she turns to show

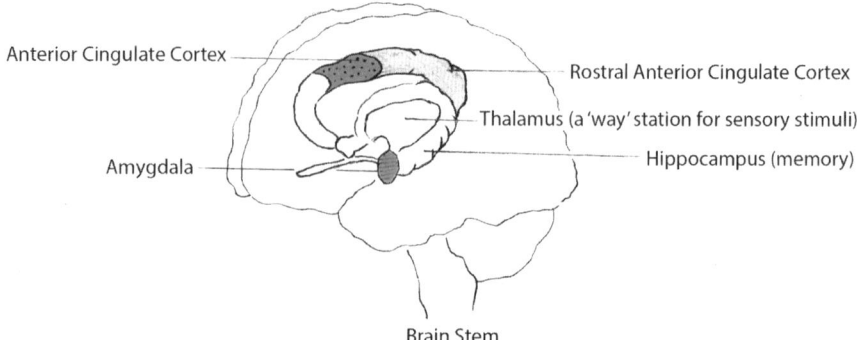

Fig. 27.1 Relevant structures of the brain

her broad-side which is a sign he can come back. When he does she watches him closely making sure he doesn't return to his mischief again.

27.5   The Neurosociology of Physical and Social Pain

We have seen that the common seat of physical and social pain in the human brain is the cingulate cortex. The top region of the front part of the cingulate cortex seen in the blue part of Fig. 27.1 is involved in both physical pain and the social pain of rejection, exclusion or ostracism. While these non-physical experiences are undeniably social, they cannot be derived from a cognitive base alone because they are also extremely emotional. The top area of the anterior cingulate cortex is associated with affective processes of isolation. In spite of the common experience of intensity of each kind of pain and the fact that sensory intensity and the subjective are experienced as coming together in pain, there are times when they can be felt as separate because they emanate from different brain circuits in the cingulate cortex. At one time surgeons treated chronic pain by disabling the anterior cingulate. Patients would report that the sensory aspects of the pain continued, but it didn't seem to bother them subjectively.

27.6   Studies of Social Pain

The sensitivity that humans display when exposed to minor cases of social pain attest to the depths of our social natures. This result has been demonstrated in numerous experiments. For example, in a frequently replicated experiment, Leary (2007) found that subjects reported feeling the pain of exclusion after being told that they would be working alone because no one in the group wanted to pair up with them. Baumeister and DeWall (2006) told participants that based on their answers to questionnaires, they would most probably end up alone in life even though they presently had numerous friends. Williams and Sommer (1997) arranged for two confederates who were waiting for an experiment to begin, to start throwing a ball to each other and include the naïve subject. Then they stopped throwing it to him and just threw it to each other. In all these experiments results included lowered self-esteem for the subjects, increased aggressiveness on their part and increased conformity to group norms. The ball-tossing experiment was then placed on line and called "cyberball". When the subject was informed that the other two players were fictional they still reported genuine feelings of social pain.

Participants who were placed in fMRI scanners to monitor brain activity showed a similar sensitivity to exclusion. In this case (implicit inclusion) persons were placed in "hyper scanners." Here, several persons simultaneously communicate with each other in other hyperscanners while their brain activities are recorded. As far as this author knows, such scanners exist only at Johns Hopkins University and at Virginia Technology's Carillon Research Institute. Using such scanners, participants were told that there was some technical difficulty that meant that they could watch, but not throw or catch the ball. This arrangement was such that no normal participant could take this exclusion personally. Yet they did experience it personally and it hurt.

In the second scan (full social inclusion) participants were told that the technical problems were fixed and they could also play catch with the other two people in scanners. For the final hyperscanner study, all participants played catch for 50 % of the game, but the other two-hyper scanner confederates excluded them for the rest of the game. Participants were then released from the scanners and asked to fill out a questionnaire assessing the degree of social pain that they experienced. The researchers also had the additional information about brain activity. Other brain circuits were also involved, but most importantly, the cingulate cortex was strongly correlated with the self-reports of social pain. Granted, correlation may not be cause, but this strongly implies that a common enabler of both social and physical pain is the cingulate cortex.

27.7 The Ubiquity of Human Isolation

Certainly science and poetry are very distinct ways of knowing the world, but they both are ways of knowing and can serve as a description of the ubiquity of our fears of being alone. In this case, we harken to the words of Thomas Wolfe who wrote about what might be called the "painful underbelly" of our social natures. In fearing aloneness, the very fear itself makes us its eternal companion.

> Naked and alone we came into exile. In her dark womb we did not know our mother's face; from the prison of her flesh we come into the unspeakable and incommunicable prison of this earth. Which of us has known his brother? Which of us has looked into his father's heart? Which of us has not remained forever prison-pent? Which of us is not forever a stranger and alone? (Wolfe 1929).

Finally we must consider the extreme contrast in intensity between the pain of rejection when research subjects are playing cyberball and the pain experienced by an individual upon discovering that his or her lover, who they trusted more than anyone one on earth, had betrayed them. A common expression of this intense experience, applicable also in the death of a loved one, is "I just can't get my head around this".

Such intense cases cannot be available for research purposes, but Meyer et al. (2013) found that the emotion of empathy, certainly an example of Anderson's (2014) "interpersonal suffering," is enabled by the very same brain areas that enabled social rejection. They also found that the empathetic pain of watching a friend's exclusion activated the same areas – the dorsal anterior cingulate and the insular. This activation was correlated with the self-reported identification with a friend. Importantly, this was not the case with strangers, which was a more distant type of experience.

27.8   Conclusions

Humans suffer from isolation and exclusion because of the depth to which we are social animals. In other words, it is our nature to do so. For those who think we have no particular natures and that human behavior is essentially cultural, this may be an unwelcome suggestion, but the research findings about the cingulate cortex as the common center of both of physical and social pain are too strong to ignore. Furthermore I have argued, that this pain is always in the background for us as it is for mammals that depend on their herd for their safety. The threats of exclusion and isolation cause us discomfort; they range in intensity from the infants in the Spitz studies to participants in a pretend game of "cyberball", but they are important parts of being human. They are also important aspects of social control insofar as violations of that control can led to sanctions and various forms of isolation. Finally, this chapter has shown how the new field of neurosociology can shed light on some strongly held beliefs about the absence of a human nature. We have also shown how neurosociology enlightens us about the reality of social pain based upon empathy with close others seen getting rejected socially. These results demonstrate the intensity and ubiquity of this kind of human pain and suffering.

References

Anderson, R. E. (2014). *Human suffering and quality of life: Conceptualizing stories and statistics*. New York: Springer.
Baumeister, R., & DeWall, C. (2006). The inner dimension of social exclusion: Intelligent thought and self-regulation among rejected persons. In K. Williams, J. Forgas, & W. Hippel (Eds.), *The social outcast: Social exclusion, rejection and bullying*. New York: Psychology Press.

Bogen, J., Dezure, R., TenHouten, W., & Marsh, J. F. (1972). The other side of the brain IV: The A/P ratio. *Bulletin of the Los Angeles Neurological Societies, 37*, 49–61.

Brothers, L. (1977). *Friday's footprints: How society shapes the human mind*. New York: Oxford University Press.

Cacioppo, J. T., & Patrick, W. (2008). *Loneliness: Human nature and the need for social connection*. New York: W. W. Norton & Company.

Franks, D. D. (2010). *Neurosociology: The nexus between neuroscience and social psychology*. New York: Springer.

Franks, D. D., & Turner, J. H. (Eds.). (2013). *Handbook of neurosociology*. New York: Springer Press.

Leary, J. M. (2007). Varieties of interpersonal rejection. In K. Williams, J. Forgas, & W. von Hippel (Eds.), *The social ostracism, social exclusion, rejection and bullying*. New York: Psychology Press.

Lieberman, M. D. (2013). *Social: Why our brains are wired to connect*. New York: Random House.

Lieberman, M. D., & Eisenberger, N. L. (2006). A pain by any other name (rejection exclusion, ostracism) still hurts the same: The role of dorsal anterior cingulate cortex in social and physical pain. In J. Cacioppo, V. Visser, & C. Pickett (Eds.), *Social neuroscience: People thinking about people* (pp. 167–187). Cambridge MA: MIT Press.

Lieberman, M. D., & Eisenberger, N. I. (2008). The pains and pleasures of social life: A social cognitive neuroscience approach. *Neuroleadership, 1*(1), 38–43.

Macdonald, G., & Leary, M. (2005). Why does social exclusion hurt? The relationship between social and physical pain. *Psychological Bulletin, 131*(2), 202–223.

Mead, G. H. (1934). *Mind, self, and society*. Chicago: University of Chicago Press.

Meyer, M. L., et al. (2013). Empathy for the social suffering of friends and strangers recruits distinct patterns of brain activation. *Social Cognitive and Affective Neuroscience, 8*, 446–454.

Nelson, E. E., & Panksepp, J. (1998). Brain substrates of infant and mother attachment: Contributions of opioids, oxytocin, and norepinephrine. *Neuroscience and Biobehavioral Reviews, 22*, 43–452.

Panksepp, J. (1998). *Affective neuroscience*. New York: Oxford University Press.

Spitz, R. A. (1966). *First year of life: A psychoanalytic study of normal and deviant development of object relations*. Madison: International Universities Press.

Turner, J. (2000). *On the origins of human emotions: A sociological inquiry into the evolution of human affect*. Stanford: Stanford University Press.

Williams, K. D., & Sommer, K. L. (1997). Social ostracism by coworkers: Does rejection led to loafing or compensation? *Personality and Social Psychology Bulletin, 23*, 693–706.

Wolfe, T. (1929). *Look homeward, angel*. New York: Scribners.

Chapter 28
Collaborative Humanitarianism: Information Networks that Reduce Suffering

Louis-Marie Ngamassi Tchouakeu and Andrea H. Tapia

28.1 Introduction

There is a strong belief among humanitarian organizations that collaboration, coordination and common projects across organizational boundaries lead to more effective and efficient service delivery. The benefits of organizational coordination and collaboration are often accepted as given, and lead to organizational resource allocation and decision-making. However, there is very little evidence that the projects actually lead to measureable benefits; or, if there is a perceived benefit, there is no evidence as to how collaborative efforts produce this change. Most importantly, there is no direct causal link between collaborative efforts and effects of the bottom line: reducing human suffering. Not only has this led to a long string of failed collaborative efforts and organizational collaborative fatigue, but it has also led to unexplained, ad-hoc, successful collaborations.

Humanitarians typically define human suffering as physical suffering due to physical deprivation (starvation or thirst), disease, or trauma from a disaster or conflict. Humanitarians attempt to reduce human suffering in two ways: first, through acute crisis response and second, through long-term development efforts. Through development efforts, humanitarians combat poverty and many of its repercussions such as disease, sanitation and food security, with the goals of increasing community resilience and capacity while reducing suffering.

L.-M.N. Tchouakeu (✉)
Faculty of College of Business, Prairie View A&M University,
519, Prairie View, TX 77446, USA
e-mail: ngamassi@gmail.com

A.H. Tapia
Faculty of College of Information Sciences and Technology,
Pennsylvania State University, State College, PA 16802, USA
e-mail: atapia@ist.psu.edu

© Springer Science+Business Media Dordrecht 2015
R.E. Anderson (ed.), *World Suffering and Quality of Life*,
Social Indicators Research Series 56, DOI 10.1007/978-94-017-9670-5_28

This physical definition of human suffering has been challenged to grow beyond the physical to include suffering caused by social issues such as repressive regimes and cultures, war and conflict. It is even stretched to include a lack of education, human rights, freedom and self expression as a cause for pain, distress or suffering. Modern humanitarianism struggles to address both the physical and social causes of human suffering.

This chapter illustrates a few collaborative paths across humanitarian organizations that eventually lead to a reduction in human suffering. We empirically explore the potential benefits of inter-organizational humanitarian networks among modern humanitarians. Specifically, we focus on large networks of organizational representatives with similar interests in humanitarian information technologies. We study the HumanaInfoNet,[1] a network of organizations engaged in humanitarian information management and exchange. The United Nation's Office for the Coordination of Humanitarian Affairs (UNOCHA) initiated the HumanaInfoNet to ensure effective and timely response to humanitarian disasters. Data were collected through multiple sources by a series of three surveys and semi-structured interviews. Our data is organized around three themes: Communication to Collaboration, Collaborative Projects and Collaborative Principles. We provide implications of our research for alleviating human suffering and designing humanitarian inter-organizational networks.

28.2   Modern Humanitarianism

The term "humanitarian" is generally associated with operations that seek to alleviate human suffering in the face of crises as diverse as armed conflicts, epidemics, famine and natural disasters. These crises often occur in fragile environments characterized by low socio-economic status, sparse infrastructure and political and environmental threats. Humanitarian relief efforts are complex responses to emergent situations where the facts and challenges on the ground can change rapidly.

Not only must modern humanitarians address new challenges in their efforts to address human suffering, but they must also work to not cause additional suffering. Modern humanitarianism is significantly different than traditional humanitarianism in five ways. First, there are a growing number of diverse participants in any response. Second, governance of these participants has become decentralized. Third, new coalitions, collaborations, and networks of participants have arisen to co-deliver response. Fourth, information itself has come to be seen as a basic need/ right in humanitarian action. Fifth, the ways in which humanitarian information is collected, shared, and analyzed has changed and continues to change, so response organizations must adapt to meet the challenge. These technical changes present both opportunities and challenges for those interested in human suffering. On one hand, humanitarians may become more effective and efficient in delivering services

---

[1] HumanaInfoNet is a pseudonym we use to protect the confidentiality of the organizations.

and goods to those under duress; however, the mechanisms to provide those services may also cause additional suffering if not done with care.

Modern humanitarianism, while possessing the same goals as traditional humanitarianism, has been greatly effected by changes in communication and information technologies. Organizations that address human suffering often operate in conditions of extreme uncertainty. This uncertainty has many sources, including the sporadic nature and lack of warning of certain types of emergencies, and the wide array of actors who may respond. This uncertainty increases the need for information, but at the same time the amount of operational information during a disaster can be overwhelming (Knuth 1999). In these circumstances, appropriate technologies and networks could make substantial improvements in the alleviation of human suffering.

According to a report from the UN entitled *Humanitarianism in the Network Age* (http://www.unocha.org/hina), there has been a fundamental shift in the ability to influence a response away from capitals and headquarters to the people aid agencies aim to assist. The authors argue that the form of the assistance and the providers of assistance are all in a state of flux due to changing technological infrastructure. Today, voluntary and private actors are taking part in humanitarian action at the local, national, regional and global levels because of extremely low barriers to entry. These new entrants ignore traditional hierarchies and their entrance is seen as decentralizing the sector. This decentralization has been seen to create new forms of collaboration between NGOs, communities, first responders and local and national governments. The widespread use of mobile technologies encourages the victims and beneficiaries to voice their own needs and participate in their own development and capacity building.

28.3 Networked Humanitarianism

Humanitarian organizations are increasingly working together through inter-organizational structures such as coalitions, alliances, partnerships, and coordination bodies (Guo and Acar 2005; Zhao et al. 2008). The international community has been putting more efforts into disaster mitigation and humanitarian assistance through the use of networks (Zhang et al. 2002; UNOCHA 2002, 2007a, b). Humanitarian inter-organizational networks are seen as a solution to duplication of efforts in assistance projects, badly planned and implemented relief efforts, and the lack of knowledge among humanitarian organizations on the actual situation in which they operate.

The benefits of inter-organizational collaboration include benefits to the individual members of the network (e.g. the ability to address shared problems more effectively, the potential for cost savings and organizational learning), benefits to the clients (e.g. victims of disasters), benefits to members of the network (e.g. the higher quality service or end product) and benefits to the community as a whole. For Jang and Feiock (2007), collaboration among nonprofit organizations has the

potential to enhance service to clients. They argue that inter-organizational collaboration is beneficiary to nonprofits because it allows them to share the risks associated with service production and delivery. Some major challenges involved in
inter-organizational collaboration in the nonprofit sector have also been intensively
documented in the literature (Gazley and Brudney 2007; Ngamassi et al. 2011;
Maitland et al. 2009). They include loss autonomy, financial instability, difficulty in
evaluating organizational results, and opportunity costs from the time and resources
devoted to collaborative activities.

Understanding networks in the field of humanitarian relief can be enhanced by
considering the content of relationships that exist among organizations. Katz and
Anheier (2005) identify the major types of relationships among stakeholders in
responding to humanitarian disasters. They include information exchange, project
collaboration, participation in meetings and forums, and joint membership in advocacy coalitions. In the field of humanitarian relief, inter-organizational networks can
be classified into two types: those oriented to project implementation and those
oriented to information sharing (Lee 2008). The purpose of the implementation
networks is to implement humanitarian relief projects. Implementation networks
are activity-focused, project-based networks that rely on partnerships to draw on
resources such as funding and skills from various partners (Unwin 2005). This type
of network applies more to the field of humanitarian relief since projects are more
often implemented by numerous project partners. Knowledge-sharing networks, on
the other hand, are often formed through affiliation to common events such as global
and regional committees, forums, conferences, and publication activities (Katz and
Anheier 2005). These networks enable organizations to be informed of their partner's and community's activities as a whole. The networks investigated in this chapter can be considered as a hybrid between these two types of networks.

28.4   Research Design

This study is part of a larger research effort that examines models of information
technology and information management collaboration among organizations in the
humanitarian relief field. Using mixed methods allowed us leverage on both the
quantitative and the qualitative research techniques. The HumanaInfoNet is spear-
headed by the United Nations Office for the Coordination of Humanitarian Affairs
(UNOCHA 2002, 2007a, b). It is made up of about 300 information technology (IT)
and IM professionals from roughly 120 international and national organizations
from the broad humanitarian community. These organizations include nongovernmental organizations (NGOs), inter-governmental organizations (IGOs), United
Nations agencies, private sectors, and academia (See Table 28.1). They vary in the
terms of missions, goals, size, and geographical location.

Table 28.1 Sample
distribution

Category	Number of Org.	Percentage (%)
Academia	7	5.88
Donor	1	0.84
Government	7	5.88
Governmental Organization	11	9.24
Inter-Governmental Organization	3	2.52
Media	8	6.72
NGO	37	31.09
Networked NGO	11	9.24
UN	24	20.17
Private sector	10	8.40

Members of the HumanaInfoNet were selected and brought together by the United Nations Office for the Coordination of Humanitarian Affairs (UNOCHA). The goals of the HumanaInfoNet were to:

1. Promote the use of humanitarian information management principles
2. Disseminate best practices of humanitarian information management
3. Improve the community's preparedness in humanitarian information management
4. Help organizations/agencies acquire resources
5. Improve the level of professionalization in the field of humanitarian information management
6. Foster collaboration on humanitarian information management projects
7. Facilitate sharing of expertise among organizations/agencies
8. Promote humanitarian information sharing
9. Strengthen relationships between organizations/agencies
10. Increase awareness of humanitarian information systems
11. Improve humanitarian information quality

We collected data through multiple sources including surveys and interviews. We conducted a series of three surveys during October 2007, May 2008, and July 2009. For questions concerning the inter-organizational network, survey participants were provided with the list of members of the HumanaInfoNet community and were asked to identify those with whom they had collaborated on humanitarian projects, and those with whom they had communicated for information seeking and/or receiving. They could also report collaborative relationships with organizations that were not members of HumanaInfoNet. We used the answers to this question to generate a multidimensional inter-organizational network in which nodes represent organizations and edges denote the relationship among organizations. Overall, representatives from 56 organizations answered the survey questions. We considered a project collaboration linkage to exist between two organizations if a survey participant from either of the two organizations reported that the two organizations had collaborated on a humanitarian information management project. Similarly, a linkage for communication on advice seeking and/or receiving exited if a survey respondent from either of the two organizations reported that one organization had provided or had received advice from the other. The multi-dimensional inter-organizational network generated was made up of about 200 organizations, some of which were not members of HumanaInfoNet. In this chapter, we only include organizations that are members of HumanaInfoNet. The total member organizations of the HumanaInfoNet reported to be part of a relationship was 119.

From September to December 2009, we conducted 19 phone-based semi-structured interviews with organizational members of the HumanaInfoNet. Interview participants were asked to state the factors that influence their organization's decision to engage in collaboration with other organizations on humanitarian IM projects. A subsequent question focusing on the implications of ICTs was also asked. Our intent was to supplement the quantitative survey data with a more detailed description and explanation of activities in the HumanaInfoNet community. Each interview lasted between 45 and 90 min. The majority of questions were taken directly from the survey with the intent to maintain a semblance for comparison between the surveys and interviews. The interviews were transcribed manually and coded both deductively and inductively (Epstein and Martin 2004).

28.5   Data Analysis and Results

We analyze and present the data from both the surveys and interviews. This data is organized around three themes: Communication to Collaboration, Collaborative Projects and Collaborative Principles. We discuss these potential benefits to collaboration and provide some implications of our research for alleviating human suffering and designing humanitarian inter-organizational networks.

28.5.1   PATH 1: Communication to Collaboration

We have found strong evidence that there is a path found in HumanaInfoNet that begins by exposing one organization to another, then provides opportunities for those organizations to interact around common interests (information management in this case). This allows for increased communication, which eventually leads to the establishment of collaborative projects. These collaborative projects then have the potential to impact human suffering. In a nutshell, the existence of an arena, such as a network, in which communication is encouraged across organizational boundaries, leads to measureable communication, information exchange and collaborative humanitarian efforts.

Our subjects acknowledged that communication plays a very important role in the formation of collaboration relationships. First, communication often precedes collaboration and serves as the basis for establishing the future collaboration relationship. This is because organizations need to communicate with acquaintances to obtain information about different joint project initiatives so that they can identify interesting projects and collaborate on them. Second, an organization's decision on whether or not to collaborate with others on a joint project is mainly based on its own evaluation of the project. However, through communication, organizations are often able to exert various levels of influence on others' decisions on collaboration.

In our study, we analyze two types of relationships between organizations: communicating for advice seeking and/or receiving, and project collaboration. In other words, we have two one-dimensional undirected networks, each of which indicates one type of relationship. An edge in the advising network means the two organizations have exchanged advice concerning humanitarian policy, technology, data, and so on. In the dimension of project collaboration, two organizations are connected by an edge if they used to collaborate on humanitarian information management projects. The project they collaborated on could be joint training of staff members, coordinated data collection, or shared database. The degree of a node is the number of edges attached to that node. Figures 28.1 and 28.2 show the networks and their

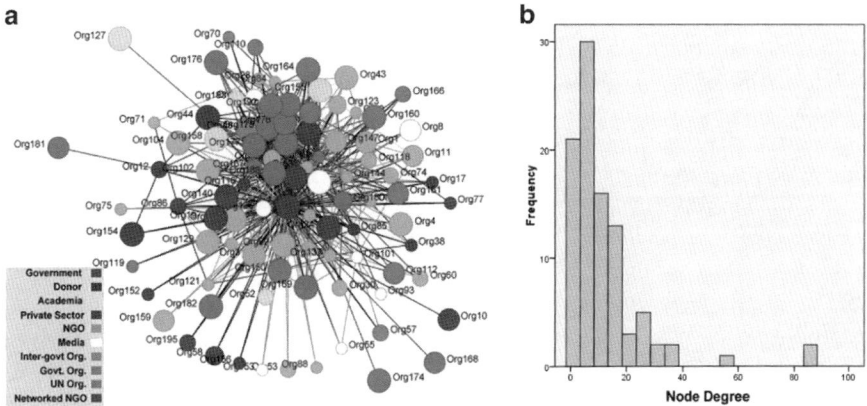

Fig. 28.1 (**a**) Inter-organizational advising network; (**b**) Advising network node degree distribution

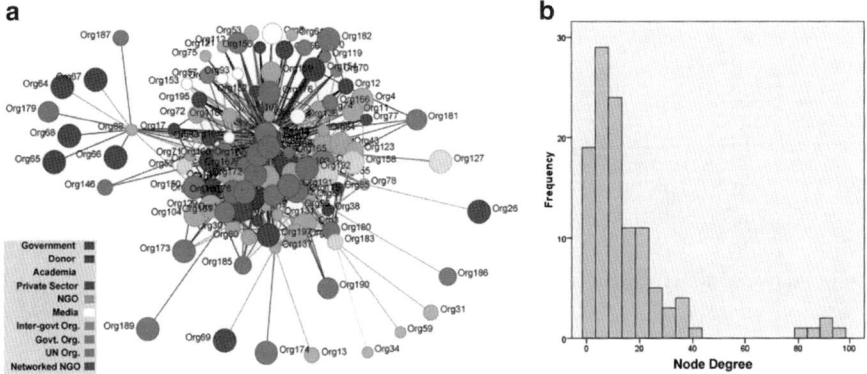

Fig. 28.2 (**a**) Project Collaboration network relationship (The size of a node is proportional to the organization's size). (**b**) Network node degree distribution

Table 28.2 Basic statistics of
the multi-dimensional networks

Network	Number of nodes	Number of edges
Advising	95	574
Collaboration	112	851

Table 28.3 Assortativity coefficients

	Degree-based coefficients	Size-based coefficients	Type-based coefficients
Advising network	−0.3896 (0.0006)	−0.0196 (0.0005)	0.0009 (0.0003)
Collaboration network	−0.4293 (0.0005)	−0.0960 (0.0004)	−0.0105 (0.0004)

Corresponding errors are listed in parentheses

degree distributions. Table 28.2 summarizes the basic statistics of the two one-dimensional networks. The cluster structure depicted in the collaboration network (Fig. 28.2) highlights the strategic brokerage position that some organizations occupy in the network, especially with regard to accessing UN agencies and certain Governments.

Assortativity describes the tendency of nodes in networks being connected with similar nodes. Assortative pattern means nodes tend to connect with those that are similar to themselves. For example, sociologists found in social networks that one tends to connect with those who are similar to oneself in demographic characteristics, such as age, gender, race, and education (McPherson et al. 2001; Kilduff and Tsai 2006). In other words, assortative patterns emerge from the homophile-based network growth. When talking about assortativity for a multi-dimensional network, one needs to be aware of the node attribute and what type of relationship the assortativity is based on. Assortativity depends on node attribute because assortativity is based on similarity between nodes and similarity can be measured by various node attributes.

In our study, we use three node attributes. At macro-level, we use the topological attribute—the node degree. At micro-level, we use two organizational attributes—the size and type of an organization. We use the number of staff as a measure of size of the organizations. Organizational size should be a scalar attributes. However, most of our survey or interview respondents were not the top-level executives of those organizations. Many of them did not know the exact number of full-time employees in their organizations. Therefore, we had to classify organization sizes into categories for them to choose. The five categories were micro (<20 full-time employees), small (21–50), medium (51–100), large (101–500), and very large (>500). Table 28.3 summarizes the assortativity coefficients and errors given by our computational analysis. As for organization type, the United Nations provide a classification scheme. Organizations in the HumanaInfoNet are classified into seven types: Academia, Donor, Government, Governmental organization, Inter-Governmental organization, Media, Non-governmental Organization (NGO), Networked NGO, UN, and Private sector.

Degree-based assortativity coefficients suggest that the inter-organizational network in the humanitarian sector exhibit disassortative patterns. This is different from the degree-based assortative patterns that researchers found in many social networks (Newman 2003). We believe the degree distributions of the networks may have contributed to the disassortativity. In the degree distributions of the two networks (Figs. 28.1 and 28.2), there are often a large number of nodes with low degrees and a small number of nodes with high degrees. However, few nodes have medium degrees. This type of polarized distribution has led to the core-peripheral structures of the network.

The core-peripheral structures suggest that several organizations are very active in this network and connect with many other organizations, thus serving as the core, or hub, of the network. Meanwhile, most organizations have low degrees, mainly connect to high-degree nodes, and are relatively peripheral to the network. This structure could potentially be explained by the nature of the community in which several general-purpose humanitarian relief organizations, such as Red Cross and Red Crescent, interact with many highly specialized organizations. Those specialized organizations include humanitarian relief organizations that focus on a specific humanitarian relief domain, such as providing shelters or protecting children; humanitarian relief organizations that work in a specific geographical area, such as Sub-Saharan Africa or Mideast; or organizations that provide specialized IT services. For example, a humanitarian relief organization may seek advice or help from a partner with expertise in landmine-detection geographic information systems. Further, these specialized organizations are less likely to work with one another in the humanitarian relief sector. For instance, the chance is relatively low for an organization working mainly in East Europe to collaborate with another one that focuses on Latin America. Similarly, a software provider may not need to interact with a telecommunication provider for the purpose of humanitarian relief.

In addition to the core-peripheral structure identified in the two networks, the analysis of the inter-organizational communication and collaboration networks also revealed the connection between communication and collaboration. Our assortativity analysis also suggests that the advising network and the collaboration network have similar assortativity patterns. The Quadratic Assignment Procedure correlation (Krackhardt 1988) between the two networks also shows that the seeking of knowledge and collaborations on humanitarian projects are correlated. The correlation is significant at the .01 level. This structural correlation is corroborated with what we heard when interviewing organizations in this community. Advising relationships often serve as the basis and prerequisites for future collaborations. For instance, one participant said:

There are people and entities we met that we are now discussing with and sharing information with just keep in touch at an informal level. I think that is very good for us. Also, with the UN being the UN, some institutions are more difficult to approach officially, or let's say institutionally. While if you have this more ad hoc, loose network where you could exchange without it becoming very formal…that is very useful. (Subject 1)

28.5.2   PATH 2: Collaborative Projects

Collectively, our research suggests that projects serve as a primary method of collaboration within humanitarian networks (see Maldonado et al. 2009; Maitland and Tapia 2007; Maitland et al. 2009; Saab et al. 2008). Here we analyze the formation of projects. Examples of actual projects formed are: a multi-organizational effort to create a common assessment tool for post-disaster damage and needs, a multi-organizational agreement to collectively buy, use, appropriate and share satellite access and imagery in the field, and the multi-organizational deployment of a device and system to collect, monitor and analyze health data from remote communities participating in maternal-child health and food security programs. All of these projects have the potential to impact human suffering.

Approximately 85 % (84.21 %) of the interviewees discussed the effectiveness of HumanaInfoNet with regards to establishing new collaborative projects, and having those projects align with their organizational goals of reducing human suffering. More specifically, as illustrated in the following quotes from the interview data, HumanaInfoNet was reported to be very effective in strengthening relationships between organizations and agencies by promoting the use of humanitarian information management project creation. Survey participants commented on this:

> Subject 11: "So I would say the HumanaInfoNet was one of the events that promoted actual projects among different partners."

> Subject 8: "I would say that there have been more information related projects and initiatives in the last two years, and, so, I mean, I think it encouraged information related projects."

Our analysis of the HumanaInfoNet data suggests an important role for sharing and pooling projects during the process of collaboration in humanitarian information management and exchange. There are two collaboration projects: sharing projects and pooling projects. Sharing projects refers to a collaboration mechanism in which the network facilitates some access to resources outside the project boundaries but inside the network. Pooling projects refers to a collaboration mechanism used by the network to facilitate some collective access to resources outside the boundaries of the organizations. Access to informational resources (e.g. large database) appears to have positive implications for the numbers of organizations interested in participating in multi-organizational projects. When project teams are created across organizations as the case in the HumanaInfoNet, the role of the participant or member (as an IT technician, an IS manager, or a CIO) may be instrumental in allowing projects to form quickly. These projects may then lead to further collaboration.

28.5.3   PATH 3: Collaborative Principles

The members of HumanaInfoNet initiated a large, network-wide collaborative project—the creation of a set of common principles and standards for information management, ratifying them as a whole body, and sending them to each member organization. The full list of principles is below (Table 28.4). While several of the principles deal directly with information management with the intent of improving information quality, accuracy, and interoperability, several others can be seen to

Table 28.4 Principles of humanitarian information management and exchange

Principle	Description
Accessibility	Humanitarian information and data should be made accessible to all humanitarian actors by applying easy-to-use formats and by translating information into common or local languages when necessary. Information and data for humanitarian purposes should be made widely available through a variety of online and offline distribution channels including the media
Inclusiveness	Information management and exchange should be based on a system of collaboration, partnership and sharing with a high degree of participation and ownership by multiple stakeholders, especially representatives of the affected population
Inter-operability	All sharable data and information should be made available in formats that can be easily retrieved, shared and used by humanitarian organizations
Accountability	Users must be able to evaluate the reliability and credibility of data and information by knowing its source. Information providers should be responsible to their partners and stakeholders for the content they publish and disseminate
Verifiability	Information should be accurate, consistent and based on sound methodologies, validated by external sources, and analyzed within the proper contextual framework
Relevance	Information should be practical, flexible, responsive, and driven by operational needs in support of decision-making throughout all phases of a crisis
Objectivity	Information managers should consult a variety of sources when collecting and analyzing information so as to provide varied and balanced perspectives for addressing problems and recommending solutions
Humanity	Information should never be used to distort, to mislead or to cause harm to affected or at-risk populations, and should respect the dignity of victims
Timeliness	Humanitarian information should be collected, analyzed and disseminated efficiently, and must be kept current
Sustainability	Humanitarian information and data should be preserved, cataloged and archived so that it can be retrieved for future use, such as for preparedness, analysis, lessons learned and evaluation
Reliability	Users must be able to evaluate the reliability and credibility of data and information by knowing its source and method of collection. Collection methods should adhere to global standards where they exist to support and reinforce credibility. Reliability is a prerequisite for ensuring validity and verifiability
Reciprocity	Information exchange should be a beneficial two-way process between the affected communities and the humanitarian community, including affected governments
Confidentiality	The processing of any personal data shall not be done without the prior explicit description of its purpose and will only be done for that purpose. Sufficient safeguards must be put in place to protect personal data against loss, unauthorized processing and other misuse. If sensitive information is publicly disclosed, the sources of such information will not be released when there is a reasonable risk that doing so will affect the security or integrity of these sources

deal more directly with alleviating human suffering. One can argue that better reliability, verifiability, accountability and accessibility may have implications for alleviating human suffering indirectly down the line in that they may allow organizations to make better decisions based on better data. For example, as organizations collect data about the effectiveness of their development projects, they can make mid-course changes in near real time that allow for better distribution of medicine and food to maternal-child health care and food security programs. Through careful data collection and monitoring of child health care statistics, outbreaks of waterborne diseases and malnutrition can be identified early and addressed, reducing current and future suffering for the mother, child and the community as a whole.

However, there are four principles that are more direct: inclusiveness, humanity, reciprocity and confidentiality. These provide direct benefits to suffering populations if employed. All four of these principles see information as a valuable asset that should not be simply taken from affected populations. Information as an asset should be controlled by its producers, shared with knowledge, used for the good of its originators and carefully managed as not to cause additional suffering. Mismanaged, stolen and sold information can cause human suffering. While information security and privacy is not often seen as an issue related to human suffering, there are many cases in which mishandled information collected by humanitarians could cause pain and duress. For example, in certain developing parts of the world, certain health-related data might carry a stigma that could result in public shaming, imprisonment, or physical punishment. Being HIV positive, and publically identified as such, carries the potential for significant human suffering. Being pregnant and lawfully unwed is information that, if exposed by a careless humanitarian worker, could lead to additional suffering for entire families and communities.

In addition, in war and conflict zones, where humanitarians often find themselves delivering services, exposed demographic information on certain populations could be used by political factions to retaliate against warring parties. Human suffering could be increased by the exposure of rebel forces receiving aid from humanitarians.

Lastly, much of the developing world has leapfrogged over the land-lined and wired telecommunications world. Mobile phones have become a core tool in conducting social and economic interaction. Mobile wallets, mobile banking and micropayments are a growing infrastructure among developing nations. This mobile infrastructure, while growing, is still fragile and easily damaged by careless exposure of economic and social information by humanitarians. For example, in several projects supported by the World Bank that included the development of robust mobile banking efforts, data was collected by evaluation teams to understand the saving behavior of participants. Mobile phone numbers, bank account numbers, demographic information and savings amounts were gathered from participants. The data was not secured and there were several incursion attempts by online predators. While the data was eventually secured before damage was caused, if it had not been, the participants could have lost all the funds they had carefully saved, and additional human suffering could have been caused.

The HumanaInfoNet held a series of conferences and workshops organized by UNOCHA. The series began in 2002 as a meeting of humanitarian information management professionals and was followed by a series of regional meetings intended to bring humanitarian information management principles and best practices to a wider range of humanitarian organizations. In particular, to bring together practitioners in the field, as opposed to only headquarters staff. The second meeting of the HumanaInfoNet was held in October 2007 and included 3 days of working group meetings designed to update the principles and best practices and identify an agenda for further development of humanitarian information management (HIM).

One of the objectives of the interviews was to assess the penetration of the principles of the HumanaInfoNet to the community as a whole. We asked the interview participants about how the HumanaInfoNet has spread to and been employed by the humanitarian community as a whole. The vast majority expressed highly positive opinions on the HumanaInfoNet's use by the community. They believed the HumanaInfoNet principles were used by the community in two ways: promoting the use of humanitarian information management principles and dissemination of best practices, and fostering collaboration on humanitarian information management projects. A couple of our participants responded:

> Subject 15: "I think the event was mostly successful in coming to an agreement among the various actors on certain standards for use of information in humanitarian response."

> Subject 8: "I think the development of the principles was useful. I think that just the working groups to address certain issues was...I think documenting the information management principles and the actual document itself that came out of the symposium I think was useful in terms of the issues of humanitarian information management."

The principles of humanitarian information management and exchange agreed upon by the members of HumanaInfoNet serve as the central backbone of this network. As humanitarian information gains recognition and purpose, these principles help to promote humanitarian objectives and foster trust and accountability among organizations. Collecting and sharing timely, reliable and accurate information during a crisis is critical to improving humanitarian response, maximizing resources and minimizing human suffering.

28.6 Discussion and Implications

Modern humanitarianism is experiencing challenges to the methods it has traditionally used to address human suffering. There are more and more diverse participants in any response, and governance of these participants has become decentralized. New coalitions, collaborations and networks of participants have arisen to co-deliver response. Information itself has come to be seen as a basic need or right in humanitarian action. The ways in which humanitarian information is collected, shared, and analyzed has changed and continues to change, and response organizations must adapt to meet the challenge.

In this new humanitarian space, we focus on a single large network of participants. Through our research we find that the participants in the network communicate with each other more, which leads to collaborative projects. One of these network-wide collaborative projects is the creation of a set of guiding principles for humanitarian information management. Projects like this, among others, create a wider, shared sense of values that considers information as a basic right, and recognizes the potential for information and information management to either cause additional suffering or alleviate suffering.

Projects are important. Collectively, our research suggests that projects serve as a primary method of collaboration within humanitarian networks (see Maldonado et al. 2009; Maitland and Tapia 2007; Maitland et al. 2009; Saab et al. 2008). Projects play a role in establishing collaborative relations among organizations (Menger 1999). Projects are governed by networks of relationships rather than traditional organizational hierarchies and well-established administrative routines (Powell 1990). Further, Bechky (2006) argues that these temporary organizations, or projects, lead to collaboration mechanisms between traditional organizations.

Our study has some implications with regards to designing effective interorganizational networks in the humanitarian relief field. Organizational members of a network must strive to keep multiple types of connections with other members. Multiplexity can be measured at the individual network member level and at the level of the whole network. A high degree of multiplexity of a member indicates high interaction of the member in a network, and signifies less liability to disruption of single relationships. A member with a large number of multiplex relations is expected to have a high potential of mobilizing different resources and information through these relations. Effective networks might have a majority of network members connected through two or more different types of relationships. In this case, multiplexity will be high, reflecting commitments among network members to one another through multiple activities.

Information is seen as a basic right, and thus needs to be treated as su--otected and secured, shared when lacking, and exposed when practices are abused. For example, beneficiaries must be guaranteed that their health information, especially if social damaging if exposed, will be kept secure. Women who are being treated for an unplanned pregnancy, a venereal disease, mental health problems or HIV would suffer more if information about their condition was carelessly leaked by the humanitarians who were offering her care, In other cases, receiving aid of any kind might threaten the status of a male member of the community who might punish his female family members who sought out aid from the humanitarian workers. Exposure of the names of those who seek benefits might again cause additional suffering. In conflict zones, humanitarians must be especially careful with information on divided populations so that political retaliation does not cause additional human suffering due to mismanaged data. Human suffering is decreased when beneficiaries are given access to and control of their personal information, information about the health and status of their community, and information about the actions taken on their behalf, as well as the effectiveness of those actions. Beneficiaries should know if a project or program has been effective at treating human suffering. Data collected by program staff about projects should be evaluated and shared with the community so that the community might continue successful practices on their own, sustain programs, and further alleviate human suffering.

28.7 Conclusion

Barnett (2005) has identified increasing politicization and institutionalization as two threats to modern humanitarianism that may derail efforts to address human suffering. Institutionalization or professionalization suggests that with time, organizational goals tend to shift toward ends that ensure organizational survival, and may not necessarily be in the best interest of the beneficiary constituents (Benini 1999). Politicization of humanitarianism threatens the overarching principles of neutrality, independence, consent and impartiality in that they are challenged by complex emergencies, conflict, war, and governmental interference. Donor intervention and manipulation may also pose threats to neutrality and independence. Even though organizations may voice the desire to remain neutral and apolitical, actions such as the promotion of democracy, human rights, peace-building and women's rights are political in themselves, and challenge the apolitical stance.

Both of these tendencies toward politicization and institutionalization could lead modern humanitarianism toward stability of organization and funding, but at the cost of reduced service to beneficiaries, fewer lives saved, and less of an impact on reducing human suffering.

Despite the pressure to institutionalize and politicize, humanitarian networks may hold the key to allowing organizations to benefit from professional networks without sacrificing principles or effectiveness. We argue that humanitarian networks provide some elements of institutionalization and professionalization, such as stability, shared risk, sets of principles, best practices and codes of ethics, and sets of standards. Humanitarian networks provide for increased communication between organizations, which lead to more collaborative action through more collaborative projects. More collaborative projects increase the strength and stability of the network and the value of the network to individual members.

Humanitarian networks also address the politicization of the humanitarian arena, especially in addressing the data collection imperative. The network provides best practices and examples of ethical data collection practices that address both upwards and downwards accountability. The network provides examples of data management, privacy and security practices for beneficiary data.

Humanitarian organizations have a variety of information gathering and processing requirements, derived in part from the need for organizational accountability and learning. These requirements necessitate information gathering from beneficiaries. The information is subsequently used to demonstrate adherence to donor-specified requirements and ideally to help improve subsequent program designs. More and more data is being taken and moved from beneficiaries and the field to headquarters. This has strong implications for ethics, privacy and the empowerment of beneficiaries. As organizations gather more data, the question must be asked: "how can this data also be seen as a social good, benefitting those communities and individuals from which it was produced?"

Several of the principles created by the HumanaInfoNet network directly addressed this tension, specifically reciprocity, addressing downward accountability and confidentiality, the ethical treatment of such data. Credible and independent information is a crucial and indispensable part of humanitarian assistance and alleviating suffering. Without communicating with and collecting data from the very people relief organizations are seeking to help, they run the risk of seriously undermining what they are setting out to achieve. It is therefore vital for humanitarian organizations to maintain a strong sense of professional ethics at every stage of humanitarian information management. Ensuring quality requires the development of, and adherence to, standards for information collection, exchange, security, attribution and use.

Networks of humanitarian organizations as discussed in this paper have the potential to address human suffering at a high magnitude through the creation of common, collaborative projects and more effective and efficient service delivery. Better humanitarian service delivery has the potential to improve and save lives. While the suffering caused by the mismanagement of data gathered by humanitarians is not of the same magnitude as suffering caused by floods, poverty and conflict, it nonetheless can add insult to injury if humanitarians cause additional suffering to those they seek to help.

References

Barnett, M. (2005). Humanitarianism transformed. *Perspectives on Politics, 3*(04), 723–740.

Bechky, B. A. (2006). Gaffers, Gofers, and Grips: Role-based collaboration in temporary organizations. *Organization Science, 17*(1), 3–23.

Benini, A. A. (1999). Network without centre? A case study of an organizational network responding to an earthquake. *Journal of Contingencies and Crisis Management, 7*(1), 38–47.

Epstein, L., & Martin, A. (2004). Coding variables. In K. Kempf-Leonard (Ed.), *The encyclopedia of social measurement* (Vol. 1, pp. 321–327). New York: Elsevier Academic Press.

Gazley, B., & Brudney, L. (2007). The purpose (and perils) of government-nonprofit partnership. *Nonprofit and Voluntary Sector Quarterly, 36*(3), 389–415.

Guo, C., & Acar, M. (2005). Understanding collaboration among nonprofit organizations: Combining resource dependency, institutional, and network perspectives. *NonProfit and Voluntary Sector Quarterly, 34*(3), 340–361.

Jang, H., & Feiock, R. (2007). Public and private funding reliance of nonprofit organizations: Implications for inter-organizational collaboration. *Public Performance and Management Review, 31*(2), 174–190.

Katz, H., & Anheier, H. (2005). Global connectedness: The structure of transnational NGO networks. In M. Glasius, M. Kaldor, & H. Anheier (Eds.), *Global civil society 2005/6* (pp. 240–262). London: Sage.

Kilduff, M., & Tsai, W. (2006). *Social networks and organizations*. London: Sage.

Knuth, R. (1999). Sovereignty, globalism, and information flow in complex emergencies. *The Information Society, 15*, 11–19.

Krackhardt, D. (1988). Predicting with networks – Nonparametric multiple-regression analysis of dyadic data. *Social Networks, 10*, 359–381.

Lee, S. (2008). The coevolution of multimodal, multiplex, and multilevel organizational networks in development communities. Doctorate dissertation, University of Southern California.

Maitland, C., & Tapia, A. (2007). Coordinated ICTs for effective use in humanitarian assistance. *Journal of Information Technology in Social Change, 1*(1), 128–141.

Maitland, C., Ngamassi, L., & Tapia, A. (2009). Information management and technology issues addressed by humanitarian relief coordination bodies. *Proceedings of the 6th International ISCRAM Conference – Göteborg, Sweden*, May 2009.

Maldonado, E., Maitland, C., & Tapia, A. (2009). Collaborative systems development in crisis relief: The impact of multi-level governance. Information systems frontiers [Special issue]. *Information Systems Frontiers, 12*(1), 9–27.

McPherson, M., Smith-Lovin, L., & Cook, J. M. (2001). Birds of a feather: Homophily in social networks. *Annual Review of Sociology, 27*, 415–444.

Menger, P. M. (1999). Artistic labor markets and careers. *Annual Review of Sociology, 25*, 541–574.

Newman, M. E. J. (2003). Mixing patterns in networks. *Physical Review E, 67*, 13.

Ngamassi, L., Maldonado, E., Zhao, K., Robinson, H., Maitland, C., & Tapia, A. (2011). Exploring barriers to coordination between Humanitarian NGOs: A comparative case study of two NGO's information technology coordination bodies. *International Journal of Information Systems and Social Change (IJISSC)*, [special issue on IS/IT in Nonprofits] 2(2), 1–25.

Powell, W. W. (1990). Neither market nor hierarchy: Network forms of organization. *Research in Organizational Behavior, 12*, 295–336.

Saab, D., Maldonado, E., Orendovici, R., Ngamassi, L., Gorp, A., Zhao, K., Maitland, C., & Tapia, A. (2008, May). Building global bridges: Coordination bodies for improved information sharing among humanitarian relief agencies. In F. Fiedrich and B. Van de Walle (Eds.), *Proceedings of the 5th International ISCRAM Conference* (pp. 471–483). Washington, DC, USA, 2008.

UNOCHA. (2002). *Symposium on best practices in Humanitarian Information Exchange: Final report*. Retrieved December 4, 2007, from http://www.reliefweb.int/symposium/2002_symposium/Symposium%20Final%20Report.pdf

UNOCHA. (2007a). *Global symposium +5 information for Humanitarian action: Draft outcomes*. Retrieved December 4, 2007, from http://www.reliefweb.int/symposium/docs/Outcomes_Symposium.pdf

UNOCHA. (2007b). *Outcome documents: Symposium on best practices in Humanitarian Information Exchange (Geneva 2002); Humanitarian Information Network Regional Workshops (Bangkok 2003, Panama 2005, Nairobi 2006)*. Retrieved October 20, 2007, from http://www.reliefweb.int/symposium

Unwin, T. (2005). *Partnerships in development practice: Evidence from multi- stakeholder ICT4D partnership practice in Africa*. Paris: UNESCO.

Zhang, D., Zhou, L., & Nunamaker, J. F. (2002). A knowledge management framework for the support of decision making in humanitarian assistance/disaster relief. *Knowledge and Information Systems, 4*(3), 370–385.

Zhao, K., Maitland, C., Ngamassi, L., Orendovici, R., Tapia, A., & Yen, J. (2008). Emergence of collaborative projects and coalitions: A framework for coordination in humanitarian relief. *World Congress on Social Simulation 2008 (WCSS-08)*. George Mason University, Fairfax – 14–17 July 2008.

Chapter 29
A New Method for Measuring and Analyzing Suffering: Comparing Suffering Patterns in Italian Society

Marco Fattore and Filomena Maggino

29.1 Introduction

The dimensions of human suffering are different; they are related to different human physical and psychological aspects and refer to different life domains. The psychological aspect of suffering can be observed through different lens, among which the subjective well-being/ill-being can represent one of the most meaningful.[1] Self-perception is, in fact, a key element in one's own personal life and may strongly contribute to personal happiness and overall life satisfaction, particularly in a "beyond GDP (Gross Domestic Product)" perspective. In this chapter, we thus adopt the subjective point of view and perform a first study of subjective suffering in Italy across the beginning of the global economic crisis.

---

[1] For a deepened dissertation of suffering, its conceptual implications, multidimensionality, and relationship with other subjective and individual characteristics, refer to Anderson (2014) and Lelkes (2013).

M. Fattore (✉)
Department of Statistics and Quantitative Methods, Università degli Studi
di Milano – Bicocca, Piazza dell'Ateneo Nuovo, 1, 20126 Milan, Italy
e-mail: marco.fattore@unimib.it

F. Maggino
Department of Statistics, Informatics, Applications "G. Parenti" (DiSIA),
Università degli Studi di Firenze, Viale Morgagni, 59, I-50134 Florence, Italy
e-mail: filomena.maggino@unifi.it

© Springer Science+Business Media Dordrecht 2015
R.E. Anderson (ed.), *World Suffering and Quality of Life*,
Social Indicators Research Series 56, DOI 10.1007/978-94-017-9670-5_29

29.1.1 Defining Subjective Well-Being

One of the most accepted and adopted definitions of *subjective well-being* conceives it as a composite construct described by two distinct components, cognitive and affective (Diener 1984). The *cognitive component* is related to the process through which each individual retrospectively evaluates (in terms of "satisfaction") her/his own life, as a whole or in different domains. The subjective evaluation is made by taking into account personal standards (expectations, desires, ideals, experiences, etc.). Consequently, the level of satisfaction is expressed as a function of the reached objectives, fulfilled ambitions, comparing ideals, experiences, other persons... In other words, satisfaction with life is the result of a cognitive process, allowing the individual to evaluate her/his present situation with reference to *standards* (Nuvolati 2002) individually defined.

The affective component refers to the emotions experienced by individuals during their daily lives and relates to the individuals' present situation. The emotions can be positive (*pleasant affects*) or negative (*unpleasant affects*), which are considered conceptually distinct and influenced by different variables (Bradburn 1969; Diener and Emmons 1984; Argyle 1987). Observing this component is particularly important because it allows obtaining information about the temperamental structure used by each individual in facing everyday life. According to some authors, such as Veenhoven, affects' determinants are universal and consequently not produced by individual response-styles or cultural differences.

The combination of the two components allows subjective well-being to be assessed. Summarizing, the concept of subjective well-being can be framed through the following dimensions:

1. "cognitive" dimension:

   - satisfaction with life as a whole;
   - satisfaction with different life domains;

2. "affective" dimension:

   - positive *affect* (happiness, serenity, etc.);
   - negative *affect* (concern, anxiety, stress, etc.);
   - *affect* related to particular situations or activities (family, work, etc.).

29.1.2 Observing Subjective Well-Being: Life Domains

Life satisfaction, as well as other relevant concepts and dimensions, has to be assessed and observed within each *life domain*. Life domains represent segments of reality in which fundamental concepts should be observed, monitored, and assessed. Typically, domains refer to households and families, income and standard of living, housing, health, transport, environment, leisure and culture, social security, crime and safety, education, labor market, working conditions, and so on. Generally, the differences concern the importance assigned to each domain. Actually, a shared list of domains and their priorities and importance does not exist, also because the list depends strictly on value judgments, valid and acceptable in a certain place and/or time (Noll 2004).

However, numerous scholars noticed that many domains recur in empirical studies (Felce and Perry 1995; Nuvolati 1997; Johansson 2002; Stiglitz et al. 2009), highlighting how human conditions lead individuals to face challenges that are common all over the world and that require collective solutions. In other words, even though different life domains can be identified, a core group of them really characterizes human lives, and through them, well-being can be observed. This could suggest that, while discomfort in specific domains is not crucial and can be compensated by well-being in others, suffering in some domains, such as health, economics, family and friendship, can turn out to be crucial for subjective well-being. Observing different combinations of well-being/ill-being levels in those domains can reveal different patterns and intensity of suffering and of risk of suffering. Monitoring the incidence across time of such combinations allows the community's conditions to be assessed especially during difficult moments, like the economic crisis. The observing and monitoring exercise should take into account that, as several scholars asserted recently (Diener 2000; Veenhoven 2004), what really regulates the intensity of subjective suffering and explains variability in subjective well-being is inequality, which represents an important additional indicator. So the analysis of what are the patterns of "suffering" and how they are changing over time should represent a crucial interest not only at scientific level.

The aim of this contribution is twofold. On one hand, we want to outline the features and the recent dynamics of suffering in Italy, comparing data from year 2007 and data from year 2010. Has the global crisis had an effect on the level of suffering in Italy? Are there any geographical differences in the distribution and patterns of suffering? Is there evidence of divergent paths across territorial areas or social groups? On the other hand, we want to pursue this goal, introducing and applying an innovative data analysis methodology, drawing on the concepts of partial order and partially ordered sets. The methodology may be applied to suffering evaluation and, more generally, to well-being evaluation, when available data are of a multidimensional ordinal kind.

The chapter is organized as follows: Sect. 29.2 describes the datasets used in the analysis. Section 29.3 provides some basic definitions of partial order theory and outlines the data analysis methodology. Section 29.4 develops the analysis of suffering data and presents the results of the study. Section 29.5 concludes.

29.2   The Data

The analysis is based on data from the "Multipurpose survey about families: aspects of daily life", held annually by the Italian National Statistical Bureau. The survey investigates a number of different aspects of daily life at individual and familiar level. Here, we consider subjective data pertaining to satisfaction on one's own economic status, health, family relationships, and friendship. In the original dataset, satisfaction is expressed on a 4-degree scale: 1 – "very", 2 – "enough", 3 – "little" and 4 – "not at all." In the following analysis, scores have been reversed, so that 1 stands for "not at all" and 4 stands for "very." To get an insight of the temporal evolution of the self-perception of well-being, we consider data from both 2007 and 2010, so as to assess suffering levels and patterns before and after the beginning of the global economic crisis. We consider data at national and macro-regional level. We also take into account sex, so as to be able to analyze data for men and women separately. In both years considered, the number of records in the datasets is about 48,000; of these, about 14 % have missing data. Since they do not appear to be systematic with reference to both sex and territorial areas, we simply deleted non-complete records from our analysis. Computations have been performed using the programming language R and the package PARSEC (Fattore and Arcagni 2014).

29.3 Partially Ordered Sets and the Suffering Evaluation Procedure

When dealing with multidimensional ordinal data, classical statistical evaluation procedures, based on score aggregation, cannot be pursued. A different mathematical language is needed, namely partial order theory. We thus give some essential definitions pertaining to partially ordered sets and provide an outline of the evaluation procedure employed in suffering assessment. We limit ourselves to the very basic concepts. Interested readers can find a more comprehensive introduction to partial orders and to the evaluation procedure in Davey and Priestley (2002), Fattore (2014), Fattore and Maggino (2014), Fattore et al. (2011a, b, 2012).

We introduce basic partial order concepts through a simplified example. Let **v** and **w** be two ordinal variables, on a four-degree and a three-degree scale respectively, coded as 1, 2, 3, 4, and 1, 2, 3 (notice that these are not numbers, but just symbols). Suppose to collect data on **v** and **w** jointly, on a statistical population. Each statistical unit is assigned a pair (x,y), where x may assume degree 1, 2, 3 or 4 and y may assume degree 1, 2, 3. The pair (x,y) is called a *profile*. There are 12 possible profiles and to each of them the number of statistical units sharing it (its *frequency*) is assigned. In a natural way we can, for example, compare and order profile (4,2) and profile (3,1), stating that the first is greater than the second, since it is greater on both components. But we cannot order profiles (2,1) and (1,3), since the first is smaller than the second on the second component, but it is greater on the first. In practice, not any pair of profiles built on **v** and **w** can be unambiguously compared and ordered, due to "conflicting" scores. The set P of 12 profiles built on **v** and **w** is in fact a *partially ordered set* (or a *poset*, for short). We can depict poset P in a simple way, by means of a Hasse diagram (Fig. 29.1). The diagram is to be read from top to bottom. Each node represents a profile. If profile **p** is greater than profile **q**, and there are no other profiles between **p** and **q**, than node **p** is put above

Fig. 29.1 Hasse diagram of poset P

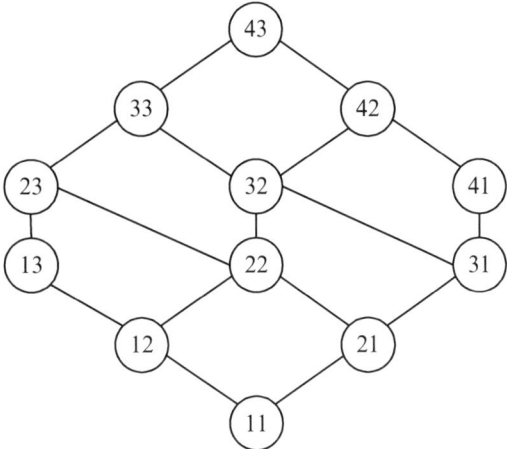

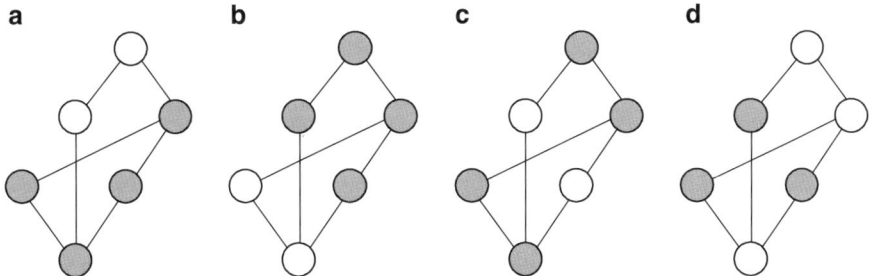

Fig. 29.2 Hasse diagram of a poset. In *grey*: (**a**) – downset; (**b**) – upset; (**c**) – chain; (**d**) – antichain

node **q** and an edge is drawn from the former to the latter. By transitivity, comparable nodes are linked by downward/upward sequences of edges.

A partial order where any two elements are comparable is called a *linear order* or a *complete order*. A subset of a poset that is a linear order is called a *chain*. At the opposite, a subset of a poset such that any two distinct elements are incomparable is called an *antichain*. Consider now node 22. The set of elements equal to or smaller than 22, i.e. profiles 22, 21, 12 and 11, constitutes the *downset* of 22. Similarly, the set of profiles 22, 32, 23, 42, 43, i.e. the set of elements greater than or equal to 22, constitutes the *upset* of 22. A profile belonging neither to the downset nor to the upset of 22 belongs to the *incomparability set* of 22. *Extending* a poset means turning some incomparabilities into comparabilities (i.e. enlarging the subset of elements that can be compared). If all the incomparabilities of a poset are turned into comparabilities, one gets a so-called *linear extension*, that is an extension that is also a complete order (see Figs. 29.2 and 29.3 for some examples of these concepts). A simple but fundamental result of partial order theory states that the

Fig. 29.3 Hasse diagram of a poset and of two of its linear extensions

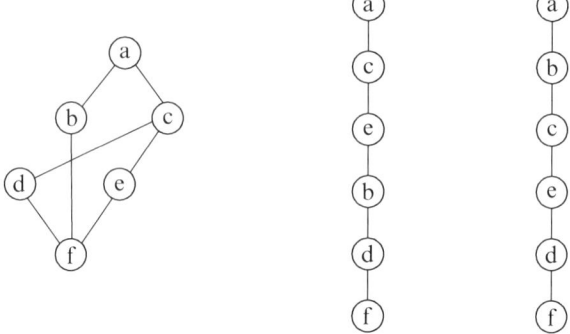

set S of all possible linear extensions of a (finite) poset characterizes the poset itself, i.e. different posets have different sets of linear extensions and given the set of linear extensions of a poset, one can reconstruct it.

Why are posets useful for suffering evaluation? The evaluation process is based on multidimensional ordinal information. Aggregation approaches, leading to classical composite indicators, cannot be applied, since ordinal scores are not numbers. Satisfaction/suffering profiles (sequences of satisfaction scores) are instead naturally described as a partially ordered set, so that synthetic suffering scores can be computed avoiding aggregative/compensative procedures. We describe the evaluation methodology as a step-by-step procedure in the following.

Step 1. Construction of the Satisfaction Poset To build the satisfaction poset, it is sufficient to apply the following partial ordering criterion to satisfaction profiles: let $\mathbf{p}=(p_1,\ldots, p_k)$ and $\mathbf{q}=(q_1,\ldots,q_k)$ be two satisfaction profiles on k ordinal *attributes* (in our study, k =4). We put $\mathbf{p}\leq\mathbf{q}$ if and only if $p_i\leq q_i$ for each i =1,…, k. We put $\mathbf{p}<\mathbf{q}$ if $\mathbf{p}\leq\mathbf{q}$ and there is at least an index j such that $p_j<q_j$. With this definition, the set of satisfaction profiles becomes a partially ordered set. The chosen partial order simply states that statistical unit **a** is more satisfied than statistical unit **b** if **a** (i.e. its profile) is satisfied not less than **b** on each attribute and more than **b** on at least one attribute.

Step 2. Threshold Selection Some profiles in the satisfaction poset may indeed represent unhappy or suffering situations. Due to multidimensionality, however, it is unlikely that a yes/no classification is effective. Some profiles could in fact represent, at different degrees, "partially" suffering configurations. Our aim is to assign a suffering score (possibly 0) to each profile in the satisfaction poset, identifying to what degree a profile may be considered as a suffering one. Since there is no natural scale against which to assess satisfaction and suffering, we address this identification problem as a multidimensional comparison issue. In practice, a set of suffering profiles that can be considered "on the edge" of suffering have to be exogenously identified, similarly to the threshold specification in classical monetary poverty studies. All of the other satisfaction profiles are then compared to the threshold, as described in Step 3, to get a suffering degree. Due to multidimensionality, more than one profile may be "on the edge" of suffering; the suffering threshold is in fact an antichain of satisfaction profiles, describing alternative suffering patterns.

Step 3. Suffering Degree Evaluation Differently from the unidimensional case, due to partial ordering not any suffering profile may be unambiguously compared with the elements of the threshold. A profile whose scores are worse (in a satisfaction perspective) than those of an element of the threshold, represents a suffering condition (since it is "worse" than a "suffering profile"). But in many cases, ambiguities arise and some profiles cannot be classified as below or above elements of the threshold, due to conflicting scores. Suffering identification must account for such ambiguities. In practice, an identification function $Idn(\cdot)$ is to be defined such that:

- elements of the threshold are scored 1 by Idn (i.e., they are classified as suffering profiles);
- profiles below an element of the threshold in the satisfaction poset are similarly scored 1 by Idn;
- profiles above *any* element of the threshold are scored 0 by Idn (i.e. they are classified as "non-suffering" profiles, since they represent situation that are better than any suffering patterns identified in the threshold);
- all other profiles are scored by Idn in $(0,1)$ (i.e. they are scored as "ambiguously" suffering profiles).

To operationally define the identification function Idn, we start by considering the set S of linear extensions of the satisfaction poset. In a linear extension (which is, in practice, a complete ranking of profiles), a profile is either above or below (or coincide with) a profile of the threshold and thus can be unambiguously identified as a "suffering profile" or a "non-suffering profile". Thus, on a linear extension one can define a 0–1 identification function assigning value 1 to profiles classified as "suffering" and 0 to all of the others. In different linear extensions, profiles classified as "suffering" are different (only profiles in the downset of the suffering threshold are scored 1 in each linear extension and only profiles in the intersection of the upsets of threshold profiles are always scored 0). All of the other profiles are scored differently on different linear extensions (see Fig. 29.4 for a simple example).

As a result, counting the proportion of linear extensions where a profile is scored 1, one gets a non-linear identification function assigning suffering values in [0,1] to satisfaction profiles. Notice that final numerical scores are directly assigned to profiles, without any preliminary transformation of ordinal degrees into numerical scores and without any aggregative procedure. The poset approach to suffering evaluation is, in a sense, a counting approach, but unlike other counting methodologies (Alkire and Foster 2011; Cerioli and Zani 1990), we count over linear extensions and not over satisfaction attributes. This leads to a much more effective way of exploiting the informative power of the data, as revealed by comparing the identification function computed by the poset-based methodology (see Fig. 29.5), to the analogous functions computed in classical counting procedures, which are usually 0–1 functions or at most linear functions.

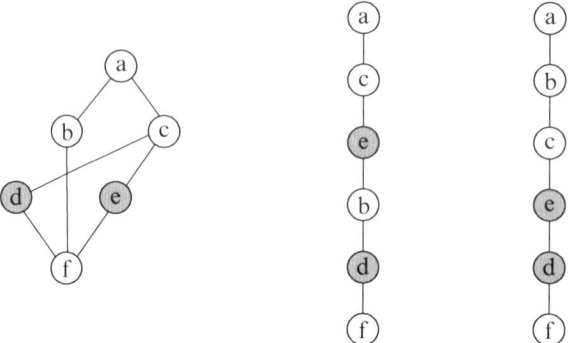

Fig. 29.4 Hasse diagram of a poset. In *grey*, the selected threshold. Node **f** is below the threshold both in the poset and in its linear extensions. Nodes **a** and **c** are above the threshold in the poset and in its linear extensions. Node **b** is incomparable with elements of the threshold. It is above all elements of the threshold in one of the depicted linear extensions, but not in the other

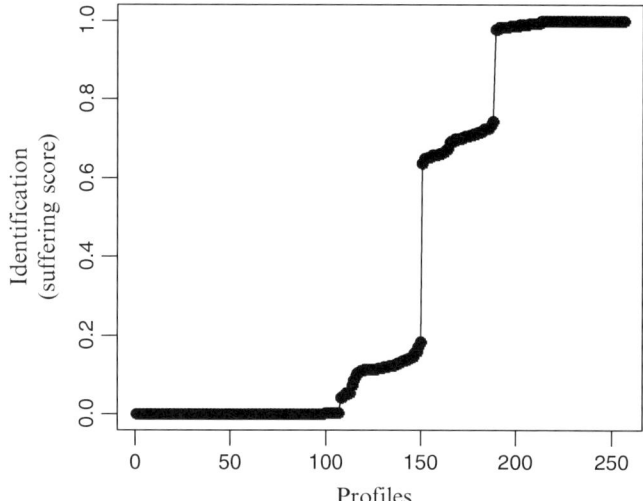

Fig. 29.5 Identification function (suffering scores), given the threshold (2223 and 2232). Profiles are numbered and listed according to increasing suffering scores

Once the identification function has been computed, each statistical unit is assigned the score of the profile he/she shares, getting a distribution of suffering scores over the population. Usual statistical indicators can then be computed to build a synthetic picture of the data.

Two final remarks are in order. First, in general terms, the evaluation methodology is designed for multidimensional ordinal data, which often arise from qualitative and subjective judgments. At the same time, the methodology is mathematically consistent and rigorous. So it may be seen as a formal way, based on "the mathematics of ordinal data," to treat qualitative information. Secondly, the methodology is descriptive in nature, in the spirit of other approaches to social measurement (e.g. that of Alkire and Foster 2011). Nevertheless, extending it in inferential terms is an important step and represents a major direction for future research.

29.4 Subjective Suffering in Italy Before and Within the Economic Crisis

In Italy, the (generically called) "crisis" and its consequences are inextricably intertwined with some historical, distinctive and often problematic features of the Italian institutional and socio-economic asset. Official regional figures reveal a complex pattern composed of different socio-economic territorial entities, coexisting within the same national context and moving on different and divergent paths. This is confirmed also by the following suffering analysis.

29.4.1 Suffering Score Computation

To make the analysis as clear as possible, we apply the poset-based evaluation methodology step by step.

Step 1. Construction of the Satisfaction Poset With four ordinal attributes, 256 subjective satisfaction profiles may be generated; each of them corresponds to a configuration of satisfactions, i.e. to a sequence of four ordered symbols chosen in the set $\{1, 2, 3, 4\}$. Partially ordering the set of profiles as outlined in Sect. 29.3, one gets the satisfaction poset. To each node, the percentage of statistical units sharing the corresponding profiles is associated, separately for year 2007 and year 2010.

Step 2. Threshold Selection The second and more delicate step is the selection of the suffering threshold. Suffering is a multidimensional experience; as such, many different suffering patterns may exist and more than one pattern may represent the "edge" between non-suffering and suffering profiles.

Identifying thresholds is always a difficult task, even in unidimensional studies; a task that should be performed according to a shared process, based on declared criteria. Here we select a threshold based on some basic considerations, briefly exposed in the Introduction, so as to show how the methodology can be put to work. We consider the economic and health attributes as the most relevant and specify the threshold as composed of two profiles, namely 2232 and 2223 (the first digit refers to the economic situation; the second to health; the third to family and the fourth to friendship). In practice to be considered as "unambiguously suffering," a profile must comprise at least three attributes scored "little," two of which must pertain to economy and health, and the fourth attribute cannot be scored higher than "enough."

It may be argued that this choice is rather strong, in that three attributes out of four must be unsatisfactorily scored. In fact, our aim is to identify relevant suffering situations. Notice that the threshold is not a function of the frequency distribution. In this sense we are assuming an "absolute" assessment perspective, rather than a "relative" one. Consistently with this remark, the threshold is the same for both years.

Step 3. Suffering Degree Evaluation The computation of the identification function would require listing all the linear extensions of the satisfaction poset. This is computationally unfeasible, due to their extremely huge number. In practice, one samples from the set of linear extensions using the Bubley-Dyer algorithm (Bubley and Dyer 1999). In this study, we sampled $5 \cdot 10^8$ linear extensions, using the R package PARSEC (Fattore and Arcagni 2014). Computing the identification function, each satisfaction profile (i.e. each node in the Hasse diagram) gets a score in [0,1], which can be interpreted as the degree of suffering of the profile. Ordering profiles according to increasing suffering scores, one obtains the graph of the identification function, as depicted in Fig. 29.5.

As expected, the identification function assumes values between 0 and 1, reproducing the nuances and vagueness of multidimensional suffering. Only profiles in the downset of the threshold are scored 1; similarly, only profiles in the intersection of the upsets of elements of the threshold are scored 0. All of the other profiles are scored strictly higher than 0 and strictly lower than 1. Notice also that profile scores do not lie on a straight line; the graph shows clusters of profiles scored similarly and might somehow remind one of a sigmoid shape. This reveals the existence of "non-linearities" that would not be accounted for properly, by aggregative or counting approaches. Notice also that the identification function does not primarily measure the intensity of suffering, but the degree of membership of a profile to the set of suffering profiles, identified by the threshold. From this point of view, it is a truly fuzzy measure of suffering.

Given the identification function, one can then proceed to computing synthetic indicators for years 2007 and 2010. In this concise study, we mainly consider two suffering measures. The first is the average identification score over the population (or subpopulations), here called *overall suffering level*, which is analogous of the Head Count Ratio adopted in classical poverty studies. However, here we are not simply counting the proportion of "suffering people" but the "average degree of membership" of individuals to the class of suffering individuals. So the average identification suffering score must be interpreted as the "relative amount of suffering in the population." The second indicator, here called *specific suffering level*, is the average identification score restricted to individuals with a non-null suffering degree. It is simply the average degree of membership to the suffering group, excluding non-suffering people. High values of the specific suffering level reveal that suffering people are likely to be "really suffering," i.e. to suffer globally from the different perspectives implied by the selected threshold. When this occurs, one can state that the population is somehow split into two groups: "completely suffering" and "completely non-suffering" people. As it will be seen in the following, this is partly the situation of Italy.

29.4.2   *Data Analysis and Interpretation*

Main results for years 2007 and 2010 are listed in Tables 29.1, 29.2, and 29.3. The average suffering score in 2007 is 0.102, basically the same as in 2010 (0.101); in practice, the fuzzy Head Count Ratio is about 10 %. In both years, Italian population appears polarized in two groups. In fact, about 90 % of the population

Table 29.1 Overall and specific suffering levels at national and macro-regional scale, for years 2007 and 2010

| | Suffering level | | | |
| | 2007 | | 2010 | |
Region	Overall	Specific	Overall	Specific
Italy	**0.102**	**0.410**	**0.101**	**0.405**
North-West	0.080	0.364	0.083	0.377
North-East	0.077	0.359	0.079	0.366
Centre	0.099	0.427	0.100	0.399
South	0.132	0.445	0.132	0.440
Islands	0.144	0.450	0.128	0.439

Table 29.2 Overall suffering levels for males and females at national and macro-regional scale, for years 2007 and 2010

| | Overall suffering level | | | |
| | 2007 | | 2010 | |
Region	Males	Females	Males	Females
Italy	**0.086**	**0.117**	**0.088**	**0.115**
North-West	0.065	0.094	0.075	0.091
North-East	0.065	0.089	0.068	0.088
Center	0.087	0.110	0.081	0.117
South	0.107	0.154	0.112	0.150
Islands	0.130	0.156	0.113	0.142

Table 29.3 Specific suffering levels for males and females at national and macro-regional scale, for years 2007 and 2010

| | Specific suffering level | | | |
| | 2007 | | 2010 | |
Region	Males	Females	Males	Females
Italy	**0.384**	**0.423**	**0.378**	**0.427**
North-West	0.336	0.386	0.356	0.394
North-East	0.336	0.376	0.338	0.390
Centre	0.414	0.437	0.358	0.431
South	0.404	0.477	0.419	0.456
Islands	0.440	0.458	0.414	0.460

has a suffering degree smaller than 0.2, while the remaining 10 % has a suffering degree greater than 0.6. Focusing only on the subpopulation of statistical units with a non-zero suffering score, the average suffering degree increases to 0.410 in 2007 and to just a little bit less in 2010 (0.405). These reveal that those who suffer in some aspects of their life are quite "globally" suffering.

At territorial level, we consider five big geographic areas, or macro-regions, namely North-West (Lombardy, Piemonte, Valle d'Aosta, Liguria, Emilia-Romagna), North-East (Veneto, Trentino Alto-Adige, Friuli-Venezia Giulia), Centre (Tuscany, Marche, Lazio, Umbria), South (Abruzzo, Molise, Campania, Basilicata, Puglia, Calabria) and Islands (Sicily and Sardinia). Both levels, overall and specific, increase moving from the north to the south of Italy, showing that, as suffering spreads, it becomes also more "global." The existence of a "north-south" axis in socio-economic performances is a historical feature of the Italian situation. Here we have evidence that the same holds for subjective suffering.

Besides territorial differences, suffering level worsens when comparing males to females. At national level, in 2007 males have an average suffering level equal to 0.086, while for females it is 0.117. Also, the specific average suffering level is greater for females (0.429) than for males (0.384). The divergence between male and female suffering levels is a common feature of Italian macro-regions, particularly in the South region, where the spread between males and females is almost 5 percentage points (males: 0.107; females: 0.154) and the specific suffering level ranges from 0.404 (males) to 0.477 (females). On the whole, the maximum overall suffering spread is between males in North-West and North-East (0.065), and females in the Islands (0.156). Analogously, the maximum specific suffering spread is between males in North-West and North-East (0.336) and females in the South (0.477). The same pattern repeats 3 years later. In 2010, male average suffering is 0.088, while for females it equals 0.120. Similarly, male specific suffering level is 0.378, while the female one is 0.427. This feature can be again invariably observed in each of the territorial areas under consideration. On the whole, the maximum spread of overall suffering level across Italy in 2010 may be observed between males in the North-East (0.068) and females in the South (0.150): a difference of more than 8 percentage points compared to an average national level equal to 0.101. Again, an even wider spread exists when specific suffering level is considered, ranging from 0.338 for males in the North-West, to 0.460 for females in the Islands macro-region.

Comparing data pertaining to 2007 and 2010, we notice that suffering levels and patterns are quite similar. The first year of the crisis does not seem to have much affected the subjective quality-of-life perception. But looking at the results, some interesting hints emerge. One can see that suffering levels (overall and specific) slightly increase over time in the northern macro-regions and slightly decrease in the southern macro-regions. These figures may be affected by approximations, due to the sampling of linear extensions, but on the whole they suggest unexpected dynamics. Why regions that historically perform better than the others show an increase in subjective suffering, while the latter do not? Might life-styles matter, in this respect? Perhaps some people living in more "developed" regions and big city areas are more affected by possible changes in their daily life and expectations than people from medium and small cities, living in a better environment. Is there any immigration process of suffering people from the south to the north? Many hypotheses can be made, but more robust statistical evidence is needed for final conclusions. In any case, these first results suggest interesting research paths to be explored using new waves of the multipurpose survey.

29.5 Conclusion

In this chapter, we have outlined a new methodology to address synthetic evaluation of multidimensional suffering and well-being in general, based on ordinal data.

Evaluation is addressed as a benchmark problem where incomparabilities between subjective satisfaction profiles play a central role, leading to fuzzy suffering measures. The methodology proves effective in accounting for nuances and subtleties of suffering evaluation, overcoming the limitations of composite indicator and classical counting procedures. The chapter has focused on subjective suffering in Italy before and just after the beginning of the socio-economic crisis, comparing years 2007 and 2010. Four subjective life satisfaction ordinal attributes have been considered, namely satisfaction pertaining to one's own economic status, health, familiar, and friendship relationships. Data have been extracted from the "Multipurpose survey on families, aspects of daily life," held by the Italian National Bureau of Statistics on a yearly basis.

The aim of the study has been to stress the relevance of subjective data about well-being and suffering and to introduce and spread a new and alternative evaluation methodology to the social scientific community. To ease computations and exposition, a limited number of attributes and covariates have been selected. Notwithstanding this, some interesting results have been obtained and deserve further research. In both years considered, data show the existence of two axes of increasing suffering: north-south and male-female. Moreover, there is some evidence suggesting that the crisis may worsen the self-perception of people in areas that are more developed from an economic point of view. This is revealed by both overall suffering level and specific suffering level.

We cannot here deepen the analysis and find out the "mechanism" behind this fact. What neatly emerges, however, is the complexity and subtlety of suffering that eludes trivial interpretations and requires more sophisticated "observational tools," that is, statistical procedures capable to capture its fundamental features. In this respect, the poset-based evaluation methodology applied in this study seems effective and opens new possibilities of describing and understanding such a complex social issue.

References

Alkire, S., & Foster, J. (2011). Counting and multidimensional poverty measures. *Journal of Public Economics, 95*, 476–487.

Anderson, R. E. (2014). *Human suffering and quality of life. Conceptualizing stories and statistics* (Series Springer briefs in well-being and quality of life research). Dordrecht: Springer.

Argyle, M. (1987). *The psychology of happiness*. London: Methuen.

Bradburn, N. M. (1969). *The structure of psychological wellbeing*. Chicago: Aldine.

Bubley, R., & Dyer, M. (1999). Faster random generation of linear extensions. *Discrete Mathematics, 201*, 81–88.

Cerioli, A., & Zani, S. (1990). A fuzzy approach to the measurement of poverty. In C. Dagum & M. Zenga (Eds.), *Income and wealth distribution, inequality and poverty* (pp. 272–284). Berlino Heidelberg: Springer.

Davey, B. A., & Priestley, B. H. (2002). *Introduction to lattices and order*. Cambridge: Cambridge University Press.

Diener, E. (1984). Subjective wellbeing. *Psychological Bulletin*, p. 95.

Diener, E. (2000). Subjective well-being. The science of happiness and a proposal for a national index. *American Psychologist, 55*, 34–43.

Diener, E., & Emmons, R. A. (1984). The independence of positive and negative affect. *Journal of Personality and Social Psychology, 47*(5), 1105–1117.

Fattore, M. (2014). "Partially Ordered Set" (entry title). In A. C. Michalos (Ed.), *Encyclopedia of quality of life and well-being research* (pp. 4627–4631). Dordrecht: Springer.

Fattore, M., & Arcagni, A. (2014). PARSEC: An R package for poset-based evaluation of multidimensional poverty. In R. Bruggemann, L. Carlsen, & J. Wittmann (Eds.), *Multi-indicator systems and modelling in partial order*. Berlin: Springer.

Fattore, M., & Maggino, F. (2014). Partial orders in socio-economics: A practical challenge for poset theorists or a cultural challenge for social scientists? In R. Bruggemann, L. Carlsen, & J. Wittmann (Eds.), *Multi-indicator systems and modelling in partial order*. Berlin: Springer.

Fattore, M., Maggino, F., & Greselin, F. (2011a). Socio-economic evaluation with ordinal variables: Integrating counting and poset approaches. In *Statistica & Applicazioni, partial orders in applied sciences* (Special issue, pp. 31–42). Milano: Vita e Pensiero.

Fattore, M., Brueggemann, R., & Owsiński, J. (2011b). Using poset theory to compare fuzzy multidimensional material deprivation across regions. In S. Ingrassia, R. Rocci, & M. Vichi (Eds.), *New perspectives in statistical modeling and data analysis*. Berlin: Springer.

Fattore, M., Maggino, F., & Colombo, E. (2012). From composite indicators to partial orders: Evaluating socio-economic phenomena through ordinal data. In F. Maggino & G. Nuvolati (Eds.), *Quality of life in Italy: Researches and reflections* (Social indicators research series). Dordrecht: Springer.

Felce, D., & Perry, J. (1995). Quality of life: Its definition and measurement. *Research in Developmental Disabilities, 16*(1), 51–74.

Johansson, S. (2002). Conceptualizing and measuring quality of life for national policy. *Social Indicators Research, 58*, 13–32.

Lelkes, O. (2013). Minimising misery: A new strategy for public policies instead of maximising happiness? *Social Indicators Research, 114*, 121–137.

Noll, H.-H. (2004, November 10–13). *Social indicators and indicators systems: Tools for social monitoring and reporting.* Paper presented at OECD, World Forum "Statistics, knowledge and policy", Palermo.

Nuvolati, G. (1997). Uno specifico settore di applicazione degli indicatori sociali: La qualità della vita. In F. Zajczyk (Ed.), *Il mondo degli indicatori sociali, una guida alla ricerca sulla qualità della vita* (pp. 69–94). Roma: La Nuova Italia Scientifica.

Nuvolati, G. (2002). *Qualità della vita e indicatori sociali.* Seminar held at the PhD degree program "Scienza tecnologia e società", aprile, Dipartimento di Sociologia e di Scienza Politica, Università della Calabria. Available on http://www.sociologia.unical.it/convdottorati/nuvolati.pdf

Stiglitz, J. E., Sen, A., & Fitoussi, J.-P. (Eds). (2009). *Report by the commission on the measurement of economic performance and social progress*, Paris. http://www.stiglitz-sen-fitoussi.fr/en/index.htm

Veenhoven, R. (2004). Happiness as a public policy aim: The greatest happiness principle. In A. Linley & S. Joseph (Eds.), *Positive psychology in practice* (pp. 658–678). Hoboken: Wiley.

Chapter 30
Hurricane Katrina, Family Trouble, and the Micro-politics of Suffering

Ara Francis and Daina Cheyenne Harvey

30.1 Introduction

> He learned that just as there is no condition in which man can be happy and absolutely free, so there is no condition in which he need be unhappy and not free. He had learned that there is a limit to suffering and a limit to freedom, and that these limits are not far away; that the person in a bed of roses with one crumpled petal suffered as keenly as he suffered now, sleeping on bare damp earth with one side of him freezing as the other got warm; that in the old days as he had put on his tight dancing-shoes he had been just as uncomfortable as he was now, walking on bare feet that were covered with sores.—Tolstoy, *War and Peace*

Recently, social scientists have picked up the early work of those who pioneered the study of suffering (Bourdieu 1999; Cassell 1982; Kleinman 1995) and have begun to treat it not as a secondary phenomenon that accompanies particular social conditions, but as a topic in its own right (Anderson 2014; Auyero and Swistun 2009a, b; Francis 2012; Harvey 2012; Smith 2011; Wilkinson 2005, and Chap. 10 this volume). Many of this volume's contributors are responsible for that initial effort and have laid important groundwork for a distinctly social orientation to the study of human woe. In our chapter, we continue this effort by examining one set of intellectual and ethical dilemmas that current scholars stand to inherit, at least in part, from previous research. Drawing from two separate studies, one on the survivors of Hurricane Katrina and the other on middle-class parents whose children have a wide array of problems, we highlight a problematic gap between scholarly and self-referential claims to suffering. We also raise difficult questions about the relationship between suffering and social stratification. To what extent should studies of social suffering include the experiences of privileged people who claim to suffer but whose hardships might seem comparatively trivial? Moreover, how should we conceptualize

A. Francis (✉) • D.C. Harvey
Department of Sociology and Anthropology, College of the Holy Cross,
1 College St., Worcester, MA 01610, USA
e-mail: afrancis@holycross.edu; dharvey@holycross.edu

© Springer Science+Business Media Dordrecht 2015
R.E. Anderson (ed.), *World Suffering and Quality of Life*,
Social Indicators Research Series 56, DOI 10.1007/978-94-017-9670-5_30

the experiences of marginalized people who appear to suffer but who are reluctant to identify themselves in such terms?

By addressing these questions, we call attention to the micro-politics of suffering and scholars' participation in the construction of what constitutes legitimate distress. By micro-politics we are not referring to state politics or public policy, though the politics of small-scale interaction shape and are shaped by macro-level politics. Rather, we are concerned with people's interpretations of suffering in dyadic and small group contexts and the dynamics of power and inequality that inform those interpretations (Clark 1997; Emerson and Messinger 1977). Likewise we note that the knowledge we produce as academics often contributes to constructions of whose suffering "counts." For better or worse, scholars of suffering operate as "moral gate-keepers" who bring attention to some cases of hardship and not others (Clark 1997: 269).

This piece also allows us to consider what scholars might gain from comparing the lived experiences of seemingly disparate groups of sufferers. Analyzing stories from the Lower Ninth Ward alongside those of the Berkeley Hills raises interesting questions about the role of symbolic and material resources in people's willingness to identify themselves as suffering. Furthermore, it highlights how strongly previous experiences and expectations for the future shape people's interpretation of tragic events. In the end, we suggest that it is possible for studies of suffering to encompass all cases of human distress, even those of privileged groups, while at the same time tailoring assertions about remediation to fit each case. However, doing so requires us to be explicitly reflexive about the moral and political assumptions that underpin our own research.

30.2 Two Cases of Sorrow

30.2.1 Middle-Class Family Trouble

Steve and Marie Davis live in a family-oriented suburb just outside of Berkeley, California. Nestled in a valley surrounded by rolling green hills, the town is idyllic. It is also expensive, home to a lot of affluent professionals who commute into the city. Steve works as a stock trader, Marie as a bank manager. Their three daughters, now 17, 20, and 24 years old, attended public schools and received excellent educations. Indeed, their local school district is considered one of the best in the region. The couple feels very much at home and well-connected in their small community. Marie, especially, has made quite a few friends over the years by being involved in her daughters' schools, sports, and other extracurricular activities. Steve is a college football fan and attends games at Stanford with his daughters and friends. By most accounts, this couple embodies the imagined "good life" in the late-modern United States. They are, without a doubt, some of the most materially fortunate people in the world. Yet I met them 6 months after they discovered that their youngest daughter, Margo, is a cocaine addict. At that time, they were suffering.

Margo had always been one to push the boundaries, her parents explained, at least more so than her sisters. But Steve and Marie had never been particularly strict with their children, and Margo had never gotten herself into any real trouble. The best athlete of the family, she was a competitive swimmer and had played water polo with the same group of girls since grade school. Her parents knew that she drank on the weekends but didn't know how much. Everything started to change during Margo's senior year of high school. She became moody and unpredictable. Despite her longstanding hopes of playing water polo at the collegiate level, she suddenly hated everyone on her team and wanted to quit. Then, one night in the midst of an argument with Marie, Margo locked herself into the bathroom and cut her wrists with a pair of scissors. As the ambulance carried her away from the house, she confessed to the EMT that she had become a daily cocaine user.

Overwhelmed by sadness, Steve and Marie cried on and off during our 3-hour conversation. In the months following their daughter's hospitalization, they lost countless hours of work and sleep. Marie had been so heartsick during the first week that she hadn't been able to eat. They came to see their daughter as someone who had been under a tremendous amount of pressure and in a great deal of pain. "No 17-year-old kid should *ever* have to go through that," Steve said. His sadness was tinged with uncertainty and fear. They were waiting for Margo to return from a therapeutic boarding school in Utah, and they had no idea what would happen when she came home. "Here's a kid that's supposed to go off to college next September, [and] we don't know if that's gonna happen, okay?"

I spent 2 years talking with parents like Steve and Marie, middle and upper middle-class mothers and fathers who identified their children as having significant problems. The problems themselves were variable, including learning and developmental disabilities, genetic and neurological disorders, mental health problems, substance addictions, and delinquency. What parents shared, however, was profound social psychological turmoil marked by feelings of anxiety, guilt, and grief.

These parents raise important questions about how we, as scholars, should conceive of privileged hardship. Do people like Steve and Marie *suffer*, or do they "suffer"? The former (italicized) word suggests that they have something in common with other sufferers, while the latter implies that their woes, however salient they might feel, are too negligible to constitute what we normally see as suffering. Of course, quotation marks also hint at the relative, constructed nature of all human experience. All situations, social constructionists argue, are rendered meaningful through language, and even suffering is a cultural product. From this point of view, the quotes are not meant to suggest that parents' suffering is fraudulent; on the contrary, their suffering is real, precisely because they identify and treat it as such. Insofar as this argument pertains to privileged and marginalized groups alike, shouldn't we conceptualize all suffering as suffering?

30.2.2 Katrina Catastrophe

Ms. Henrietta pointed to the abandoned homes of her neighbors. The house across the street, which Ms. Henrietta spent hours staring at each day as she sat on her porch, listed to one side, only half of it visible from behind nearly ten feet of overgrown grass and stringy trees that popped up everywhere after Katrina. The other two, a brick house and a shotgun on the other side of the street, had neat, trimmed lawns, but neither of their former occupants had returned since being forced to evacuate. Their belongings sat inside, covered in a toxic coating of silt, waiting on their owners.

I first met Ms. Henrietta in 2010, more than 5 years after Hurricane Katrina and the federal levee failures had decimated the Lower Ninth Ward. I lived in the Ninth Ward for a little over 14 months, working with a consortium of nonprofits, community groups, and neighborhood associations to help rebuild the neighborhood. From April 2010 to June 2011, I attended close to 200 community and neighborhood meetings, formally interviewed 38 residents of the Lower Ninth, and informally spoke to hundreds more. I worked on large-scale community projects and was frequently called on for smaller things, such as replanting a garden or helping paint a room. For the most part I worked with a nonprofit, lowernine.org, and helped rebuild houses—like Ms. Henrietta's neighbors.

Ms. Henrietta had spent the last 4 days watching a group of us work on a house down the street—a complete rebuild. On the first day she watched curiously from her front porch. On the second she ventured out into the street. By the fourth day she came over into the yard and spoke with us. She had a few small jobs she wanted to know if we could attend to. For the next 3 days I worked at Ms. Henrietta's house, fixing her doorbell and a sewage leak under her house. While always guarded, we eventually spent most of a day talking on her porch. In addition to talking about her long-gone neighbors, she told me how much her life had changed since her home had been flooded 5 years earlier.

Ms. Henrietta used to spend most of her days checking in on her neighbors, walking down Egania toward Claiborne. She would spend hours talking with friends on their porches, exchanging pleasantries with any passer-by, and welcoming folks into her home for coffee and gossip. Five years later she barely left her yard. After spending a few days watching me ride my bicycle through the neighborhood and walk down the streets, she said she worried about my safety. She no longer welcomed anyone into her home for fear they might carelessly tell others how well she was doing.

On the last day we spoke she told me her "Katrina Story." She had evacuated with her daughter and granddaughter and had returned to find most of her possessions gone and her home covered in mud. She had insurance and a bit of money given to her from the Road Home Program—a program administered by the U.S. Department of Housing and Urban Development to assist homeowners in rebuilding their homes. A contractor approached her and told her if she would write a check to him for half of the rebuilding estimate, she could move to the top of the rebuild list. Wincing as she told me this, she motioned the sending off of the check.

The contractor never returned; she lost $20,000. She told me of long walks while she stayed with her daughter; she regularly passed a gun shop. One day she ventured inside and held a handgun, thinking of the contractors who stole her money. She told me what she thought it would be like to kill them. Weeping, she told me she was glad she didn't do anything drastic. And yet Ms. Henrietta refused to see herself as someone who was suffering. She would explain how people living down the street were suffering; people living elsewhere in the neighborhood, south of Claiborne or around Florida, were suffering, but not her.

New Orleans' Lower Ninth Ward, where Ms. Henrietta lived, was ground zero for Hurricane Katrina and the federal levee failures. One hundred percent of the homes were declared uninhabitable by the EPA, and close to half of all the fatalities there were neighbors and family members. More than 5 years later, there was no police or fire station, no grocery store, no health clinic, and only one school where before there had been seven. Only one in four residents had returned. The murder rate post-Katrina was creeping up to where it had been when, in the 1980s, the Lower Ninth had the unfortunate moniker of the murder capital of the murder capital (Landphair 2007).

Ms. Henrietta was suffering and yet she refused to see herself as someone who suffers. She described particular neighbors as suffering and assumed others in the community suffered, and yet like for many others in the Lower Ninth Ward, for Ms. Henrietta suffering existed elsewhere. In the 14 months I lived in the Ninth Ward, I met many residents like Ms. Henrietta. Residents either blamed themselves for what happened in the immediate or long-term aftermath, empathized with disaster victims elsewhere and thus discounted their own experiences, or simply refused to see the effects of Hurricane Katrina as extraordinary or exceptional, as if Katrina and the destruction of their community was simply to be expected, part of a larger pattern and hence normal.

The questions raised by residents of the Lower Ninth Ward and by troubled parents are both conceptual and political. What is suffering? Whose suffering counts? However strong the constructionist position, placing quotes around or questioning the indignities borne by Ms. Henrietta is a tricky proposition. We take her suffering for granted and assume that deconstructing it would diminish it.

A critical analysis of Steve and Marie's suffering seems more palatable, not because of the quality of their experiences, but because they occupy a position of relative privilege. Yet, neither of these assessments aligns with how these individuals make sense of their own circumstances. When taking account of others' suffering, how do we strike an analytical balance between objective conditions and subjective experiences?

30.3 The Micro-politics of Suffering

To say that someone is suffering, or to denote a structural or social condition as causing suffering, is a moral act. And while these moral dealings are influenced by macro-level politics, small group interactions are often where the rubber meets the proverbial road. Hence, while politics suffuse social life at multiple levels, people serve their own interests by exercising power over others in dyadic and small group interactions. Scholars of micro-politics point out that suffering is necessarily about making moral and political claims. This is because asserting that something is wrong or that someone is suffering suggests that remediation is called for (Emerson and Messinger 1977). Moral questions about responsibility are central to remediation: Who is at fault? Who is obligated to help? Such questions are tightly bound to dynamics of power and inequality, particularly in our late-modern, neoliberal context where people are often assumed to be responsible for their own suffering (Wolf 2011). Suffering can confer vulnerability and potentially mark someone as a social liability. Moreover, sympathy can render the sufferer indebted to those who display concern (Clark 1997).

The contentiousness of claims of suffering played out in interesting ways when news outlets featured stories about the financial woes of affluent families following the 2008 economic downturn. In an online piece titled, "Don't Think the 1 % Aren't Suffering Too (True, Not Satire)," one reporter wrote about financiers who could no longer afford home renovations, children's private educations, or extravagant vacations (Abelson 2012). In a similar vein, the *New York Times* ran a piece on a family whose sole breadwinner lost his job as a technology analyst for a Manhattan investment firm. Now earning $150,000 per year instead of the $800,000 they'd grown accustomed to, the couple had to cut back on childcare and travel expenses, and they argued frequently about how to further curb their spending (Tyre 2009). Readers had strong, sometimes vitriolic responses to these pieces. In the readers' comments section beneath the first segment, someone posted: "This reads like propaganda for a pity the rich campaign. Seriously? […] you poor, suffering things. I'm sure you'll figure out how to steal the difference back from those less fortunate than you, you soulless, absolutely deluded, empty machines." Similarly, *New York Times* journalist Judith Warner (2009) criticized her paper's attention to wealthy families' woes: "Wealthy families may be downsizing somewhat, but many others are living right on the edge […] So let's make sure we remember who's really suffering."

When it comes to the relationship of suffering to social stratification, scholars in sociology and anthropology focus largely on marginalized groups. Given our disciplines' critical attention to social inequality and stratification, it makes sense that we would foreground the experiences of those who are, from Warner's point of view, "really" suffering. This focus serves an important political purpose, but we worry that by narrowing our attention in this way, we are unable to fully theorize the role of symbolic and material resources in the lived experience of suffering. We also miss out on an important opportunity to create an analytical space in which to consider the positive aspects of human suffering and the resources that people need in order to suffer meaningfully and with dignity.

It is essential to place people's own sense-making at the center of scholarly analysis. The failure to do so risks a misrecognition of suffering. For example, many residents of New Orleans, particularly in the long-term aftermath, suffered from the same "Katrina Fatigue" (Peek 2012) as did folks elsewhere. They similarly did not want to talk about, think about, or see the effects of Hurricane Katrina. They simply wanted it to be over. They wanted to move on. While most residents of the Lower Ninth Ward, where only a quarter of the population had returned, were nonetheless still dealing with the aftermath of Katrina 6 years after their neighborhood flooded (see Harvey, this volume), there were residents there who sought to minimize the suffering attributed to them and claimed by other members of the community. Here the past, present, and future were joined as a seamless experience of exploitation and trouble.

Many of Ms. Henrietta's neighbors likewise did not see themselves as sufferers. As a resident of the Lower Ninth Ward remarked after being asked about the aftermath of Katrina immediately after the BP oil disaster and an explosion at a nearby petro-chemical plant that covered the neighborhood in toxic pollution, "That ain't nothing, we use to it." Another resident said of Daina's disbelief of how the explosion at the petro-chemical plant was being perceived by residents, "just wait till tomorrow." The resident was not implying that eventually others would come to understand the potential for toxic suffering (Auyero and Swistun 2009a) caused by the explosion and dusting, but that they had already made sense of it and were waiting for something worse to happen in the near future. An 80-year-old woman, whom Daina met at a potluck dinner at her house, summarized the effect of Katrina in her newly rebuilt kitchen by exclaiming, "Yeah, she messed up my yard!"

Andre, a 70-year old former Black Panther, reminded Daina that while Katrina may have had life lessons for some, for those whose life already held similar lessons, Katrina was simply "one more obstacle, one more road block." And Betty, who was almost 90 and trying to repaint her kitchen, said Katrina was "just one more thing on my plate." These comments seem shocking, especially in light of Andre still being without his home and Betty, whose home was being rebuilt, was nonetheless far from living in it. While many of Ms. Henrietta's neighbors would disagree with their neighbors, many others made similar comments.

Ms. Henrietta and the others present a problem for portraying suffering—mainly that they claim to be outside of the frame. While they would say that their neighbors who were living in similar conditions were suffering, they equated suffering with claiming a status of victim and were reluctant to do so. Being someone who suffers meant being someone who was still in the process of recovering from or attributing meaning to the aftermath of Hurricane Katrina.

Ms. Henrietta and the others likewise did not want to be seen as sufferers because they did not want to be understood or identified as a social problem. For them, Hurricane Katrina and the federal levee failures represented a turning point for their community, one in which they could alter their futures by becoming agents for social change rather than waiting for change to occur. For them, then, talking about suffering seemed accusatory; it was as if they had not done enough or were failing their community. Likewise, suffering for residents of the Lower Ninth Ward was a normative state (see Chap. 20 by Harvey in this volume). They could scarcely remember a time their community was not in peril; distinguishing between pre- and post-Katrina problems was difficult.

For the residents of the Lower Ninth Ward, suffering, while quite evident to the casual tourist or volunteer, needs to be voiced and acknowledged by others.

It has to be placed into the realm of suffering by the other. Neoliberalism, history, race, pride, culture—all prevent residents from acknowledging their particular suffering while nonetheless seeing it elsewhere. Suffering in the Lower Ninth can only be placed into a micro-politics of suffering by interrogating how residents attribute (and perhaps more importantly how they *fail* to attribute) meaning to suffering.

In contrast with residents of the Lower Ninth Ward, privileged parents like Steve and Marie laid claim to their suffering quite directly. Many women and men cried openly when talking about children's problems and used words like "devastation" and "trauma" to describe what had happened to them and their families. Tim, whose son was diagnosed with a genetic condition when he was just 2 years old, recalled how shattered and adrift he felt when doctors told him his child would never be more capable than a 10-year-old. "… [it] burns your life to the ground in a figurative sense," he said. "I just didn't understand why this had happened and why it had been laid on us…"

Parents' suffering had an embodied quality. In addition to talking about the acute upheaval of sleeping and eating habits, some parents described a slow deterioration of health over time as anxiety, sadness, and intensive caretaking wore away at their bodies. Lauren has twin 10-year-old daughters with Pervasive Developmental Delays and, as a result, has been very active in the local special-needs community. When I met her for breakfast, she approached the restaurant leaning heavily on a cane. Her degenerative arthritis had spun out of control because she didn't have time to take care of herself. "…You can make yourself sick over this," she said, "and I've made myself sick over it."

These parents' troubles might seem small when measured against those of the residents of the Lower Ninth Ward, but in our child-centered era, where middle-class parents premise large swaths of personal life upon raising "normal," "healthy" children, their losses are real and salient (Francis 2012). A father named Seth explained how his children are his life. "Everything else, you can buy a new car, a new house, who cares? All that stuff. Your kids, that's the one thing, that's the most important thing. So if something is really wrong, significantly wrong … there's no worse trouble in our family than kid trouble." Seth and his wife were crushed when their 14-year-old daughter ran away from home and was living on the streets. Seth tried to convey how painful it was to drive his daughter, against her will, to an out-of-state therapeutic boarding school. "It was the hardest day of my life. Everything else paled in comparison. I've never done anything before or since that was a tenth as difficult for me."

Several parents echoed Seth's sentiment that managing and making sense of children's problems was the most difficult thing they'd ever experienced. Relative to the residents of the Lower Ninth Ward, many of whom had biographies characterized by oppression and disruption, the middle-class parents I interviewed had led privileged lives. Most had homes, college educations, and white-collar jobs that positioned them firmly among the American middle class. Thus, children's problems were a clear *departure* from what participants were accustomed to. Their suffering, it seemed, was proportional to their unmet expectations.

Parents also had little to lose by narrating their own experiences in terms of hardship and woe. Yes, some people saw them as "bad parents" and blamed them for children's problems; here, neoliberalism casts its shadow over privileged and marginalized groups alike. However, unlike Ms. Henrietta, the parents I talked to were fluent in a psychotherapeutic language of loss and grief. In the worlds they occupied, articulating emotion and embracing one's own pain is the mark of a "healthy" person. The failure to do so signifies "denial" and, possibly, psychological "dysfunction." The women I interviewed promoted this view. Many had sought counseling for how to cope with children's problems, and they sometimes encouraged their spouses to grieve openly for the loss of the "normal" child. Bill, whose 16-year-old son has a seizure disorder and developmental disabilities, explained, "I didn't understand the grief cycle for a long time. My wife had some counseling help … and she kept saying, 'You've gotta grieve. You've gotta grieve…' and it wasn't until I heard it three and four and five times that I finally said, 'Oh, I understand it now. Yeah, okay.'"

Thus, parents' willingness to embrace the discourse of suffering makes sense in light of their perceived losses, relatively privileged biographies, and adherence to an emotional culture that prizes the ability to embrace and express one's grief. To analyze their experiences through the lens of suffering is political insofar as it recognizes their deep sorrow and designates them as deserving of sympathy. Such an analysis also invites comparisons with marginalized groups, such as the residents of the Lower Ninth Ward. Nonetheless, to place quotation marks around parents' feelings of woe would be, in our view, to misunderstand suffering. This is not to suggest that their suffering is somehow proportionate—or disproportionate—to that of other groups. Rather, our argument is that any analysis of suffering must take into account how people experience and narrate their own hardship. Though social location *must* inform our analysis, marginality and privilege cannot by themselves guide our assertions about who suffers.

30.4 Conclusion

In this chapter we sought to begin a conversation with those who wish to take up a study of social suffering. It was not our intention to exhaust the political ramifications of suffering. We merely wished to use two very different case studies to underscore common problems in studying suffering: *What is suffering? Whose suffering counts?* The contrast between Hurricane Katrina victims and the middle-class parents of problem children highlight a set of dilemmas associated with the relationship of suffering to social interaction and also the gap between scholarly and self-referential claims to suffering.

To be sure there are many other ethical dilemmas in the study of social suffering. First and foremost, social suffering is experienced differently in various parts of the world. While our two cases are very different, the suffering presented here sharply contrasts from the sexual violence in war-torn countries in the chapter by Féron in this volume. How do we justify a focus on suffering *here* when so much more suffering occurs *there*? Another dilemma that our research raises is how to pick apart and analytically prioritize certain causes of suffering. Expectations about norms of family dynamics or the interaction among community members might fail to get at larger structural or racial or class-based sources of suffering. How do we interrogate these different causes and yet simultaneously write about suffering in a holistic way?

Our analyses of these two cases suggest that focusing on micro-politics offers a partial solution to some of these dilemmas. Harvey (2013) usefully examines the former as a case of how a community avoids certain interactions to minimize their suffering. Francis (2012), on the other hand, analyzes Steve and Marie's woes as a case of "family trouble," highlighting the cultural elevation of children among middle-class families and its consequences for how parents construct their identities. In our view, both pieces of research are case studies in suffering. As these cases imply, assertions about whose suffering deserves public attention or state-supported remediation are *moral assertions*. We should not shy away from making these judgments. Our work always and inevitably has political implications; it is simply a matter of how openly and reflexively we acknowledge those politics.

References

Abelson, M. (2012). Don't think the 1 % aren't suffering too (true, not satire). *Signs of the Times*. Retrieved March 28, 2014. http://www.sott.net/article/242288-Don-t-Think-the-1-Aren-t-Suffering-Too-True-Not-Satire-

Anderson, R. (2014). *Human suffering and quality of life: Conceptualizing stories and statistics*. Dordrecht: Springer.

Auyero, J., & Swistun, D. (2009a). *Flammable: Environmental suffering in an Argentine shantytown*. Oxford: University of Oxford Press.

Auyero, J., & Swistun, D. (2009b). Tiresias in flammable shantytown: Toward a tempography of domination. *Sociological Forum, 24*, 1–21.

Bourdieu, P. (1999). *The weight of the world: Social suffering in contemporary society*. Cambridge: Polity Press.

Cassell, E. J. (1982). The nature of suffering and the goals of medicine. *The New England Journal of Medicine, 306*(1), 639–645.

Clark, C. (1997). *Misery and company: Sympathy in everyday life*. Chicago: University of Chicago Press.

Emerson, R. M., & Messinger, S. L. (1977). The micro-politics of trouble. *Social Problems, 25*, 121–135.

Francis, A. (2012). The dynamics of family trouble: Middle-class parents whose children have problems. *Journal of Ethnography, 41*, 371–401.

Harvey, D. C. (2012). A new geography of trouble. In L. A. Eargle & A. M. Esmail (Eds.), *Black beaches and bayous: The BP Deepwater Horizon oil spill disaster* (pp. 119–133). New York: University Press of America.

Harvey, D. C. (2013). Disasters as hyper-marginalization: Social abandonment in the Lower Ninth Ward of New Orleans. In C. C. Yeakey, V. S. Thompson, & W. Anjanette (Eds.), *Urban ills: Post-recession complexities of urban living in the twenty-first century, in global contexts*. Boston: Lexington Books.

Kleinman, A. (1995). *Writing at the margin: Discourse between anthropology and medicine.* Berkeley: University of California Press.

Landphair, J. (2007). The forgotten people of New Orleans: Community, vulnerability, and the Lower Ninth Ward. *Journal of American History, 94*, 837–845.

Peek, L. (2012). They call it "Katrina Fatigue": Displaced families and discrimination in Colorado. In L. Weber & L. Peek (Eds.), *Displaced: Life in the Katrina diaspora* (pp. 31–46). Austin: University of Texas Press.

Smith, D. (2011). A sociological alternative to the psychiatric conceptualization of mental suffering. *Sociology Compass, 5*, 351–363.

Tyre. (2009, January 11). Daddy's Home, and a Bit Lost. *New York Times*, p. ST1.

Warner, J. (2009). Families to care about. *New York Times, The Opinion Pages Blog*. Retrieved March 27, 2014. http://opinionator.blogs.nytimes.com/2009/03/19/families-to-care-about/

Wilkinson, I. (2005). *Suffering: A sociological introduction.* Malden: Polity Press.

Wolf, J. B. (2011). *Is breast best?: Taking on the breastfeeding experts and the new high stakes of motherhood.* New York: New York University Press.

Chapter 31
Emotions, Empathy, and the Choice to Alleviate Suffering

Caitlin O. Mahoney and Laura M. Harder

31.1 Introduction

In the age of neuroscience, emotion and empathy tend to be viewed as *processes* rather than as *states of being* (Franks 2008). The principal phases of empathy include recognition of emotion, emotional resonance, self-regulation of emotion, and role-taking. Together, these components have the potential to incite compassion and altruistic action. Each occurs within the contexts of mental abilities, valued cognitions, and social settings. Emotion is not the sole determinate of desires or attempts to reduce suffering. Nor is empathy the sole component of the experience of suffering. However, both play major roles in individuals' choices to reduce suffering. In particular, they can help clarify the personal value of relieving suffering as a principal source of meaning in life. The nature of emotions in conjunction with the experience of pain and suffering is reviewed first. Then we identify and discuss phases of the processes of empathy to clarify the important role empathy plays in the human response to suffering.

C.O. Mahoney (✉)
Faculty of Psychology, Metropolitan State University,
700 E 7th Street, St Paul, MN 55106, USA
e-mail: Caitlin.Mahoney@metrostate.edu

L.M. Harder
Department of Psychology, Metropolitan State University,
700 E 7th Street, St Paul, MN 55106, USA
e-mail: hardla@metrostate.edu

© Springer Science+Business Media Dordrecht 2015   413
R.E. Anderson (ed.), *World Suffering and Quality of Life*,
Social Indicators Research Series 56, DOI 10.1007/978-94-017-9670-5_31

31.2 The Emotions of Suffering

As noted by Anderson (2014), certain types of suffering are primarily associated with specific emotions. Anderson's (2013, 2014) taxonomy of suffering is guided by those types of suffering, which can be distinguished from combinations of answers to questions in standard health surveys. He interprets results from the 2010 National Health Interview Survey (NHIS) as indicators of the prevalence of different types of suffering in the United States population. Among the types of suffering in the taxonomy are physical suffering (e.g., pain every day or most days in the past 3 months); mental suffering (subsuming depression, anxiety, grief, and hopelessness); social suffering (structural or institution-produced pain from stigmas such as poverty, racism, and disability); and combinations of these. According to Anderson, "using these indicators, about one third of American adults (70 million) were seriously suffering at any one time."

Using narratives from several of his investigations, Anderson (2013, 2014) also identified common experiences, many of them emotional and all of them negative, associated with each category of pain or suffering. He asked respondents to report their "most extreme suffering" and "a recent calamity in which they suffered." Findings suggest that the experience of physical pain evoked a sense of hurt, torture, or agony. Mental pain took several forms: depression was linked with melancholy, misery, and desolation; anxiety with agitation and obsession; grief with loss or sorrow; social suffering with shame, humiliation, guilt, or low self-worth; and existential suffering with hopelessness, despair, and purposelessness. Other studies have shown that such psychological pain can register in much the same way as physical pain (Eisenberger et al. 2003). Thus, Anderson (2014) notes that emotions may be sources of suffering (e.g., the pain of loneliness) or outcomes of suffering (such as fear of further pain).

Cassell (2004) has claimed that what distinguishes suffering from pain is a perceived threat to personal identity. So, whether one *suffers* as a result of pain depends, in large part, on how one makes sense of one's situation. The meanings we assign to an experience are enmeshed with our emotional experiences, and, since emotions are more than simple physical and physiological manifestations, they entail directions to act in a particular way. They transform our way of being in the world (de Rivera 2006). Thus, emotions are an apt barometer of relationships with others, objects, and one's own situation at any given moment. Here are examples of three separate emotions that may arise from suffering and demonstrate three distinct ways of relating:

Anger While anger is commonly understood to be "negative" in valence, it is not necessarily unpleasant. In fact, it can be associated with feeling "good" and "powerful" (de Rivera 2006). Anger is evoked when "there is a challenge to what (one) assert(s) ought to exist" (de Rivera et al. 2007). Thus, it entails an implicit belief that something about the situation "ought" or "should" be different and, in fact, might be (de Rivera 2006). Anger's power may temporarily buoy one against pain.

Depression Although it is a type of mental suffering, depression is often an outcome of physical suffering. As explained by de Rivera (2006), "whereas anger instructs the person to remove the challenge, the instructional transformation of depression is to 'remove the self'." Depression is "the powerless feeling that nothing can be done" and may occur when there are "forces which prevent the challenge from being removed." Here the action impulse is *inaction*. Action is deemed futile.

Fear One may be immobilized by fear of his or her pain. For de Rivera (2006), fear is equivalent to "a wish" to "escape from something that is dangerous" and likely "unalterable." At the individual level, fear is experienced as a "constrictive movement that moves people to pull into themselves" (de Rivera et al. 2007) and away from the perceived threat.

Each of the above responses to pain has negative connotations. Fredrickson (2001) has suggested that negative emotions serve to narrow one's "momentary thought action repertoires". That is, they focus our attention, thoughts, and actions on the immediacy of fight or flight. We know, too, that certain types of psychological pain prime one toward defensiveness against impeding threat. Hawkley et al. (2003) found that the pain of loneliness is associated with "higher stress appraisals and poorer social interactions," including a tendency to be less understanding and more distrustful. Trapped in one's own pain, a person who suffers may be less likely to notice and understand the pain of others.

Anderson's (2013, 2014) research further suggests that the emotional experience of suffering is largely linked to the meaning one constructs around one's experience, which is embedded with socially defined meanings. Thus, the emotional correlates of different types of pain are not simply defined by personal meaning-making, but also by each individual's socio-cultural context. For instance, in a society that stigmatizes mental illness, one may suffer from a painful bout of depression as well as from the shame or humiliation attached to suffering the condition itself.

With all this taken into consideration, we propose that some emotional experiences are more motivating and more sustainable than others when it comes to addressing suffering. Further, the suffering of singular others or larger collectives of people may have the potential to sway moral and emotional senses, indeed begging for compassionate response. However, one's capacity to respond to the suffering of another is largely anchored in one's capacity to empathically connect with another's experience and to regulate one's feelings so that they are not incapacitating or demotivating. An appropriate response to the distress of another requires an understanding of what response will alleviate, rather than compound, that suffering and an ability to turn personal motivation into social relief.

31.2.1 Empathy

Cassell (2004) has claimed that to accurately recognize that another is suffering (rather than simply experiencing pain) is challenging, but not impossible. Batson (1990), Wiseman (1996), Pinker (2011) and others have proposed that the primary pathway by which we attend to another's suffering is through empathy. Those others may be close to us (e.g., kin) or quite far away (e.g., victims of natural disasters), but the processes by which we make sense of their experience are quite similar. It follows from Cassell's (2004) description that the better we know another, the better our empathic accuracy.

Empathy, which tends to be defined as a process rather than as emotion, is the key component to understanding how emotions lead to pro-social behavior. According to Eisenberg, empathy is "an affective response that stems from the apprehension or comprehension of another's emotional state" (2002: 135). In other words, empathy is role-taking or vicarious enactment of another's experience. The sight of someone in need can serve as a stimulus to an empathic response. Those with greater empathetic abilities will relate more strongly and experience a stronger emotional response to the suffering of others.

Empathy is so important that it has been referred to as the "indispensable ingredient" in psychotherapy (Kitron 2011) and is consistently cited as the essential key to helping change behavior. Paciello and her colleagues (2013) conducted a study observing helping behavior in youth. They found that high levels of empathy led to more altruistic responses, while self-centered behaviors were derived from higher personal distress levels. Stocks et al. (2009) garnered similar results regarding the role of empathy in helping. Their study examined whether people high in empathy helped others for altruistic reasons, or more as a means to escape psychological discomfort. They found that people who are empathically aroused by seeing someone in need were more likely to offer help, regardless of whether or not physical escape was available. Their findings also demonstrated that helping behaviors evoked by empathy were elicited by altruistic motives to alleviate suffering – not by an egoistic need to reduce psychological distress. Empathic capacity or role-taking is at the core of whether one will seek to alleviate the suffering of others and it is, to some extent, limited by personal suffering.

Table 31.1 gives a detailed, 10-phase description of the mental processes embedded in empathy, ending with empathic action. The phases emerge from the three conceptual models and each phase appears in at least one of the three. The first model (Decety and Jackson 2006) draws heavily from social neuroscience research on empathy and is not concerned with follow-up action. Ekman's (2008) model, the second, is influenced by both empirical psychology and Buddhist philosophy, and it highlights how the empathic process can end in compassion and altruistic action. The third model, from Morton (2013), draws upon psychological research and is a philosophical analysis of the meaning of emotions, including those involved in empathy processes.

As shown in Table 31.1, empathy is preceded by external stimuli, self-awareness of emotions, ability to associate new emotional experiences with past ones, and the core processes of emotional resonance and emotional self-regulation. Empathy and the ability or willingness to empathize are shaped by all of these emotion-related mechanisms (phases 1–7). We can see the chain of events that will lead emotions to elicit a response to suffering by tying these concepts together.

Morton (2013) offers a useful distinction between empathy and sympathy, which are often conflated in both normal discourse and the scientific literature. He notes

Table 31.1 Components of empathy in three conceptual models

Phase	Phase/Process	Decety and Jackson (2006)	Ekman (2008)	Morton (2013)
1	Cognitive intervention or perception	Unique affective experiences of another		
2	Awareness of own emotions	Ability to self-monitor emotions		
3	Emotion and emotion history recognition	Shared emotional states	Recognition of other(s) emotions	
4	Emotion resonance – affective interaction	Shared representations	Emotion resonance – from cues of others	Emotional resonance
5	Maintaining agency and distance	Agency as crucial in empathy		
6	Emotion regulation	Emotion regulation		
7	Role-taking perspective	Capacity for role-taking perspective		Emotional identification
8	Recognition of choice to relieve suffering			Emotional appropriateness
9	Choice/desire to relieve suffering		Compassion	
10	Action (potentially-altruistic)		Altruistic actions	

that empathy refers to vicarious experience, while sympathy means to feel regret or sorrow for another's suffering or experience. Sympathy often implies pity, which is characterized as an authoritative or superior feeling. Neither sympathy nor empathy necessarily encompasses actions that relieve another's suffering. For this reason, phases 8–10 are depicted (by a dotted line) as *potential*, but not determined, outcomes of the empathic process.

While the neuroscientific elements of Decety and Jackson's (2006) model detail the perceptual and affective states of emotion in empathic processes, only Ekman's (2008) model addresses the phases that follow the role-taking function. Partly because of the emphasis of compassion within Buddhism, Ekman discusses how compassion develops and then is transformed into action by individual choice. The four phases identified by Ekman represent the sequential steps of empathy. Morton (2013) also expands upon the influence of empathy on the choice to take action, but he clouds the process by labeling it an assessment of "emotional appropriateness."

31.2.2   Emotional Regulation

Self-regulation is a monitoring and control process that begins in infancy and allows us to moderate our reactions as we mature (Geangu 2011). Habits of emotional response emerge from genetic pre-dispositions and social learning and are intimately linked to our emotional reactivity. To the extent that emotions become consistent ways of responding, they may be more difficult to regulate (Lerner and

Keltner 2001). Well-trod patterns (which include resonance and regulation) have a great deal to do with one's physical and mental well-being.

While it is challenging to establish causal relationships between emotional patterns and negative health outcomes, research seems to support the notion that certain ways of being predispose one toward risk while others more reliably serve a protective function. According to Kabat-Zinn (1990), "feelings you experience toward yourself and toward other people and how you express or don't express them seem to be particularly important" to health outcomes. For instance, those whose personalities are vulnerable to anger and who regulate their emotions by internalization rather than sharing are more likely to develop cancer. Likewise, hypertension (high blood pressure) coincides with unregulated anger and hostility (a lack of "basic trust") correlates with heart disease. Finally, internalization and rumination are linked with the experience of depression (Seligman 2011), which is linked with decreases in immunological function (Kabat-Zinn 1990).

Since self-regulation ultimately filters whether we engage in helping, it is vital to consider how different regulatory styles bring forth varying responses. Carlo et al. (2012) explain, "To engage in caring actions toward others requires effective regulation of one's own emotions." Consider what occurs when we engage in too little or too much regulation. If we are highly regulatory, we might regulate our emotions and behaviors to such an extent that we do not engage at all with someone who is suffering. Studies have shown this type of response when people are faced with needs of large populations. They see the need as overwhelming and regulate themselves as to prevent an emotional response (Cameron and Payne 2011).

The flip-side comes when we fail to sufficiently regulate our emotions and experience personal distress, defined by Eisenberg as the "aversive, self-focused reaction to others in need or distress" (Eisenberg 2000: 668). If we are focusing on our own experience, we are unable to effectively tend to the needs of others. For this reason, personal distress and low levels of self-regulation have been shown to decrease helping behaviors (Eisenberg 2000).

Empathy and self-regulation can help us to understand how emotions lead us to alleviate the suffering of others. Equilibrium between the two is equally important. To be most effective in tending to the needs of others, we must be able to see their perspective and "feel for them," but also regulate our reactions so as to maintain a healthy boundary between our own experience and theirs.

31.2.3 Mindfulness

Mindfulness is not necessarily an emotion, but it closely relates to the recognition and regulation of emotion. Training in mindfulness (meditation) centers largely on enhancing one's attention and awareness, grounding in present experience without attempting to flee or to change it. Affiliative trust and seeing the basic goodness in others and in ourselves hold intrinsic healing power, so developing an awareness of one's emotional patterns presents the possibility of mitigating the negative and cultivating the positive. Kabat-Zinn (1990) and his associates claim that, through mindfulness meditative practices, we can learn to attend humanely to our own suffering and grow our capacity to trust others. He has collected empirical evidence that a mindful approach to pain management (whether that pain is physical or mental) improves one's quality of life.

Holzel and colleagues (2011) have outlined four pathways by which mindfulness training (meditation) alters one's experience. First, attention is regulated and may serve as a building block for other mechanisms of change. For instance, to attend to our own pain, we must recognize that we are in pain. Kabat-Zinn notes that this attention helps us to notice what enhances our pain, what diminishes it, and how we relate to it. Furthermore, we become aware of how our behavior impacts our experience and our relationship to others. According to Holzel et al. (2011), what follows then is a stronger awareness of one's own bodily experience, a "pre-condition" for emotion regulation. In this regard, attention and awareness bring often-unconscious self-appraisals to the fore, allowing for conscious and continuous reappraisal.

Through attending to our pain rather than denying it, we become attuned to it. Negative arousal—what we might call clinging to or dwelling on the pain—loses its power and interest. We understand the pain and, in a way, are asked to accept our own pain in order to act to lessen others'. Finally, mindfulness seems to alter the perspective of the self. Those who practice mindfulness meditation believe the self is (and all things are) inconstant and changing and believe that all beings are connected (Kabat-Zinn 1990). These feelings may enhance feelings of self-compassion, including kindness toward oneself (see Neff 2011). Mindfulness fosters acceptance; counteracts the "should and ought" implicit in the experience of anger, depression, and fear; and enhances the tendency to be gentle and compassionate toward the self and others (Siegel 2010).

Mindfulness also asks the individual to find balance in all things, including empathy. Over-attention to others may lead to burnout (Miller et al. 1995) and compassion fatigue (Figley 1995). The rubric of self-compassion provides a set of practices that make it possible to empathically address the suffering of others without succumbing to self-suffering.

Kabat-Zinn explains, "by changing the way we see ourselves in relationship to stressors, we can actually change our experience of the relationship and therefore modify the extent to which they tax or exceed our resources or endanger our well-being" (1990: 240). Mindfulness practices are meant to foster the development of "new ways of seeing and being in the world" (Kabat-Zinn 1990: 218). Thus, in addition to better noticing, regulating, and responding to our own experiences, these practices have important implications for how we relate to others. As mindfulness training grounds us in awareness and understanding of our own bodily experience, it inadvertently grows our capacity to understand others (Decety and Jackson 2004), increases our empathic engagement (Dekeyser et al. 2008), and enhances our inclination to take compassionate action on behalf of others (Condon et al. 2013).

31.3   Social Suffering

Beyond the suffering of a single other, we are faced (perhaps daily) with news of larger scale suffering. The term "social suffering" encompasses the human consequences of war, famine, depression, and disease, and torture – "the whole assemblage of social problems" caused by social norms and institutions (Kleinman et al. 1996).

Cassell (2004) argues "most ideas about the suffering of others are really beliefs about the seriousness of what threatens them – pain, hunger, isolation, or loss, for example" (1991: 3). Pinker (2011) highlights the need to grow systems of morality and reason to address public ills, as empathy is inherently limited by one's history of experiences and one's social identity. If empathy is a channel by which we may experience another's pain or joy, that channel is not immediately open to all.

Globally, we seem to recognize suffering through "expressions, gestures, and behaviors" (Cassell 2004). However, it seems that we are particularly attentive to cues regarding kinship, age, and gender in defining our circle of empathic and moral regard and when allocating our attention and concern to others' pain (Pinker 2011; Höijer 2004). Further, while Elfenbein and Ambady (2002) found evidence to support cross-cultural accuracy in emotion recognition, they also concluded that one's ability to accurately judge another's emotional experience is improved when that other is part of one's in-group. Thus, "the match between the cultural background of the expresser and judge is important." Socially and developmentally, we learn which physical cues correspond with which emotional experiences. Cross-cultural exposure (physical proximity and verbal contact) seems to eliminate much of the in-group advantage. So, to some extent, empathic accuracy can be improved through acquaintance. Of course, this naturally means that social suffering can be deepened through acquaintance, too.

Specific cases of social suffering test the bounds of empathy along these lines. Such suffering is often geographically distant, and Slovic (2007) has noted that statistical and aggregate renderings of suffering (e.g., genocide counts) are counterproductive to appeals for aid because of empirical findings regarding the earlier mention of being overwhelmed: the larger the number of suffering others, the less likely one is to give to a cause (Small et al. 2007). Slovic believes that "the statistics of mass murder or genocide, no matter how large the numbers, fail to convey the true meaning of such atrocities. The numbers fail to spark emotion or feeling and thus fail to motivate action." Barbalet (2001) argued that emotional energy is important to social action, above and beyond the necessity of reason. And "Even if social action does result from the individual actors' calculus of their interests, the emotional basis of interest remains crucial" (Barbalet 2001).

To the extent that action on the part of the observer may have utility, it seems that personal engagement with an issue and emotional energy are important (de Rivera et al. 2007). How do we make social suffering a personal issue? Historically, institutions like slavery were viewed as a public sin and it was not until a cultural paradigm shift made it a *personal sin* that individuals were motivated to eradicate it (Young 2001). Certainly attempts to grow the circle of empathy may alter the sense of personal relevance. We might also consider which emotions serves greater motivational roles. Barbalet (2001) has championed the historical utility of vengefulness and resentment in driving social movements. Moral outrage may be partially predicted by a combination of anger and disgust (Salerno and Peter-Hagene 2013) – emotions that often bypass our attempts at regulation.

Even if this is true, those who hope to alleviate suffering at the largest scales are urged not to follow Barbelet's advice. Habitual anger is simply not good for one's health, and may exceed our ability to control its behavioral outcomes (Dalai Lama 2003). When imagined, vengeance is experienced as "sweet," but when enacted it leaves a "bitter" taste; is often unsatisfying and has the potential to spur cycles of violence (Jaffe 2011). Appeals for aid or involvement may also be less welcomed if the appeal maker is perceived as angry. Newer research suggests that negative stereotypes associated with activists (that they are "angry," for instance) reduce their target audience's willingness to cooperate (Bashir et al. 2013).

Still, while it is tempting to conclude that negative emotions are detrimental, as evolved capacities, they have served historically adaptive functions and may have some pragmatic and motivational utility. If we did not have an aversive reaction to suffering, we would not be motivated to relieve it. Some research suggests that negative moods may make us more equitable and that working to accept negativity may make us *feel* less negative (Jaffe 2012). Sylvia Boorstein, quoted by Tippett (2013), has argued that one may

> need (anger) just to alert you to what needs attention, but you don't need to carry it along with you to keep refueling you. As a matter of fact, if you keep nurturing the flame of anger, it confuses the mind and maybe we don't respond as wisely as we ought to. But I need the anger as if I had 104 fever; it would be a sign that I need to do something about it.

More recent work in neuroscience brings these ideas together, demonstrating how mindful awareness grows one's ability to recover from and release negative emotion more quickly (Davidson and Begley 2012; Vago and Silbersweig 2012). Thus attempts to foster emotional balance and stability – our degree of comfort with and what we *do* with negative emotion – may be more important predictors of effective response than a singular focus on type or valence of affect alone, (Jaffe 2012).

31.4 Relief of Suffering

A growing body of literature in the past 10 years has touted the importance of what one might call "global compassion". The distinction between compassion as a value orientation, as a cognitive set, and as an emotional experience is unclear. However, some theoretical triangulation leads us to understand that compassion entails empathy, concern, and responsibility. Compassion may rival the energy and power of anger, but allow for more emotional and behavioral control (Mahoney 2008).

Höijer (2004) suggests that global compassion (a moral sensibility or concern for remote strangers) may be aroused by media exposure, but that individuals are more compassionately roused by images of "worthy" victim groups such as children, women, and the elderly. Media consumers show less sympathy for those whom we may readily blame for their plight. The nature of images seems also to be important. For example, a tearful, direct gaze reduces ambiguity and focuses emotion recognition (and meaning-making) on pain. It also places responsibility on the observer, whose reactions may include feeling tenderhearted, blame-filled, shame-filled, or powerless (Höijer 2004). Mixed emotions may be common: one may feel tenderhearted toward victims, indignation toward perpetrators, and powerless to help. Appeals to the public, then, are tricky.

Consider that compassion is far from the only reaction one may have toward distant others. Methods of "distantiation" from compassion may include denying the "truth claim" of news reports, dehumanizing victims, becoming numb, and criticizing reports as sensational. These manifestations can actually be a demonstration of emotional sensitivity – someone who feels deeply may attempt to guard against all feeling. Beyond the possibility that the observer feels too much or too little, emotional responses are socially learned. Thus, there seem to be gendered differences in compassion. Women may choose to "turn (their) back" on suffering because of compassion fatigue or as a function of feeling too much, too often. A diminished inclination to "let oneself be moved" by the suffering of another or to display those feelings may be more common among men. We might consider the moral and pragmatic quandary of arousing concern without active behavioral outlets to dispel uncomfortable sentiments. If one is incapable of acting to relieve the suffering of distant others and that feeling of helplessness is actually warranted, perhaps the pragmatic response *is* inaction and disengagement. Breaking a distant and large-scale suffering into ways an individual can take action may make an emotional appeal much more effective in the relief of suffering.

31.5 Conclusion

Contemporary Western thought, especially that which is sympathetic toward humanitarianism, generally assumes that relief of suffering is a widely accepted human value. Our model certainly centers on this assumption. While there is some truth to this presumption, there remains a sizable subpopulation of postmodern societies that derives enjoyment from suffering (Van Dijk et al. 2012). This paradoxical cultural genre is even demonstrated though the word "schadenfreude" found in the German language Alternatively, suffering has been considered in other modern cultures as an opportunity to ignite change, hope, and the development of compassion. The very act of helping others altruistically has transformed the experience of personal suffering (Johnston 2015). Thus, cultural and social norms accurately map the bounds of when and for whom empathy is appropriate, as well as the meaning that suffering holds.

Our analysis of the importance of role-taking and emotional regulation suggests potential foci for educational initiatives that may prove challenging. We identified that the negative emotions of anger, fear, depression, and anxiety can be learned by individuals who empathize and identify intensely with others suffering from severe types of distress. Empathy, resonance, and regulation require balance – a balance that may be consciously fostered through mindful attention and socio-emotional learning.

We can see that the automatic processes that can create negative emotions and barriers to helping others are the same processes that allow us to connect with one another. Through understanding how our emotions lead to our willingness to alleviate suffering in others, we can continue to progress towards a peaceful society. Compared to only a few centuries ago, some forms of suffering (like, public executions and torture) have greatly subsided. A major force behind this reduction in cruelty seems to be a growing commitment to humanitarian ethics of care (see Chaps. 3 (Wilkinson 2015) and 4 (Sznaider 2015), in this volume). In addition to promoting the ethic of care, improving institutions such as poverty, racism and inequity, radical reduction of suffering could become reality.

References

Anderson, R. E. (2013, August). *The emotions of suffering.* Paper presented at the International Society for Research on Emotion meetings in Berkeley, CA.

Anderson, R. E. (2014). *Human suffering and quality of life: Conceptualizing stories and statistics.* New York: Springer.

Barbalet, J. M. (2001). *Emotion, social theory, and social structure: A macrosociological approach.* Cambridge: University Press.

Bashir, N. Y., Lockwood, P., Chasteen, A. L., Nadolny, D., & Noyes, I. (2013). The ironic impact of activists: Negative stereotypes reduce social change influence. *European Journal of Social Psychology, 43*(7), 614–626.

Batson, C. D. (1990). How social an animal: The human capacity for caring. *American Psychologist, 45*(3), 336–346.

Cameron, D. C., & Payne, B. K. (2011). Escaping affect: How motivated emotion regulation creates insensitivity to mass suffering. *Attitudes and Social Cognition, 100*(1), 1–15.

Carlo, G., Crockett, L. J., Wolff, J. M., & Beal, S. J. (2012). The role of emotional reactivity, self-regulation, and puberty in adolescents' prosocial behaviors. *Social Development, 21*(4), 667–685.

Cassel, E. (1991, May-June). Recognizing suffering. *The Hastings Center Report, 21*(3), 24–32.

Cassell, E. J. (2004). *The nature of suffering and the goals of medicine.* Oxford: Oxford University Press.

Condon, P., Desbordes, G., Miller, W. B., & DeSteno, D. (2013). Meditation increases compassionate responses to suffering. *Psychological Science, 24*(10), 2125–2127.

Dalai Lama. (2003). *The compassionate life.* Boston: Wisdom Publications.

Davidson, R. J., & Begley, S. (2012). *The Emotional Life of Your Brain: How its unique patterns affect the way you think, feel, and live–and how you can change them.* London: Penguin.

de Rivera, J. (2006). Conceptual encounter: The experience of anger. In C. T. Fischer (Ed.), *Qualitative research methods for psychologists: Introduction through empirical studies* (pp. 213–245). Available online: http://www.clarku.edu/faculty/derivera/PDFs/Ch.8_Conceptual_Encounter-_The_Experience_of_Anger.pdf

de Rivera, J., Kurrien, R., & Olsen, N. (2007). The emotional climate of nations and their culture of peace. *Journal of Social Issues, 63*(2), 255–271.

Decety, J., & Jackson, P. L. (2004). The functional architecture of human empathy. *Behavioral and Cognitive Neuroscience Reviews, 3*, 71–100.

Decety, J., & Jackson, P. L. (2006). A social-neuroscience perspective on empathy. *Current Directions in Psychological Science, 15*(2), 54–58.

Dekeyser, M., Raes, F., Leijssen, M., Leysen, S., & Dewulf, D. (2008). Mindfulness skills and interpersonal behavior. *Personality and Individual Differences, 44*, 1235–1245.

Eisenberg, N. (2000). Emotion, regulation, and moral development. *Annual Review of Psychology, 51*, 665–697.

Eisenberg, N. (2002). Empathy related emotional responses, altruism, and their socialization. In R. J. Davidson & A. Harrington (Eds.), *Visions of compassion* (pp. 131–164). Oxford: Oxford University Press.

Eisenberger, N., Lieberman, M., & Williams, K. (2003). Does rejection hurt? An FMRI study of social exclusion. *Science* (New York, N.Y.), *302*(5643), 290–292.

Ekman, P. (Ed.). (2008). *Emotional awareness, overcoming the obstacles to psychological balance and compassion: A conversation between the Dalai Lama and Paul Ekman*. New York: Times Books.

Elfenbein, H. A., & Ambady, N. (2002). On the universality and cultural specificity of emotion recognition: A meta-analysis. *Psychological Bulletin, 128*(2), 203–235.

Figley, C. R. (Ed.). (1995). *Compassion fatigue: Coping with secondary traumatic stress disorder in those who treat the traumatized* (Psychology, 39, pp. 649–665). London: Brunner-Routledge.

Franks, D. D. (2008). The neurosociology of emotions. In J. E. Stets & J. H. Turner (Eds.), *Handbook of the sociology of emotions* (pp. 38–62). New York: Springer.

Fredrickson, B. L. (2001). The role of positive emotions in positive psychology: The broaden-and-build theory of positive emotions. *American Psychologist, 56*(3), 218–226.

Geangu, E. (2011). Individual differences in infant's emotional resonance to a peer in distress: Self-other awareness and emotion regulation. *Social Development, 20*(3). doi:10.1111/j.1467-9507.2010.00596.x

Hawkley, L. C., Burleson, M. H., Berntson, G. G., & Cacioppo, J. T. (2003). Loneliness in everyday life: Cardiovascular activity, psychosocial context, and health behaviors. *Journal of Personality and Social Psychology, 85*(1), 105.

Höijer, B. (2004). The discourse of global compassion: The audience and media reporting of human suffering. *Media, Culture & Society, 26*(4), 513–531.

Holzel, B. K., Lazar, S. W., Gard, T., Schuman-Oliver, Z., Vago, D. R., & Ott, U. (2011). How does mindfulness meditation work? *Perspectives on Psychological Science, 6*(6), 537–559.

Jaffe, E. (2011, October). The complicated psychology of revenge. *Observer, 24*(8). Available online: http://www.psychologicalscience.org/index.php/publications/observer/2011/october-11/the-complicated-psychology-of-revenge.html

Jaffe, E. (2012, November). Positively negative: Research shows there's an up side to feeling down. *Observer 25*(9). Available online: http://www.psychologicalscience.org/index.php/publications/observer/2012/november-12/positively-negative.html

Johnston, N. E. (2015). Healing suffering: The evolution of caring practices. In R. E. Anderson (Ed.), *World suffering and quality of life*. New York: Springer.

Kabat-Zinn, J. (1990). *Full catastrophe living*. New York: Bantam Dell.

Kitron, D. (2011). Empathy – The indispensable ingredient in the impossible profession. *Psychoanalytic Inquiry, 31*, 17–27.

Kleinman, A., Das, V., & Lock, M. (1996). Introduction. *Daedulus, 125*(1), 1–5.

Lerner, J. S., & Keltner, D. (2001). Fear, anger, and risk. *Journal of Personality and Social Psychology, 81*(1), 146–159.

Mahoney, C. O. (2008). *Transcending the limits of compassion: The influence of joy on reactions to the suffering of distant others*. Unpublished doctoral dissertation, Clark University, Worcester.

Miller, K., Birkholt, M., Scott, C., & Stage, C. (1995). Empathy and burnout in human service work: An extension of a communication model. *Communication Research, 22*(2), 123–147.

Morton, A. (2013). *Emotion and imagination*. New York: Polity.

Neff, K. (2011). *Self-compassion: Stop beating yourself up and leave insecurity behind*. New York: HarperCollins.

Paciello, M., Fida, R., Cerniglia, L., Tramontano, C., & Cole, E. (2013). High cost helping scenario: The role of empathy, prosocial reasoning and moral disengagement on helping behavior. *Personality and Individual Differences, 55*, 3–7.

Pinker, S. (2011). *Better angels of our nature: Why violence has declined*. New York: Penguin.

Salerno, J. M., & Peter-Hagene, L. C. (2013). The interactive effect of anger and disgust on moral outrage and judgments. *Psychological Science, 24*(10), 2069–2078.

Seligman, M. E. P. (2011). *Flourish: A visionary new understanding of happiness and well-being*. New York: The Free Press.

Siegel, R. D. (2010). *The mindfulness solution – Everyday practices for everyday problems*. New York: Guilford Press.

Slovic, P. (2007). "If I look at the mass I will never act": Psychic numbing and genocide. *Judgment and Decision Making, 2*, 79–95. Retrieved April 24, 2007, from http://journal.sjdm.org/vol2.2.htm

Small, D. A., Lowenstein, G., & Slovic, P. (2007). Sympathy and callousness: Affect and deliberations in donation decisions. *Organizational Behavior and Human Decision Processes, 102*, 143–153.

Stocks, E. L., Lishner, D. A., & Decker, S. K. (2009). Altruism or psychological escape: Why does empathy promote prosocial behavior? *European Journal of Social, 39*, 649–665.

Sznaider, N. (2015). Compassion, cruelty and human rights. In R. E. Anderson (Ed.), *World suffering and quality of life*. New York: Springer.

Tippett, K. (Host/Executive Producer). (2013, May 9). *Sylvia Boorstein – What we nurture*. [Audio podcast]. Retrieved from http://www.onbeing.org/

Vago, D. R., & Silbersweig, D. A. (2012). Self-awareness, self-regulation, and self-transcendence (S-ART): A framework for understanding the neurobiological mechanisms of mindfulness. *Frontiers in Human Neuroscience, 6*(296). doi:10.3389/fnhum.2012.00296 – See more at: http://journal.frontiersin.org/Journal/10.3389/fnhum.2012.00296/abstract#sthash.oZ9jzDyZ.dpuf

Van Dijk, W. W., Ouwerkerk, J. W., Van Koningsbruggen, G. M., & Wesseling, Y. M. (2012). "So you wanna be a pop star?" Schadenfreude following another's misfortune on TV. *Basic and Applied Social Psychology, 34*, 168–174.

Wilkinson, I. (2015). Social suffering and critical humanitarianism. In R. E. Anderson (Ed.), *World suffering and quality of life*. New York: Springer.

Wiseman, T. (1996). A concept analysis of empathy. *Journal of Advanced Nursing, 23*, 1162–1167.

Young, M. P. (2001). A revolution of the soul: Transformative experiences and immediate abolition. In J. Goodwin, J. M. Jasper, & F. Polletta (Eds.), *Passionate politics: Emotions and social movements*. Chicago: University of Chicago Press.

Chapter 32
How Suffering Challenges Our Future

Ronald E. Anderson

32.1 Introduction to Considerations for the Future

In an uncertain world with increasing climate calamities, a worst-case scenario leaves little time for research and effective policy. If the world were to become a failed state, research would be a luxury. But even as we see a slow rise of large-scale disasters swirling around, it is not too late to spend time and resources on research that can help us understand if not alleviate the inevitable suffering that follows these crises.

Suffering of all types takes a heavy toll. If our goal is to relieve and contain suffering, or even substantially reduce suffering, then we have no choice but to continue the best paths of research and practice related to suffering. This type of knowledge must serve as a foundation for improved decisions of both individuals and global institutions on the essential steps necessary to solve the systemic problems underlying world suffering.

Given these possibilities for the future, this final chapter asks some general questions about the future and gives some tentative answers: What priorities should guide exploration and research related to suffering and its reduction? What social policies and political actions might be necessary to reduce global suffering? How can we improve our conceptual frames for suffering and its social contexts? To what extent do human rights violations shape world suffering? From all this analysis, can we guide our generation—or the next—to learn how to better alleviate suffering?

I selected chapters for Part V because they describe an approach, a new method, or a field of research that seems to have the potential for improving the study of suffering and advancing knowledge related to suffering. The next section briefly summarizes these papers, then shows their interrelationship and implications.

R.E. Anderson (✉)
Department of Sociology, Emeritus Faculty of Sociology,
University of Minnesota, Minneapolis, MN 55455, USA
e-mail: rea@umn.edu

© Springer Science+Business Media Dordrecht 2015   427
R.E. Anderson (ed.), *World Suffering and Quality of Life*,
Social Indicators Research Series 56, DOI 10.1007/978-94-017-9670-5_32

32.2   Capsule Summaries of Part V Chapters Related to the Future

David Franks (Chap. 27) starts with evidence of the social dependency of the human brain. Unusually strong affirmation comes from the Spitz (1966) study between infants with and without human contact. Isolation of the infants deprived of mothering and cuddling created interpersonal suffering, which ruined their physical health. The discovery that the same general brain areas enable both physical pain and social isolation casts light on the plight of isolated infants. Neuroscience and neurosociology research show how both physical and social pain share the cingulate cortex as a common center for core functioning. Franks shows how the new field of neurosociology demonstrates the intensity and ubiquity of social rejection and suffering. Recent experimental research found that seeing others being rejected socially could produce the same effect on the brain. Future neuroscience research may well revolutionize our understanding of suffering even more.

Louis-Marie Ngamassi Tchouakeu and Andrea H. Tapia (Chap. 28) explore how networks of organizations collaborate and share information about humanitarian activity. They analyzed data collected through multiple members of the HumanaInfoNet, a community of organizations engaged in humanitarian information management and exchange. Modern humanitarianism combines the traditional focus of unconditionally alleviating human suffering with the need to operate in an arena of providers that is increasingly crowded, heterogeneous, and technologically enabled. This chapter illustrates some collaborative paths across humanitarian organizations that eventually lead to less human suffering. Major advances in risk management for relief agencies, have in the past decade, often increased the organizational effectiveness in organizational response to disasters by paying immediate attention to priority actions that can result in reducing casualties (Haddow et al. 2010). More of both types of research that improve practice can continue to increase the efficiency, as well as effectiveness, of aid organizations.

Marco Fattore and Filomena Maggino (Chap. 29) propose a novel analytic technique using survey methodology for transforming and interpreting the responses. They analyzed data from the annual survey, the Multipurpose System, collected by the Italian National Institute of Statistics, from 48,000 adults in 2007 and again in 2010, corresponding to the year before the world recession began and again, 3 years later. Their survey asked for self-reports of life satisfaction. They applied a measurement procedure based upon *partially ordered sets*, or *posets* for short, in order to assess the overall proportions of people who were highly dissatisfied with life and hence were suffering. They referred to this as "overall suffering," but they also calculated the degree of suffering for those who expressed any suffering, and labeled this "specific suffering." Using the poset-based procedure, Fattore and Maggino found that, in 2007 and 2010, overall and specific suffering levels increased from north to south and were higher for women than for men. While more research is needed, these findings indicate a tendency in Italy for many women, particularly in the south, to face social suffering due, perhaps, to gender discrimination. Both the analytical technique and the possibility that gender bias produces social suffering among women are topics that deserve further attention.

Ara Francis and Daina Harvey (Chap. 30) contrast the suffering of the Lower Ninth Ward in New Orleans with the suffering of parents with troubled children in an upper-middle-class California neighborhood. They interviewed parents of children who suffered from addictions, self-injury, disability, or mental illness. The parents and others tended to attribute blame to the parents themselves for the problems of their children, even though many had been "model parents." This *social suffering* was accompanied by *interpersonal suffering* in that some of their friends and family members became less likely to choose to interact with them, leaving the bewildered and depressed parents more isolated and lonely. Francis and Harvey found it perplexing that the well-to-do California parents tended to attribute severe suffering to themselves, while many of the poor, discriminated, and vulnerable residents of the Lower Ninth Ward in New Orleans refused to think of themselves as suffering. The researchers concluded it was an important lesson in the politics, or micropolitics, of suffering, not just an anomaly in social status. They ask how public policy could deal with the two types of suffering and conclude that the people of the devastated Ninth Ward are more deserving of assistance. Of course, there still remains the question of the type of assistance needed, because given the elevation of the "Lower Ninth," the long-term habitability of the geographical area is controversial. Also, mental illness most often is considered a matter of personal, not public, responsibility. Thus, these issues are as much a question of ethics as of politics. If we feel a responsibility to reduce world suffering, we must set priorities for taking corrective action–a choice that may be even more difficult in the future. Priority setting should not preclude provision of some relief for all types of severe suffering.

Caitlin O. Mahoney and Laura M. Harder (Chap. 31) offer conceptual frameworks for evaluating the role of emotions and empathy in the desire and choice to alleviate suffering. Because the locus of the suffering (self, other, or social) may change the role of emotions in suffering, they are discussed collectively and separately. The structure of the empathy process is outlined in 10 steps or phases, including emotional resonance and self-regulation. This larger perspective on empathy encompasses shared experience as well as the potential for compassion and altruism. Mindfulness and other such self-interventions offer strategies for building resilience in coping with different types of suffering. Better understanding of emotional processes holds great potential for decision-making on how best to contribute to solutions for a wide mix of needs for relief.

32.3   Implications and Relevance of Part V for the Future

The work underlying these chapters in Part V offers a diverse blend of approaches. Not all directions will be fruitful, but some may be wildly so. The proposed work on emotions already has begun, e.g., experimental studies on perceptions of "worthy victims," what factors underlie withdrawal from compassion, and the relationship between social characteristics such as social status and gender on willingness to take compassionate action (Piff et al. 2010, 2012). All hold great potential for advancing knowledge about human suffering and how to eradicate preventable suffering.

Contemporary Western thought, when sympathetic toward humanitarianism, generally assumes that relief of suffering is a widely accepted human value. While this assumption carries some truth-value, there remains a sizable subpopulation of contemporary societies that derives enjoyment from watching others suffer (Van Dijk et al. 2012). The German word *schadenfreude* best captures the essence of this paradoxical cultural genre. Alternatively, suffering has been considered in other modern cultures as an opportunity to ignite change, hope, and the development of compassion. The very act of helping others altruistically has transformed the experience of personal suffering (See Chap. 8). Thus, cultural and social norms accurately map the bounds of when and for whom empathy is appropriate, as well as the meaning that suffering holds.

Through better understanding how emotions lead to willingness to alleviate suffering in others, we can continue to progress toward a relatively peaceful society. Compared to only a few centuries ago, public executions and torture have greatly subsided. A major force behind this reduction in cruelty seems to be a growing commitment to humanitarian ethics of care (See Parts I and II of this book.) In addition, systemic changes like reductions in poverty, racism and inequality could radically reduce suffering, as does the ethic of care.

32.4 Illustrative Conceptual Framework

Because most of the writing about suffering has been philosophical or religious, the positive or scientific understanding of suffering's roots and outcomes has been relatively neglected. While normative theories of suffering play a very important role in society, questions relating to what results in and from suffering – social science questions – deserve concerted effort now and in the future. In moving toward building an empirical base of knowledge about suffering, the following diagram (Fig. 32.1) depicts some possibilities.

If a conceptualization were to try to explain suffering by focusing on factors that influence the occurrence and amount of suffering, then its structure would look something like the left side of the flow model diagram in Fig. 32.1. The whole diagram not only illustrates the link between suffering and its roots but also maps suffering and its effects on the right side of the figure. This flow diagram does not attempt to represent normative, including religious or philosophical, theories of suffering.

Keep in mind that the influences and outcomes listed in the flow diagram originate in many (mostly qualitative) studies. Importantly, this flow model applies as a tool for both qualitative and quantitative studies. The suffering research does not yet

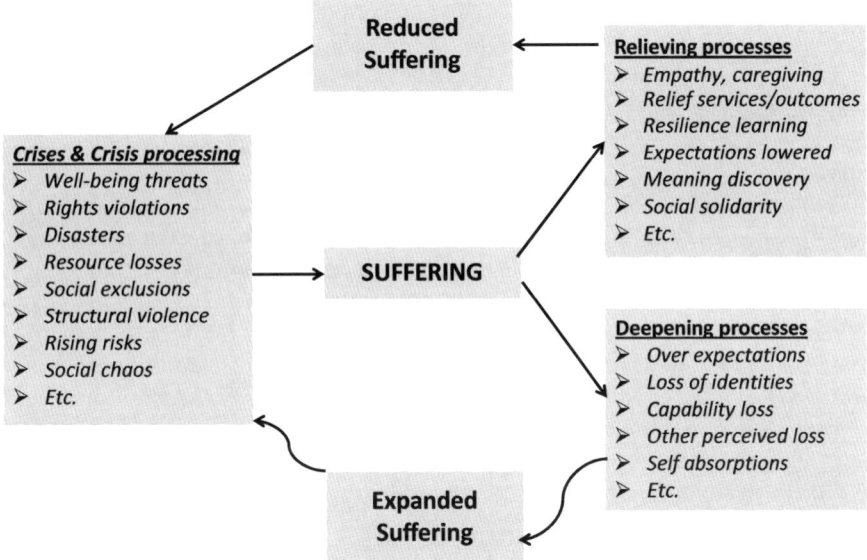

Fig. 32.1 A model of cycles of relieving and deepening suffering

specify the precise conditions under which suffering would or would not occur, or produce a specific effect or not. Furthermore, we do not know from existing research the magnitude or severity of suffering required to produce any particular effect in question. This is the type of knowledge needed to improve both our humanitarian and research objectives more effectively in the future.

As noted in earlier chapters, human rights violations produce a large share of preventable suffering. In fact, the greatest atrocities generally come up for discussion with an emphasis on human rights as it provides a frame for discussing the seriousness of the atrocity as well as alternate tactics to cope with their consequences. Human rights declarations are works in progress, and other types of victimization and social exclusions produce suffering as well.

Structural violence, a label coined by Galtung (1969) and popularized by Farmer (2013), points to indirect or institutionalized violence as a major source of suffering. This phenomenon appears in the flow model in the left-hand box labeled *Crises & Crisis Processing*. This title for suffering antecedents in the model, conveys that those factors shaping suffering include both external events like disasters and systemic forces but also internal or mental (including affective) states like fear or serenity, which all may lead to diverse states and increments of suffering.

The boxes on the right-hand side of Fig. 32.1 list outcomes (effects) of suffering or suffering relief. Like the producers of suffering, these elements include external events but mostly consist of internal states having to do with cognitive processing. These elements that contribute to the reduction of suffering include resilience, lowered expectations, meaning discovery, and social support through social solidarity. Those outcome elements that contribute to the deepening or expanding of suffering include identity loss, rising expectations, and so forth. These two sets of outcomes appear in two separate lists on the right side of the flow diagram.

The most interesting feature of the model appears as two feedback loops, one reducing suffering and the other expanding it. These two loops can be conceptualized as two cycles of suffering, in which one relieves suffering and the other exacerbates it. Exacerbation or expanding can either deepen the intensity or variety of suffering. For example, suffering might start out as social suffering only, but then cycle into mental suffering through erosion of self identity, which then evolves into physical suffering as well. The relieving and deepening cycles may operate simultaneously as in the sabotage of a major disaster relief effort.

Perhaps the most notable feature of this model accrues from the potential to apply it to an infinite variety of suffering situations. Its principal utility can be to help the researcher or analyst frame their problem and identify the most important elements. Keep in mind that any number of factors can be added to each type of input (e.g., crisis) or outcome. Both qualitative and quantitative researchers can use this model as a tool for evaluating their priorities for each stage of their research.

32.5 Clarifying the Compatibility of Human Rights and Suffering

While humanitarianism provides a philosophical and ethical rationale for the reduction of suffering, the human rights movement addresses concrete human abuses that result in suffering and identifies moral obligations to deduce such violations of human rights. Both humanitarianism and human rights place high priority on the premise of common humanity or universalism. Thus, human rights, and humanitarian assistance for those who need it, apply in principle to every human being (Baxi 2012; Farmer 2013; Schulz 2002; Wronka 2008). International Human Rights Law (IHRL) applies not just to warfare or emergencies, as does International Humanitarianism Law (IHL), but to any situation in which humans encounter violations. Human rights hold profoundly radical potential, by contesting power and asserting equality and dignity (including non-discrimination) for every person.

As originally codified in late 1948 by the UN, the Universal Declaration of Human Rights (UDHR) remains the primary declaration of human rights. It alludes to, but does not encompass, the full range of proposed human rights, beginning with political and civic rights, and then moving on to health, economic well-being, cultural, and solidarity rights. More recent declarations and treaties have attempted to be more specific about rights outside the political and civic domains. Because some categories of human rights are less institutionalized than others, the UDHR rights are listed here in two tables. Table 32.1 lists the commonly accepted political and civic rights (from articles 1 to 21), couching many in terms of freedom, while Table 32.2 designates those rights labeled "social, economic, cultural, and solidarity" (from Articles 22 to 30). "Solidarity" rights include rights to social order including

Table 32.1 *Political and civil* human rights with associated indicators of human rights violations

Human right	UDHR[a] article no.	Violation	Indicators of violations
Freedom from discrimination	1,2,7	Gender & other bases of bias	Gender and other types of discrimination
Life & security of persons	3	Killing	Deaths from civil war
Life & security of persons	3	Killing	Homicides
Justice for all	3, 25	Insecurity	Failure to provide citizen safety, e.g., traffic fatalities
Right to food	3, 25	Killing	Starvation
Freedom from slavery	4	Slavery	Human trafficking, enslavement
Freedom from persecution	5	Torture	Incidents of torture
Freedom from persecution	5	Violence	Assaults, sexual and otherwise
Justice for all	6, 9	Unfair trials	False imprisonment
Right to equality access to law	9	Injustice	Inequality-based injustice
Fair trial, justice	10, 11	Injustice	Subversion of justice, e.g., bribery, corruption
Freedom of movement	13	Lacking mobility	Refugee blockage
Property rights	17	Loss of place	Internally displaced persons
Freedom of speech	19	Lack freedom	Violations of freedom of speech

[a]Universal Declaration of Human Rights

environmental preservation. Some rights issues, such as the rights of the elderly, are not listed here even though there are groups within the UN and elsewhere working on them.

32.5.1 Aligning Suffering and Violations of Human Rights

To date, suffering tends to be defined in terms of distresses and calamities, which has unique advantages for purposes of caregiving practitioners. But for purposes of global and comparative research, suffering might more usefully be defined in terms of violations of human rights. Components of an operationalized definition of suffering from the standpoint of human rights would include the rights, and their associated violations, listed in Tables 32.1 and 32.2. Note that associated with each human rights violation is a UDHR article number or numbers, indicating that the violation links to one or more of the original principles of the 1948 Declaration.

This approach benefits from each violation's association with a particular source or type of human suffering. Some of the indicators can easily be translated into quantifiable measures, e.g., the count of homicides and deaths from warfare

Table 32.2 *Social, economic, cultural and solidarity* human rights with associated indicators of violations

Human right	UDHR[a] article no.	Violation	Indicators of violations
Safe working conditions	23	Unsafe work	Unsafe working conditions
Right to medical care	25	Lack of healthcare	Non-infectious illnesses & injuries
Right to medical care	25	Lack of healthcare	Deficiency in end-of-life care
Access to basic health resources	25	Lack of healthcare	Death from HIV/AIDS, tuberculosis, and other diseases
Access to other basic resources	25	Lack of healthcare	Number without health coverage
Protection of children	25	Lack of healthcare	Infant deaths
Right to an adequate living standard	25	Lack of resources	Survival risks due to poverty
Access to basic food resources	25	Lack of resources	Hunger & nutrition deprivation
Freedom from income-gaps	25	Major inequality	Gross inequality
Right to education	26	Illiteracy	Inaccessibility of education
Right to mental healthcare	27	Lack healthcare	Suicide & untreated mental illness
Right to cultural participation	27	Loss of culture	Inaccessibility to cultural heritage
Right to social international order (cooperation)	28, 29	Environmental Damage	Inadequate policies to preserve ecology; death from pollution
Right to international order	28, 29	Warfare	Number of civil wars
Right to local & global order	28, 29	Disorder	Social or civil disorder
Respect & care from others	29	Disorder	Instances of cruelty & hurtful acts
Right to enforcement of UDHR	30	Disorder	Failure to recognize legitimacy of human rights

[a]Universal Declaration of Human Rights

represent the degree to which the human right to life and security have been ignored or violated. Note that some human rights and their associated violations represent more than one row in the tables, because of the multidimensionality of some rights and their violations.

Importantly, the violations listed in Table 32.2 did not receive much credence as human rights until recent decades. The human rights perspective points us to the inhumane, horror-generating violations that mock notions of empathy and humanity. Violations of torture and warfare produce the most heinous suffering imaginable. Thus, the human rights perspective definitely offers an advantage in terms of capturing or representing the full spectrum of human suffering.

32.6 Using Human Rights Violations to Measure Suffering

Now that a human rights perspective on suffering has been outlined, how different does it function from perspectives or classifications not associated with human rights? Last year, I created two separate global indexes of suffering (Anderson 2014). One was based upon self-reported dissatisfaction with life, and the other was a composite of key demographic variables, specifically HIV mortality, infant death rates, prevalence of hunger and of poverty. Most of these indicators have roots in public health except perhaps for the poverty rooted in economic well-being.

Further refinements are needed to develop better national and community indicators of both subjective and objective suffering. Using indicators of human rights violations has considerable promise for either predicting suffering or at least representing the miserable conditions of suffering. These indicators offer the potential for greater objectivity, validity, and precision. As Tables 32.1 and 32.2 suggest, aligning human rights violations of different types with available, official statistics might require considerable effort because of the many different components or types of human rights.

The Fund for Peace already compiles data annually on indicators of human rights violations for 178 countries and releases this information as the Fragile State Index (Fund for Peace 2011, 2014). Formerly called the "Failed States Index," this index combines thousands of reports daily on each of 178 countries, using a combination of automated and manual syntheses of the information on human rights policies and practices in each country. The Fund for Peace also provides sub-index estimates and one of these sub-indexes captures political/civil rights; another measures social human rights. The two were added together for the analysis below.

Figure 32.2 shows the scatterplots of the 122 countries, which had both the subjective suffering data and the human rights data. This inter-relationship depicts a moderately high degree of correlation.[1] The co-variation between suffering and a rough measure of political and social human rights violations constitutes a sign that further work on using human rights violations as indicators of suffering has a strong likelihood of yielding greater understanding of major elements of global suffering. In addition, it might lead to a more robust and reliable indicator of "objective" suffering.

---

[1] The correlation depicted in Fig. 32.2 is 0.8, although if you take away either the political or the social sub-indices, the degree of correlation declines to 0.6.

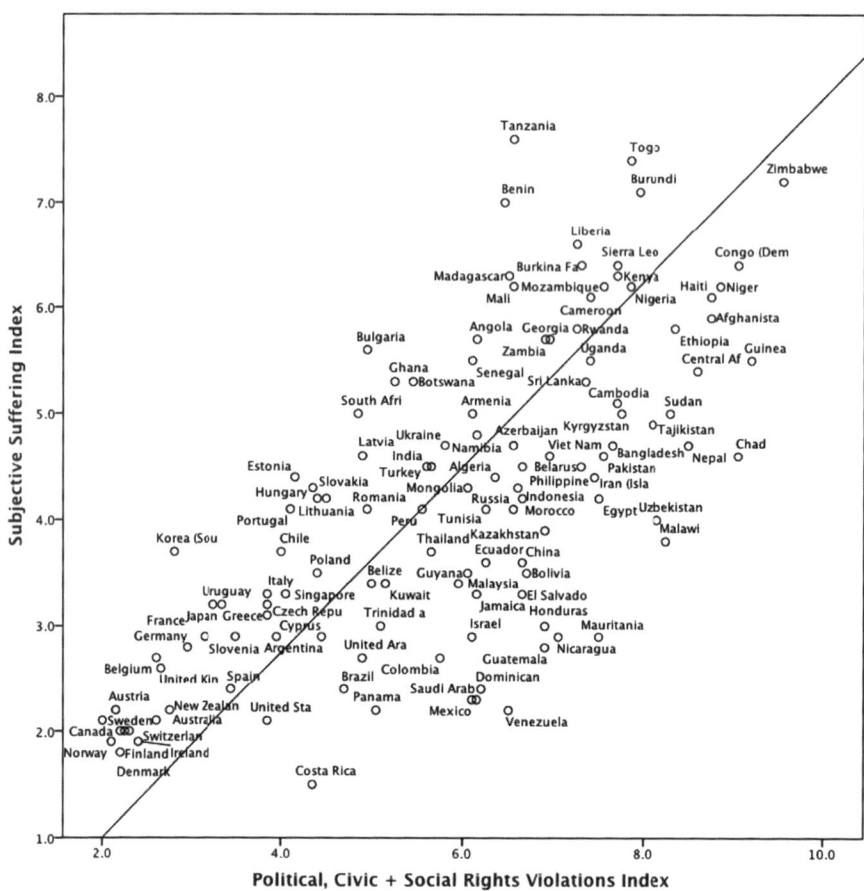

Fig. 32.2 Subjective suffering as a function of political and social human rights violations (Sources are UNDP (2010) for suffering data; Fund for Peace (2011) for human rights data)

32.7 Progress in Qualitative Research

Several major chapters in this volume use qualitative methods, principally ethnographies and case studies. This research strategy yields in-depth understandings of individual and social behavior. Not only does qualitative methodology tend to give a deeper description of the processes of suffering, but also it provides clues of the precipitating conditions and typical outcomes of these social events. These approaches to the compilation of such data provide ways of helping to answer such questions as: How did this person(s) get to be a victim of suffering? What are all the ways that people experience suffering? Under what conditions do they suffer? And how does it affect their lives? Mostly importantly, qualitative methods offer the most valid ways to answer any question that has to do with how and what a person experiences, feels or thinks with regard to what s/he considers suffering.

When suffering has not previously been studied in any given situation, qualitative methods turn out to be the most cost-effective way to begin to understand the key elements of the situation. The examples earlier in this chapter emphasize quantitative approaches, but qualitative research usually comes first for such work to be successful. This is particularly true with the construction of measuring techniques with adequate validity and other dimensions of measurement quality. Thus, the future of suffering research depends upon the future use of both qualitative and quantitative research methods.

32.8 Conclusions

In Chap. 1, my estimate of global physical suffering or pain in 2010 put sufferers of physical pain at over one billion people—at least a seventh of the worldwide population. This global community of pain victims includes only those suffering from major, persistent physical or mental suffering. In the United States alone, the IHIS[2] survey in 2010 gave an estimate of 62 million adults (27 % of the national population) enduring either physical or mental suffering. Obviously, suffering is not distributed equally across the globe.

Globalization has not only given new life to the humanitarian and the human rights sectors, but it has channeled world suffering to home television screens, computers, and cell phones around the world. This technology-based revolution, giving new visibility to global suffering, may lead to unexpected public opinion on suffering and actions, positive or negative, around the globe.

However, as noted by Wilkinson in Chap. 3, Chouliaraki (2013) and others make a strong case for the negative effect of contemporary campaigns for donations to humanitarian relief and development. These campaigns presumably create the impression that the public should give aid to make themselves feel better rather to improve the well-being of others. Another implied media message is that the existing institutions take care of the problems of global suffering. Critical theorists, Boltanski (1993), Chouliaraki (2013) and Fassin (2012) argue that humanitarianism corrupts society because it undermines the arguments that global problems cannot be solved without a replacement of the global power structure and without repudiation of backward ideologies like neoliberalism and post-colonialism. Critical humanists view humanitarian work as largely misguided because they believe that the global crisis is not so much a matter of suffering as it is a hijacked global power structure and humanitarian aid system overcome by the greed for donations.

Some even oppose humanitarian development assistance because it has resulted in so many disappointing projects (Easterly 2006). While a critical analysis of development projects or the role of the media in shaping the public view of suffering provides a useful service, any conclusion to largely ignore suffering until the media

---

[2] IHIS is the Integrated Health Interview Series, a periodic survey of adults in the United States, and was accessed on 7 June 2014 at https://www.ihis.us/ihis/.

or global power are restructured is not consistent with the inherent inclination to empathize and help other humans in distress. Furthermore, to neglect world suffering rejects humanitarian values and perpetuates human rights violations. Reflecting back on the 32 chapters of this book, written by highly qualified academics, readers are left with the sense of an enormous degree and variety of suffering, some of which may not yet have come to light.

Suffering and negative quality of life are complex constructs and deserve more conceptual attention. Some chapters imply that current suffering relief efforts tend to be superficial, not addressing the underlying human, community, and societal weaknesses that are the principal cause or source of the problems. While funding is a prerequisite to solving many problems of human suffering, changes in basic social and political institutions also are needed for long-term solutions to the enormous amount of human suffering.

Obviously, some people cannot shed their suffering on their own, but much suffering remains preventable and relievable, whether with self-care, professional health care, the help of informal caregivers, or by the humanizing of societal institutions. However, the amount of the world's preventable suffering is enormous. To achieve the goals of alleviating suffering and improving the quality of life of those trapped by suffering, social institutions will have to change, and the culture of interpersonal caring will have to greatly expand. If researchers, health care professionals, activists, and ordinary citizens help each other arrive at common solutions to suffering as well as the means by which to alleviate it, we will move forward toward reaching a solution to this global challenge.

References

Anderson, R. E. (2014). *Human suffering and quality of life: Conceptualizing stories and statistics*. New York: Springer.

Baxi, U. (2012). *The future of human rights* (3rd ed.). New York: Oxford University Press.

Boltanski, L. (1993). *Distant suffering – Morality, media and politics*. New York: Cambridge University Press.

Chouliaraki, L. (2013). *The ironic spectator: Solidarity in the age of post-humanitarianism*. Cambridge, MA: Polity Press.

Easterly, W. (2006). *The white man's burden: Why the west's efforts to aid the rest have done so much ill and so little*. New York: Penguin.

Farmer, P. (2013). *To repair the world*. Berkeley: University of California Press.

Fassin, D. (2012). *Humanitarian reason: A moral history of the present*. Berkeley: University of California Press.

Fund for Peace. (2011). *The Fragile States Index 2010*. Washington, DC: Fund for Peace (FP). Accessed on 5 June 2014 at http://ffp.statesindex.org/

Fund for Peace. (2014). *Conflict assessment framework manual*. Washington, DC: Fund for Peace (FP). Accessed on 5 June 2014 at http://ffp.statesindex.org/

Galtung, J. (1969). Violence, peace, and peace research. *Journal of Peace Research, 6*(3), 167–191.

Haddow, G., Bullock, J., & Coppola, D. P. (2010). *Introduction to emergency management* (4th ed.). Philadelphia: Butterworth-Heinemann.

Piff, P. K., et al. (2010). Having less, giving more: The influence of social class on prosocial behavior. *Journal of Personality and Social Psychology, 99*(5), 771–784.

Piff, P. K., Stancato, D. M., Cote, S., Mendoza-Denton, R., & Keltner, D. (2012). Higher social class predicts increased unethical behavior. *Proceedings of the National Academy of Sciences, 109*(11), 4086–4091.

Schulz, W. (2002). *In our own best interest: How defending human rights benefits us all*. Boston: Beacon.

Spitz, R. A. (1966). *First year of life: A psychoanalytic study of normal and deviant development of object relations*. Madison: International Universities Press.

UNDP. (2010). *Human development report 2010*. New York: Palgrave Macmillan for the United Nations Development Program.

Van Dijk, W. W., Ouwerkerk, J. W., Van Koningsbruggen, G. M., & Wesseling, Y. M. (2012). So you "wanna be a pop star?" Schadenfreude following another's misfortune on TV. *Basic and Applied Social Psychology, 34*(2), 168–174.

Wronka, J. (2008). *Human rights and social justice*. Los Angeles: Sage.

Printed by Printforce, the Netherlands